One Peaceful World

Creating a Healthy and Harmonious Mind, Home, and World Community

Michio Kushi
with Alex Jack

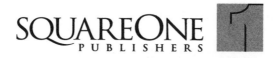

SQUAREONE
PUBLISHERS

COVER DESIGNER: Jeannie Tudor
EDITOR: Caroline Smith
TYPESETTER: Gary A. Rosenberg

Square One Publishers
115 Herricks Road
Garden City Park, NY 11040
(516) 535-2010 • (877) 900-BOOK
www.squareonepublishers.com

Library of Congress Cataloging-in-Publication Data

Names: Kushi, Michio, author. | Jack, Alex, 1945- author.
Title: One peaceful world : creating a healthy and harmonious mind, home, and
world community / Michio Kushi, Bestselling author of The Book of
Macrobiotics, with Alex Jack, President of Planetary Health.
Description: Garden City Park, NY : One Publishers, [2017] | Originally
published: 1987. | Includes bibliographical references and index.
Identifiers: LCCN 2016032664 | ISBN 9780757004407
Subjects: LCSH: Macrobiotic diet—Social aspects. | Mental health. | Peace
(Philosophy)
Classification: LCC RM235 .K876 2016 | DDC 613.2/64—dc23
LC record available at https://lccn.loc.gov/2016032664

Printed at Nutech Print Services - India

10   9   8   7   6   5   4   3   2   1

Contents

Part IV Practical Steps

Appendices

To the memory of Teru and Keizo Kushi,
my mother and father,
who taught me a love of peace.

To the memory of Homer and Esther, Alex's parents,
who have devoted their lives to reconciliation
and a world without war.

To Ann Purvis and the memory of her parents,
Harry and Virginia, true world citizens.

To the memory of Rev. Dana McLean Greeley,
a tireless promoter of peace and justice
within the world religious community.

To all the people who have died in battlefields
since ancient unknown times and to all those past,
present, and future who have devoted their lives
to creating a more healthy, peaceful world.

Acknowledgments

I am deeply grateful to George and Lima Ohsawa, Rev. Toyohiko Kagawa, Professor Shigeru Nanbara, Professor Toyohiko Hori, and my other teachers in Japan; and to Pitirim A. Sorokin, Albert Einstein, Thomas Mann, Upton Sinclair, Norman Cousins, Robert M. Hutchins, and other seniors in the United States for inspiring and encouraging me to devote my life to peace and the health and happiness of endless generations.

I am grateful to Alex Jack for his help in preparing this volume. *One Peaceful World* is the third in an ongoing series of books, including *The Cancer Prevention Diet* and *Diet for a Strong Heart,* which we have written on the greatest challenges to modern humanity's continued evolution. I am thankful to my wife, Aveline, for her tireless devotion and support. Christian Gautier provided the graceful artwork, and Florence Nakamura did the lovely musical score for the song.

To our other family members, staff, and co-workers, including Lucy Williams, Gale Beith, Edward and Wendy Esko, Donna Cowan, Sherman Goldman, Ann Fawcett, and Julie Coopersmith, we are thankful for their encouragement and advice. In sections entitled "Peace Promoter" that are found throughout this book, we look briefly at selected profiles of men and women around the world who are spreading the way of health, happiness, and peace. They are truly pioneers of the future world community, and we thank them for sharing their stories with us.

To all of my friends and associates around the world, as well as people everywhere who are true peace promoters, I am grateful for your heartfelt efforts and for the opportunity to be together with you on this beautiful planet with all of its wonderful difficulties. I pray that we can always love and help each other and together realize One Peaceful World.

Michio Kushi
Becket, Massachusetts

Foreword

Then the angel showed me the river of life-giving water, shining like crystal, flowing from the throne of God and the Lamb through the middle of the city's main street. On each side of the river is the tree of life, which produces twelve crops of fruit, bearing its fruit each month. The tree's leaves are for the healing of the nations.
                                                                    –Revelation, 22:1

Although he was born in Japan and made his home in Boston, Michio Kushi was actually a citizen of the world. Although he spent eighty-eight years enjoying life on this planet, Michio was also here as an ambassador of the universe.

Michio spoke often about cosmic cycles and their influence on human destiny, both individual and social, and indeed on the future of humanity itself. Looking at the vast sweep of geological, biological, human, and cosmic history, Michio identified two crucial star dates that will arrive soon. The first of these milestones is set to occur in the year 2036. This date marks the conclusion of a spiral of human history that began millions of years ago within the vast whirling motion of the Milky Way.

Human history was set in motion when our ancient ancestors began to eat cereal plants and started to walk upright, precipitating human brain development and the ability to see and imagine the entire universe. Further development took place when our ancestors started to use fire both in cooking and for warmth. The mastery of fire is what separates human beings from all other species. The use of fire enabled human ancestors to range across the planet and led to the development of technology, including the technological advances we see today. It also made it possible for humanity to destroy the planet and, along with it, to destroy itself.

The second pivotal date is to occur around 2100. This marks an important milestone in the great cycle above the North Pole. The earth is like a spinning top or gyroscope. It spins on its axis and also "wobbles" in a slow circular motion that is difficult for us to perceive. It takes about 26,000 years for the earth to make a complete wobble; more precisely, 25,800 years. Known in ancient times, the Greeks named this cycle the "Great Year."

As Michio explains in this book, the star Polaris, in the small dipper constellation, will come directly over the North Pole around 2100. From Polaris, the Pole will continue on its journey toward the constellation Cepheus, the king, married to the constellation Cassiopeia, and father of the constellation Andromeda, en route to its rendezvous with the great belt of the Milky Way that stretches across the north sky. Once it appears directly overhead, the energy of the Milky Way begins charging the earth, vegetation (especially cereal plants), and human beings with vibrant life force. The energy of the Milky Way bathes the planet in spiritual force, making health, peace, and elevated consciousness an everyday reality. A similar era, animated by galactic energy, occurred in the remote past. This era is referred to in myth and legend as the Golden Age, the Age of Paradise, and the Garden of Eden. At the same time, a similar era has been prophesied for the future. For example, in the Book of Revelation, in the quotation cited above, the coming influence of the Milky Way is referred to as "the river of life-giving water, shining like crystal, flowing from the throne of God." In Japan the Milky Way is also referred to as a river. The Japanese word for the galaxy is *Ginga*, or "silver river."

The inexorable march toward this epochal transformation will begin in earnest in 2036 with the completion of the Spiral of History and continue to the passing of Polaris in approximately 2100. We refer to the period from 2036 to 2100 as *Convergence*. It is during this period that all the positive and negative trends of human evolution and development will converge at the center of history. We see these two opposite trends gathering force today. During Convergence, humanity will choose between its current path of decomposition, unsustainability, and almost inevitable destruction, and a new path of healing, sustainability, and regeneration.

As Michio points out in this book, food will play a critical role in that choice. The ideograms that make up the Chinese and Japanese language offer a clue as to how this will take place. The ideogram, or *Kanji*, for "peace" is pronounced *Wa*. It is made up of images for "cereal plant" and "mouth." We usually interpret this to mean that a peaceful society is made up of people who eat grain, rather than meat, as their primary food. However, a deeper meaning is also revealed in this concept.

In their original state, cereal grains share a common characteristic. Tiny hair-like structures project from each grain. These are called "awns." The awns point toward the universe; they point upward toward heaven. They function as tiny antennae. During the day, the awns channel energy directly from the sun. At night, they channel energy from the cosmos, including from the Milky Way. When we eat whole grain as our main food, we are receiving stored energy and information coming directly from the universe. That is why eating grain was understood to be essential for developing consciousness and spirituality.

Those who eat a plant-based macrobiotic diet centered on brown rice and other whole cereal grains are already receiving the energy of peace, light, and harmony emanating from the Milky Way. They intuit that the coming world is one of health and peace, and they are capable of leading humanity toward that positive destiny. In *One Peaceful World*, Michio Kushi and Alex Jack provide a practical roadmap for the realization of that timeless vision and universal dream.

–Edward Esko
Pittsfield and Stockbridge,
Massachusetts

Preface

Following Michio Kushi's death at the end of 2014, his family, students, and colleagues started to gather, preserve, and make available his voluminous writings, audiotapes, videos, and other teachings. Foremost among them is *One Peaceful World*, a book originally published in 1986. Among all his books, it was Michio's favorite. As he relates in the autobiographical chapters that comprise the first part of this text, he had been inspired as a young man to devote his life to world peace after visiting Hiroshima just one month after the atomic bombing in August 1945.

In macrobiotics—the universal way of health, happiness, and peace—Michio found the practical means to this end. After coming to the United States in 1949, he devoted himself heart and soul to realizing the goal of a world of enduring health and peace. "One Peaceful World"—a world founded on a balanced, natural food and agriculture system with justice, equality, and freedom for all—became his mantra. In thousands of lectures, seminars, conferences, consultations, and personal conversations over the next half-century, Michio put forward this ideal. After it came out, *One Peaceful World* was translated into French, German, Japanese, and many other languages. In the early 1990s, it was cited by the United Nations' Society of Writers when it awarded Michio the Award of Excellence, its annual literary award for his outstanding contribution to peace and international understanding. Previous recipients included Norman Mailer, Arthur Miller, Mikhael Gorbachev, Gloria Steinem, and Stephen Hawking.

As the new millennium dawned, the Smithsonian Institution established a permanent Michio Kushi Collection at the National Museum of American History in Washington, D.C. Michio's books, macrobiotic foods, and Aveline Kushi's pressure cooker were exhibited, and a gala was held in the Rotunda and attended by hundreds of people. On behalf of the United States Government, the Smithsonian cited the contribution of Michio and Aveline and the macrobiotic community not only to personal health and well-being, but also to peace and the problems of society. The U.S. House of Representatives unanimously passed a resolution honoring Michio and Aveline on this occasion for their pioneer leadership.

Following his death, the Kushi Institute decided to honor Michio by celebrating One Peaceful World Day on his birthday, May 17. By coincidence, this was the day the original preface of this book was penned and delivered to St. Martin's Press, the original publisher (see page xv). The Kushi Institute also decided to give an annual Kushi Peace Prize to an individual or organization that embodied the universal ideals he taught, especially health, peace, and sustainability. The first prize was awarded posthumously to Shizuko Yamamoto on May 17, 2015. Shizuko, a student of George Ohsawa's (as were Michio and Aveline), moved to New York in the late 1960s and passed away just before the prize was awarded. She introduced Shiatsu massage to a generation of students, as well as taught cooking, health care, and philosophy. She was particularly active at the end of her life in the campaign to protect rice, wheat, and other whole grains from GMOs and environmental threats. A gala dinner was held at the Kushi Institute on One Peaceful World Day, and around the world macrobiotic friends, families, organizations, and businesses commemorated Michio's life and dream in a multitude of personal and public ways. It is our hope that this macrobiotic holiday spreads and the Kushi Peace Prize becomes internationally recognized. In 2016, the Kushi Peace Prize was awarded to Dennis Kucinich, the Congressman, presidential candidate, and leader of the peace caucus in Congress.

For this new edition of *One Peaceful World*, I have lightly revised the original text, completing Michio's biography and adding new material to bring up to date the sections on the Spiral of History, Nine Star Ki, and historical cycles. There is also a new chapter on increased violence in the early twenty-first century as a result of the spread of nuclear weapons and power, the introduction of GMOs and SSRIs, the impact of the information and digital revolutions, and global warming and climate change.

While weapons of mass destruction and the threat of terrorism continue to increase, the actual rates of violence and deaths in war have continued to decline sharply in recent decades. From the macrobiotic view, this is directly linked to the change from a meat-and-sugar based diet to a plant-centered diet over the last generation. Since adoption of the Food Guide Pyramid in the U.S. and similar dietary models in other countries (e.g., the Food Pagoda in China), the incidence of crime, violence, rape, cruelty to animals, and other major indices have all fallen. This trend is explored in a new chapter entitled "Diet and the Decline of Violence."

Several profiles have been added to the sections on Peace Promoters, including Lidia Yamchuk and Hanif Shaimardanov, medical doctors in Russia who pioneered in the macrobiotic dietary treatment of radiation sickness; Dennis Kucinich; Bill Spear, whose Second Response emergency teams have been helping children traumatized by natural disasters and war; and Baydaa Laylaa, a Kushi Institute graduate teaching macrobiotic cooking in war-torn Syria. Many new illustrations, tables, and charts have also been added.

Sachi Kato, an accomplished macrobiotic cooking teacher based in California, has prepared the menus and recipes for One Peaceful World Day. Edward Esko, my longtime colleague and associate director of Kushi Institute, has also contributed several new appendices, including material on Planetary Commonwealth and a peaceful new model of the universe based on the cosmological teachings of George Ohsawa and Michio Kushi. Edward is also profiled in a Peace Promoters section for his pioneer research into the quantum conversion of elements and new renewable sources of energy and materials. The resource and suggested reading/viewing sections have also been completely redone.

I am grateful to Rudy Shur, publisher of Square One Publishers, for bringing out this new edition, and to Caroline Smith and the rest of the staff for their hard work and dedication to this project.

I hope that this edition of *One Peaceful World* will appeal to both new and old macrobiotic friends, as well as all peace-minded individuals, families, and communities, and contribute to a more harmonious and joyful planet.

Alex Jack
Founder and President, Planetary Health, Inc.
Becket, Massachusetts

Preface to
the First Edition

We all share and are nourished by one common planet, the earth. For thousands of generations, most of the human family has lived together in relative harmony on this small sphere as it spirals through space. Before the spreading rays of the dawn and under the revolving canopy of the Northern Sky, millennia of parents, children, and grandparents have shared the harvest and saved seeds to plant the following spring. From the earliest campfires in the Ice Age to the fertilization of the Tigris-Euphrates River Valley, from the caravans winding along the Silk Road to China to the Pilgrim ships landing on Cape Cod, humanity's traditional food has consisted largely of wild and domesticated whole cereal grains, vegetables and roots, seeds and nuts, local fruit in season, and a small amount of fish, game, and other animal food. Through times of plenty and peace, and seasons of war and want, human beings have learned to adjust to their natural surroundings or move on in quest of a secure and more joyful future. Only in the last century have we run out of new land to settle and cultivate. Only in the last couple of generations have we devised a technology to extinguish the flame of life itself.

In the twenty-first century, there is a growing sense of impending collapse. Cancer, heart disease, diabetes, Ebola, and other chronic and immune-deficiency diseases are spreading. Terrorism, regional conflicts, and lack of meaningful arms control and disarmament agreements have resulted in widespread pessimism and despair. The pollution of the environment and the spread of biotechnology pose serious threats to the continued existence of many species, including our own.

Years ago, the elders of the Hopi nation prophesied that a "gourd of ashes" would fall from the skies and destroy the North American continent unless we learned to live in harmony with the land. In the Bible and the writings of Nostradamus and other prophets, others see signs of coming apocalypse. Yet every prospect of doom and destruction is accompanied by the opportunity for reconciliation and rebirth. Prophecies of war and strife are warnings to humanity to awaken before it is too late. They are not irrevocable. They will be fulfilled only if we continue to shun a natural way of life, especially a natural way of eating, which is the foundation of human culture and civilization.

Macrobiotics—the way of peace through biological and spiritual evolution—does not require legislation, treaties, demonstrations, violence, power politics, or ideological battles. Peace does not begin with any political party, religious movement, or social platform. It begins in kitchens and pantries, gardens and backyards, where the physical source of our daily life—food, the staff of life, our daily bread or rice—is grown and prepared. From individual hearts and homes, peace radiates out to friends and neighbors, communities, and nations.

Whoever takes charge of the cooking is our general, our pilot. We need no weapons, no shields, no offensive and defensive powers, just will and self-reflection. Brown rice, millet, miso soup, whole grain bread, beans and bean products, fresh vegetables and fruits, sea vegetables—these and other whole, unprocessed foods are our "weapons" to turn around the entire world. The energies of nature and the infinite universe are absorbed through the foods we eat and are transmuted into thoughts and the actions that spring from them. By becoming one with our larger environment and observing the universal laws of change and harmony, we are quite capable of restoring balance and order to our planet.

Michio Kushi
Becket, Massachusetts

PART I

Journey to Health and Peace

Win without fighting.
Convince without speaking.
Send for without calling.
Realize without instruments.
That is the pathway of one who lives
the Order of the Infinite Universe

—Lao Tzu

1.

Memories of Hiroshima and Nagasaki

My interest in macrobiotics began while I was living in Japan after World War II. After seeing firsthand the devastating effects on the environment and human lives that war brought, I devoted myself to figuring out how to bring about world peace. Initially, I thought a world government—in which all countries participated and cooperated—was the answer. However, after the war, I met George Ohsawa. His teachings about how the food we eat could lead to inner and worldly peace initially were strange to me. As I spent more time with him, I began to see how he was right; observations and personal experience showed me that daily food was truly the most important factor in our health and peace of mind. My roots in Japan supported this belief, although I did not yet know it at the time.

ANCESTRY AND EARLY UPBRINGING

My ancestors came from Wakayama Prefecture in the southernmost part of Honshu, Japan's central island. It is an earthly paradise. The black sea current flows offshore and is home to many fish and whales. Oranges and tangerines flourish in the orchards, and the land is bathed by clear water and crystal waterfalls, including Nachi Falls, the highest in Japan. Many shrines and temples dot the largely mountainous landscape. From ancient times, this Kumano area of southern Wakayama has been known as the sacred place of Japan.

According to legend, my family's ancestors descended from the heavens and settled in the Kumano area, long before the beginning of Japan as a country. The Kushi tribe was also related with the Kushians in ancient Pakistan and the Kushites in the Upper Nile region of ancient Africa. Later, more than 2,000 years ago, the troops of the present Imperial family invaded from Kyushu Island in the west, passing through the Kumano area and beginning the present country of Japan under the first emperor, Jimmu, in the current line of imperial succession. For about the last 1,200 years, my ancestors engaged in farming, as well as trading by boat, maintaining family headquarters in Ohtamura. The family temple in this village is named Dai Taiji, or Temple of Great Peace. Since the arrival of Buddhism into Japan, the temple's main symbol has been Ya-Kushi-Nyorai, the Buddha of Medicine and Salvation.

During the Buddhist era, family members continued to engage in farming and trading. Some forebears died on the ocean. Others became Buddhist priests and chiefs of the villagers. Legend also has it that the treasure of the family is hidden in the east where the sun rises. This has been interpreted to mean that descendents of the Kushi family are destined to journey east.

About 100 years ago, as the country began to modernize under the Meiji Emperor, the family's power declined and economic difficulties arose. My grandfather Jisaburo Kushi, the head of the family, and his wife, Kiku, bore five children. The eldest son, Hyakumatsu, worked very hard, reconstructing the economic and social power of the Kushi family. The second son, Kikusuke, served as an apprentice in the store of a merchant in Nachi, a nearby town. As a result of his honesty and hard work, he married the daughter of the family of the owner and became a successful merchandiser. The third son, Eijiro, married into a family of pharmacists in Shingu, the largest town in the Kumano area. The fourth child, Ine (a daughter whose name means "rice"), married a farmer of a nearby fishing town named Taiji and lived more than ninety years. The fifth and last child, Keizo, was the intellectual of the family. Supported by his elder brothers, he entered into teachers' college, then Tokyo Educational University. After teaching in Wakayama Teachers' College for a short while, he went on to graduate work at Kyoto Imperial University, majoring in Western history, especially the Renaissance. Before he entered Kyoto University, he arranged to marry Teru Toji, who also hailed from Ohtamura, and who was a daughter of a banker and enterpriser, Shunzo Toji. Although it was very rare for a woman from such a small rural village at that time to receive the highest education, Teru had excelled in her studies and entered Tokyo Women's Teachers' University. Inevitably, Keizo and Teru, the two young scholars nurtured from the same soil in central Japan, became engaged.

In Kokawa in 1923, a son was born to the young couple. His name was Toshio, which means Man of Discipline or Man of the Country of Wakayama (Ki no Kuni). Three years later, I was born and given the name Michio—Man of Tao, or Man of Righteousness, or Man of the Order of the Universe. Kokawa is the site of the Kokawa Temple, one of the prominent Buddhist temples in Japan, and I lived in this town for the first three years of my life. After completing graduate work in nearby Kyoto, my father was named assistant professor of Western history at Hiroshima University. Our family moved to Hiroshima and lived in a house near Yamanaka Girls' High School, where my mother taught. Once, when I was about four years old, I came down with very severe pneumonia and suffered almost forty days. Because both parents were educators, my brother and I received very careful attention and were brought up to observe a very simple way of life. The doctor, however, advised ice cream for my overheated condition. Ice cream was very new to Japan at that time, and my sickness took a long time to heal.

When I was five years old, our family left Hiroshima because my father's position shifted to Ishikawa Province Teachers' College. We moved to Tsubata and later to Kanazawa, in Ishikawa Province, facing the Japan Sea. In primary school, I won first prize in a speech contest among all primary school students in the province. However, my accomplishments were soon overshadowed. The next year we moved to Akita, and the girl with whom I shared a desk in the fifth and sixth grades was named Japan's number-one healthy child. We were brought up together through the elementary school attached to Akita Women's Teachers' College by the same teacher, Kenzo Sasamura, who inspired our entire class with his lively mind, gentle strength, and sportsman's spirit.

The strongest influence on my early development, however, came from my mother. Large in body structure, possessed of an ethical mind and keen insight, she constantly encouraged us to become persons of the world, not persons of the city, province, or even the country. She encouraged us to dream of going anywhere in the world without hesitation: America, South America, Europe. She was also devoted to her home, and when not teaching history and social science at the Catholic Holy Ghost Women's High School, she taught her young sons to clean house, sew, cook, and receive and serve guests. In Akita in 1936, when I was ten years old, Teru gave birth to a third son. He was named Masao—Man of Righteousness. Akita was to remain our family home until after the war, when my parents moved farther east and mother became a judge of the Family Court in Tokyo.

During this period, from about age fourteen, I was very much attracted to the invisible world of spirit and began to visit a local shrine. There, I would sit, meditate, and pray by myself about a half-hour each day—sometimes in the morning, sometimes on the way home from school, sometimes in the evening. One day, in my sixteenth year, while meditating in the front of the shrine, I experienced a golden and silver light enveloping me. It was shining, with many radiant spirals. Surprised, I looked around, and in this glowing atmosphere felt one with the whole universe. Gradually the brilliance faded. I stood up, climbed down the steps, and went outside. Then again the light returned, and I experienced all the trees, rocks, stones, and clouds around me as part of one universal spirit. At that moment, I understood that everything has life and is a manifestation of God or one eternal infinite being.

I went back home and then to school, but from that day on I spent most of my time wondering and marveling at the universe. My grades all went down. My parents worried, and one night I told them about my experience at the temple: "Everything is spirit, everything is God. I have to teach this." They were very surprised, but did not object. Gradually I resumed my ordinary studies, but the experience of the one shining light continued to inspire and guide me.

COLLEGE AND UNIVERSITY STUDIES

After the fourth grade of Akita Middle School, I entered Yamagata College, majoring in literature and philosophy, and began intensive studies of English, German, and French. I had always been attracted to poetry, novels, plays, and the arts, rather than to science and math. It was natural for me to emphasize liberal arts in college in preparation for serving society in the future from that dimension. Life at this time was dominated by the war in East Asia, which had intensified with the bombing of Pearl Harbor. Since I had been a small child living in Hiroshima, Japan had been at war—first in Manchuria and then in China. As a result, education was oriented to developing self-discipline. In addition to regular classes in literature, science, math, physics, chemistry, history, foreign languages, arts, and music, we received instruction in the martial arts in grammar school and in military training while in middle school. After fighting with the United States broke out, everyone's preoccupation with news and events of the war heightened. The possibility of being drafted put our daily studies under much tension.

In college, I lived in a dormitory with 600 other students. During the second year, I was chosen to be chairman of the dorm, and in this position I was responsible for taking care of, and managing, the students living in the dorm as well as serving as liaison with the school administration. To carry out my duties, I had to be the first one up in the morning and the last one to sleep at night.

As the situation in the Pacific intensified, more and more students began to be drafted. One by one, the third-level students—and then some in my own second level—were drafted. They would come to me and say, "You are young, Michio. I may die on an unknown battlefield. If you survive, please work for world peace." Many died, but I never forgot their departing words.

As the war progressed, food became scarce and rationing began. Every morning, we would awaken to the sound of drums and go out to the training and exercise fields before breakfast. Then after cleaning the dorms, we would enter the dining hall and, following the ringing of bells, bow to a small altar dedicated to soldiers who died in the war. The meal consisted of grains and vegetables, and we chewed every piece very, very well because the amount of food was very limited. Also, about once a month, we would march to a shrine commemorating those who died in battle.

In March 1945, I was accepted at Tokyo Imperial University. I moved to Tokyo and arranged to stay with one of my uncles who worked in a bank and lived in a small house in Saginomiya, in the Nakano area of the city. In April I began my studies in the political science department of the University's Faculty of Law, which had traditionally produced the nation's political, social, and governmental leaders. I went to school by public transportation, but because of air raids, sometimes I would have to seek refuge along the way in nearby shelters with hundreds of other people. In addition to my books, I always carried roasted rice, umeboshi plums, and sea salt for emergency use. At school, too, the air raid sirens would sometimes warn of imminent attack, and we would leave our lectures and hide in an arcade or basement until the all-clear was sounded. On several occasions, the public rapid transit could not run because of bombing damage, and like other students I would have to walk miles to and from class, often not returning to my uncle's home until after midnight.

That spring, large areas of Tokyo were burned away in massive air raids. Waves of B-29s struck on March 10 and again in April. The major part of the capital was destroyed in this carpet bombing, and fires raged out of control for several days in many areas. Yet studies at the University continued. Like everyone else, I slept at night with a helmet on and by my futon kept packs of roasted rice, along with my books, notes, and pencil, in case I had to escape immediately if the bombers returned.

In the middle of May, the government forced the University to send the majority of students to factories to assist in the war effort. The University wanted to continue studies with a small number of students in order to maintain traditional educational values, even under emergency circumstances. Unexpected examinations were held to determine which students would stay and which would be sent to the factories. To my relief, I was one of thirty students in my class of 600 to pass the exam. But ironically, one month later, I received a notice to report for army duty from my draft board in my native province of Wakayama. I was nineteen years old.

MILITARY TRAINING AND SERVICE

I returned immediately to Akita to arrange my things and bid goodbye to my parents and friends. At the railroad station, less than twenty-four hours later, I prepared to leave from my hometown for Osaka. About 300 people came to see us off. More than 200 were young women and girls from the Catholic Holy Ghost Women's High School. In the front square of the station, they saw us off with a concert. They sang a few army songs, a few beautiful folk songs, and one song of peace. Everyone waved their hands and flags as we departed, and I waved my student cap in return until the station vanished in the distance.

The next day, I reached Osaka and joined several hundred young men drafted from various provinces. In the underground arcade of the station, we gathered with draftees from other parts of Japan and received our military designations. Soon we were back on a train, headed west, but no one knew our final destination since all the windows were kept shaded. In the June heat and artificial darkness, the air was suffocating. Densely packed together, we passed the time half-sleeping, half-talking, half-sitting, half-lying on the floor, and half-standing. The train traveled fast, occasionally slowing down and stopping completely. After many hours, rice balls and water were distributed and many men grew drowsy and fell asleep. Several hours later, the train suddenly stopped, and we were allowed to open the windows briefly for some fresh air. Awakening from a shallow sleep, I saw that the train had stopped at Hiroshima Station. I could see many buildings and crowds of people—businessmen, families, school children, soldiers—going about their daily lives. After a short period, the shades were lowered and the train began to move farther west. I peeked out and watched the suburbs of Hiroshima and Ujiyama, a small suburban mountain, recede into the distance. Warm memories of my childhood in Hiroshima welled up in my mind.

Night came and the train continued west. By now, almost everyone knew that we were bound for Kyushu. Rice balls and water were given out again. The next morning, we arrived in Kurume, a city in the northern part of Kyushu, where a large military base was located. There, we were inducted into an infantry regiment and given army clothes. Like the others, I was in the lowest class of soldiers. That afternoon, military training began, and several sergeants and senior officers supervised the training of newcomers. Every day we dug holes, made shelters, and received one-hour lectures on military discipline. We also cleaned the barracks, took care of blankets and bedding, and made order among equipment assigned to each of us individually as well as to all collectively. We ate red Manchurian millet as our main food, along with miso soup, salty pickles, cooked vegetables (sometimes), and, once a week, salty cooked fish. Many soldiers had diarrhea for several days in the beginning because of the coarseness and hardness of the millet. By evening, almost everyone was completely exhausted. The discipline was exacting. If some minor faults were discovered, such as dust remaining on the table or a cloudy spot on a weapon after polishing, the sergeants would strike all soldiers. At these times we received strong blows on one cheek or both cheeks.

After many days and nights of hard training, I felt confident enough to disobey the rules and read after everyone fell asleep. Deeply hidden in my bag, I had brought two books into the army base: the Bible and a Japanese classic of strategy. My thoughts centered not on the outcome of the war, but how I should die and whether my death would really serve the cause of world peace. Like many soldiers, in the deep bottom of my heart, I felt that through this war, the world might become more peaceful (however small my own contribution).

After a month's training in Kurume, my section was dispatched to Tosu Station. Tosu Station was a junction between the main Kyushu railroad (running north to south) and the eastern line, branching off to Nagasaki. About thirty soldiers were assigned to guard the station. During the days we patrolled the platform carrying guns, controlled traffic, collected information, and from time to time went into town for petrol. At night we slept in nearby buildings and warehouses. Every day we saw U.S. bombers flying high in the sky toward the north, the industrial heartland of Kyushu. From time to time, Japanese fighters flew up to challenge the bombers. But in most cases, these small fighters were no match for the mighty Super-Fortresses and were shot down.

One day, about forty planes, including both bombers and fighters, attacked Tosu Station from an aircraft carrier in the Pacific. The anti-aircraft batteries surrounding the station were destroyed immediately, sending up huge balls of fire and smoke. Then the fighters came in and strafed the platform. The machine gun fire was like a thunderstorm. I had just reported for duty on the railroad platform with several others. Nearby, two soldiers screamed; their lifeless bodies tumbled down from the platform to the ground while their guns fired in different directions. I instinctively jumped down to the side of the platform as the bullets streaked by. The machine gun spurts, spaced about an inch apart, narrowly missed my body, which was pressed against the side of the platform. By the time I tried to shoot back, the plane had already pulled away. Shortly, a second plane came, and again I dove for cover as the bullets raced by. In a few minutes, the American airplanes started to rendezvous in the sky in a southeast direction and turn back toward sea. I jumped up to the platform. Some of my soldier friends were injured; others were dead. Continuing on, I ran to the entrance of the staircase of the nearby access road, where many passengers—ordinary citizens—had gathered to hide during the raid. I shouted, "Now you are all right. You may come out. The air attack has ended." All eyes showed sudden relief and ease.

Several days later, the station was attacked again. The rail line was damaged and several nearby warehouses and buildings were destroyed. I lost some more of my soldier friends. Among the survivors, everyone's face reflected deep tension. No one knew how long he might live and whether he would be alive tomorrow.

THE BOMBING OF HIROSHIMA AND NAGASAKI

In the guard compound, we received communications from military headquarters. On a small desk attached to the wall, there was a radiotelegraph machine that received and transmitted messages. Taking turns, soldiers in our unit would sit at the desk with the receiver to their ears, listening to military headquarters. One day we received news of the widespread destruction of the industrial area in northern Kyushu. Another day came word that the U.S. naval fleet, with several aircraft carriers, was approaching Kyushu. Then one day—an unforgettable day, the morning of August 6, 1945—a sudden bulletin came from headquarters to all military bases. In a deeply anxious voice, the announcer reported, "Hiroshima is attacked. We don't know what kind of bomb, but terrible misery has resulted. All communication with Hiroshima has stopped."

Several hours later, we received another bulletin. "If you see an enemy airplane, immediately hide. Even if only one plane, hide deeply, in shelters or behind hard, solid walls, buildings, or basements." Before, that was not the rule. If an enemy airplane came, we had orders to go out and shoot back. But now those orders had abruptly changed.

The next day, whispers spread among the soldiers that Hiroshima must have been attacked by an atomic bomb. The rumor was based on the hope that Japan someday soon would invent and develop a nuclear weapon and the war would turn toward victory. But now the face of every soldier betrayed deep anxiety and uncertainty, lest the United States had developed an A-bomb before Japan. Several days later, it became clearer this was an atomic bomb—the world's first.

Details of the bombing gradually became known, though the full extent of the tragedy was not fully comprehended for many days, weeks, months, and even years. The atomic bomb exploded over Hiroshima about 8:15 a.m. on August 6. At that time, the total population of Hiroshima City was about a half-million, including those living in the suburbs. The blast and firestorms of the bomb instantaneously killed and injured about 300,000 people. Another 30,000 people died from radiation sickness within the next few days. Today, several decades later, people in and around Hiroshima who survived the bombing are still dying from leukemia and other forms of cancer every year.

Eyewitness accounts soon brought the magnitude and horror of Hiroshima's annihilation into focus. For example, that morning, a group of 200 soldiers were standing in military training formation in the infantry regimental yard in Hiroshima. When the flash came, they were all changed into ashes—standing ashes—in a moment. Some other people were standing in front of a concrete wall. When the bomb burst they disappeared totally; only their shadows remained, imprinted on the wall. Many people were facing the flash, which has been described as brighter than 10,000 suns. Their front half exploded so that their flesh and their organs changed to blood running out, while their back side still remained. In that form, they staggered ten to twenty meters before they died. Many people who survived sought water. Hiroshima has many rivers and they went there. But as soon as they drank the water they died. Along the riverbanks, thousands of bodies lay lifeless, while thousands of other bodies floated in the water. Practically 90 percent of all the buildings collapsed, as fires burned out of control. The skeletons of a few concrete buildings remained, their iron and steel frames twisted like matchsticks. Under such conditions radioactivity continued to fall, and rescue units from the outside could not get in for about three days.

On August 9, the second atomic bomb fell, on Nagasaki. Once again, several hundred thousand people were killed or injured, though the city itself was only partially destroyed. My station, itself half in ruins, received many trains directly from Nagasaki, which is located on the western side of Kyushu. Every day, the trains brought thousands and thousands of survivors, including many people riding on the roofs of the trains. Nearly all of them were badly injured. Many of them died on the train, and many others reached our station barely alive. Of course, families, children, and parents were separated and did not know what had happened to each other. Many individuals stayed in Nagasaki searching for their loved ones. But the fallout was very heavy there, and one by one, many of them died. Along with other soldiers and civilians, I helped the Nagasaki survivors down from the trains and carried them to hospitals and nearby houses to rest. We arranged transportation to farther locations for other survivors, since Karume could not possibly care for everyone. While helping out, I looked up to Heaven from time to time, gazing far to the northeast in the direction of Hiroshima and then turning my head to the western sky toward Nagasaki. I wondered why the human mind and human society could give rise to such tragic things under this clear blue sky.

THE WAR ENDS

Following the Potsdam Declaration, the Soviet Union entered the Asian war and attacked Japanese forces in Manchuria on August 8. On the morning of August 15, all soldiers received orders to gather in front of the radio for an important announcement to be made by the Emperor himself. Standing silently, we gathered in the guardhouse, saluting a small radio. Following the voice of the announcer, a very deep, solemn, and very sad voice came through. At times it was difficult to hear, and the words were sometimes incomprehensible. The Emperor told the nation that Japan had surrendered. The Potsdam Declaration had been accepted and the war was over.

Everyone was stunned. For an hour, no one could utter a word. We just stood or sat looking at each other. Tears welled up and lined the eyes of many soldiers as they fumbled to inquire of each other whether it was really true that the war had ended. Suddenly, through the window, several Japanese airplanes were sighted overhead scattering papers. One of the soldiers dashed out and brought back a leaflet. It said, "We shall never surrender. We will continue to fight. Do not believe Japan's surrender." Meanwhile, from the wireless came news of Japanese pilots flying away toward Saipan with bombs, making a last attack on the U.S. naval fleet. They never returned.

Despite isolated instances of disobedience, order and discipline were generally maintained throughout the armed forces. In Karume, military headquarters ordered us to maintain security at Tosu Station for ten more days and then return to our infantry regiment at the base. There, we inventoried the weapons, stored the equipment, fixed the machinery, and generally put things in order, as well as kept patrol in nearby cities to maintain peace until further orders came from National Headquarters, which was preparing to receive the U.S. Occupation.

One by one, nearby regiments were discharged, but my unit was kept mobilized for these administrative tasks. I began to feel that it was totally unnecessary to remain in the army. I had to prepare to contribute to the future of Japan and the world as soon as possible. For that, I had to return to the University and continue my studies. I knew, however, that I would now have to concentrate on *international* political science and international law to achieve world peace. I anxiously awaited the date of my discharge, but the order would not come. Finally I began to organize a group of soldiers with the idea of escaping the regiment. With my best friend, Kohei Yamanoi, a student at Kyoto University who was drafted at

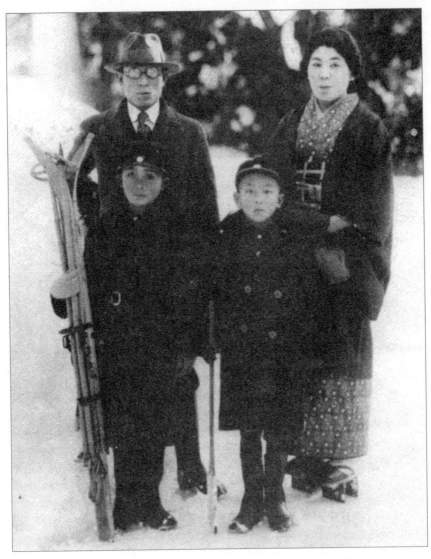

Keizo and Teru Kushi with their sons, Toshio (left) and Michio (right),
on a skiing trip.

the same time as me, I mapped a plan of mass escape. Sergeants and even a few officers wanted to join. As the day of our breakout neared, however, a third of our regiment was discharged, including me and all the others who wanted to leave.

It was October, already two months after the end of the war. I packed my bag containing several days' provisions, a few socks, and my two books from East and West—the Bible and the Oriental classic of strategy. I boarded a train for the return journey to Akita, where I knew my parents must be anxiously waiting. The train was crowded with tired, weary people, but this time the windows were open. At length, the train arrived at Hiroshima Station.

From the barren wooden platform, I surveyed the area of the atomic bomb explosion. As far as the eye could see, burned ashes and melted steel extended from the epicenter of the explosion, miles and miles toward the north, far to the mountains, as well as toward the east and west. I could make out fields of burned ashes, twisted steel structures, and graves containing untold souls and spirits. The barren landscape was broken occasionally by a burned tree, but there were no houses or buildings standing. There was no sign of life: no people, no animals, no birds singing. Silence prevailed.

From deep within, tears and anger welled up. Tears for the spirits and souls of the hundreds and thousands of dead who received this unexpected misery. Anger with the senseless human greed and violence which lies deeply within all of us, including myself. Sadness for the failure of humanity to realize the shining world of spirit that had been revealed to me while meditating in the shrine. I decided somewhere deep in my heart, and without knowing how I would proceed, to devote my life to realizing peace—peace for the world, peace for all people, peace for all humanity, peace for all animals, peace for all living beings. However difficult the endeavor, whatever the sacrifice it would cost, however long it would take—perhaps tens and hundreds of generations— I resolved to dedicate myself to universal understanding and the creation of One Peaceful World.

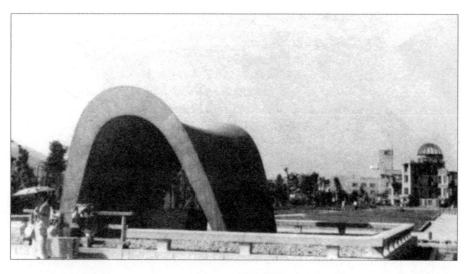

The Hiroshima Peace Memorial, containing the names of all who perished from the explosion, is modeled on the ancient house in which people lived in an early era of peace and harmony. To the right is the A-Bomb Dome.

PEACE PROMOTER

Tatsuichiro Akizuki, M.D., Japan

Around the world, thousands of individuals and families are promoting peace through macrobiotic activities, including organic farming and natural foods distribution, home and family care, community service, teaching and counseling, writing and publishing, medical and scientific research, and technology and the arts. In these Peace Promoters sections, we shall look at a few of the ways people and communities in different countries have been transformed by whole foods and a deeper understanding of the Order of the Universe.

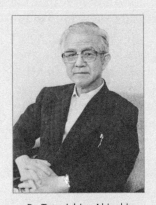

Dr. Tatsuichiro Akizuki

In August 1945, Nagasaki experienced a hot spell, punctuated by constant air-raid alarms and the rush to air-raid shelters. Starting in April, the city had been bombed and strafed once or twice, but it had generally escaped the damage suffered by other cities as the bombing of Japan intensified.

Located in a mountainous bay on the southwest coast of Kyushu, Japan's southernmost island, Nagasaki was a famous seaport and site of the largest Christian community in Japan. In the sixteenth century, European merchants, missionaries, and doctors first entered Japan through Nagasaki. From the maze of dockyards and shipping facilities in the port, the city's industrial and residential areas stretched up two fertile valleys. The giant Mitsubishi Company dominated local commerce. Shipyards, steelwork facilities, and munitions factories were contributing directly to the war effort, and some war-related industries had been dispersed and relocated in schools and municipal buildings as well as in tunnels underground.

In September 1944, Tatsuichiro Akizuki, M.D., age twenty-nine and a native of Nagasaki, was appointed director of Urakami First Hospital, a small medical facility that had been established in a Franciscan monastery on the northern edge of the city. Toward the end of the war, very few priests, monks, or seminarians remained in the large three-storied structure, and the hospital housed mostly tuberculosis patients.

On the morning of August 7, 1945, Dr. Akizuki opened the newspaper as usual to find out what regions of Japan had been bombed the day before. The front page headline drew his attention: "New type of bomb dropped on Hiroshima—Much damage done." Dr. Akizuki was alarmed. Normally the papers described all bombs as "incendiary" and announced damages, however big, as "slight." The article was a bad omen.

On the morning of August 9, the skies over Nagasaki were clear. The cicadas were chirping, and it looked like it would be another hot and sultry day. At 8:30 a.m., Dr. Akizuki began seeing outpatients. During the morning, he stopped to chat with Mr. Yokota, whose daughter was an inpatient. Yokota, who worked as an engineer at the Mitsubishi Ordnance Factory where the torpedoes used in the attack on Pearl Harbor had been made, said: "I hear Hiroshima was very badly damaged on the sixth."

Dr. Akizuki and Mr. Yokota despaired over the future of Japan. The engineer said that he didn't think the explosion was caused by any usual form of energy and speculated that it was "an atomic bomb, produced by atomic fission."

Just then, the air raid sirens sounded. Mr. Yokota hurried back to his factory. It was 10:30 a.m. Some of the hospital attendants were making a late breakfast, filling big bowls with brown rice and miso soup and distributing them to patients in the wards. Nagasaki residents had grown so accustomed to warnings that they often failed to take precautions. Besides, outside, the familiar formation of B-29 bombers could not be seen in the clear sky. The all-clear sounded a half-hour later and the hospital returned to its normal activities.

A few minutes later, shortly after 11 a.m., Dr. Akizuki was attending to a patient when he heard the low droning sound of a distant aircraft. The sound grew louder and seemed to be almost directly overhead. He shouted: "It's an enemy plane! Look out—take cover!" He dived for cover by the bed.

A blinding flash of white light lit up the room, followed by a gigantic "bang" and "crack." A violent shock shook everyone. There was maybe only a second or two between the strange drone of the aircraft and the impact of the hit. Dr. Akizuki lay flat on the floor. Some debris fell tumbling down on his back.

"Our hospital has been struck!" he thought. He started to have fits of giddiness and his ears rang. About ten minutes later, he got up staggering and looked around. There was nothing but a yellow smoke, with a white powder hanging in the air and a certain darkness.

"Thank God, I'm not hurt," he thought. After recovering from the shock, he thought of his staff and patients. Miss Murai, a nurse who had been assisting him, appeared unhurt, though she was completely covered with dust. Dazed, he wandered into a consulting room and looked out over the rubble. "Out in the yard dun-colored smoke or dust cleared little by little. I saw figures running. Then, looking to the southwest, I was stunned. The sky was as dark as pitch, covered with dense clouds of smoke; under that blackness, over the earth, hung a yellow-brown fog. Gradually the veiled ground became visible, and the view beyond rooted me to the spot with horror.

"All the buildings I could see were on fire: large ones and small ones and those with straw-thatched roofs. Farther off along the valley, Urakami Church, the largest Catholic church in the East, was ablaze. The technical school, a large two-storied wooden building, was on fire, as were many houses and the distant ordnance factory. Electricity poles were wrapped in flame like so many pieces of kindling. Trees on the nearby hills were smoking, as were the leaves of sweet potatoes in the fields. To say that everything burned is not enough. It seemed as if the earth itself emitted fire and smoke, flames that writhed up and erupted from underground. The sky was dark, the ground was scarlet, and in between hung clouds of yellowish smoke. Three kinds of color—black, yellow, and scarlet—loomed ominously over the people, who ran about like so many ants seeking to escape. What had happened? Urakami Hospital had not been bombed—I understood that much. But that ocean of fire, that sky of smoke! It seemed like the end of the world."

After a long while, he could at last identify the bomb: "That's it! It was the new type of bomb—the one used on Hiroshima." The fire from the hospital spread little by little. It was strange that the main roof had burnt first. The temperature of the atmosphere at the time of the detonation was several thousand degrees at the epicenter and several hundred degrees near the hospital. The wooden structures, located less than a thousand yards from the epicenter, burnt immediately, and a huge fire ensued. At the interior of 1,000 yards around the epicenter, even steel was burning! The hospital was located about a mile from it. The fire had started with a few flames around the roof.

Fortunately, all seventy inpatients at the hospital were alive and uninjured. Two severe tubercular cases had been pinned under fallen beams but had been rescued. Most of the medical equipment, however, including modern X-ray machines, medication and drugs, and 10,000 volumes on religion and medicine, had been destroyed in the blast. Dr. Akizuki found himself practically unprepared, with only a pain reliever, some gauze, and Mercurochrome to treat his patients. Meanwhile, the hospital was besieged by survivors from other parts of the city. Many had widespread and deep burns. Others had fragments of shattered glass deeply encrusted in their bodies. Outside, processions of groaning, half-naked people sought relief in banks of a stream. No one knew what had happened to bring out their terrible injuries. Each felt that the bomb had fallen only on them. Making do as best he could, the doctor spread zinc oxide oil over extensive burns with a writing brush.

Dr. Akizuki had no idea at all of atomic radiation. Among the patients who had not been burnt, many were having stomachaches and inflammation of the mouth. He thought it was because they were cramped living in the shelter from the time of the explosion. But as days passed, they began to suffer from diarrhea and bloody stools. The stomatitis (inflammation in the mouth) brought about gum bleeding, and subcutaneous hemorrhages followed. Then, the inside of the mouth became purple.

The doctor thought at first it was dysentery, but it proved to be much worse. At the time, no one knew how terrible it would be. For one year, Dr. Akizuki had been assistant in the Department of Radiotherapy of the hospital of the Faculty of Medicine of Nagasaki. This had given him the opportunity to discover that catarrh (excessive mucus buildup in the nose or throat) was frequently brought on by the continual irradiation of persons suffering from uterine or breast cancer. He himself had administered X-ray exams daily, and had also experienced symptoms of catarrh. This experience proved very useful. Around August 15, he finally realized that the symptoms he was now feeling after the bombing corresponded exactly to this type of catarrh.

From the point of view of classical physics, X-rays are very short electromagnetic waves which can go through the cells of the human body and even destroy them in the case of intense irradiation, like radium. The cells destroyed by this type of radiation are the ones where frequent divisions arise. The most fragile cells (the sexual cells, marrow cells, and all cells that have a vital function) are destroyed by radioactivity. It was the only thing he could guess about the "atomic disease."

When Dr. Akizuki took care of cancer patients suffering from roentgen catarrh (radiation-induced catarrh) or suffered from it himself, he would drink or give to them to drink a salty solution which contained a little bit more salt than the regular application, and it turned out to be very effective. He decided that salt would be good also for those who had been exposed to this bomb. Although he had no knowledge of nuclear physics or atomic biology, he became convinced that a dietary method offered the only effective treatment against atomic radiation. He also knew that while salt or sodium ions gave back to the blood its vitality, sugar in turn was toxic and would aggravate the condition.

This acid/alkaline principle of balance corresponded to the patients' treatment by doctors and staff at the Faculty of Medicine of Nagasaki. Applying the same mineral method to atomic survivors proved very effective. Dr. Akizuki noted, "I felt something like confidence welling up in my chest. I gave the cooks and the staff strict orders that, when they made the unpolished-rice balls, they must add some salt to them, and make salty, thick miso soup at every meal, and never use any sugar. When they failed to follow my instructions, I scolded them remorselessly, saying: 'Don't ever take any sugar, nothing sweet!'"

Some time before the bombing. Dr. Akizuki, influenced by macrobiotic dietary principles, had regularly fed his co-workers brown rice and miso soup, and they had been forbidden to eat sugar, which was generally unavailable anyway. After the bombing, rice balls, seaweed, salt, and other good-quality yang foods were distributed to all patients and staff as well as to neighbors and other people who had managed to reach the hospital yard before collapsing.

"What's so bad about sugar? Why is salt so effective in the cure of atomic disease?" people asked him. It was time-consuming explaining yin and yang to everyone in detail, so he replied, "Sugar is bad for you—you have my word for it! Sugar will destroy your blood."

This macrobiotic dietary method enabled Dr. Akizuki to remain alive and go on working vigorously as a doctor while other medical personnel who survived, including Dr. Tsunoo, President of the Medical College Hospital, succumbed to atomic disease. Thanks to his method, Brother Iwanaga, Reverend Noguchi, Chief Nurse Miss Murai, other staff members, and inpatients all kept on living in the lethal ashes of the bombed ruins.

Other people in Nagasaki—most of whom were no longer eating a macrobiotic or traditional diet—said it was a miracle that everyone at the hospital survived. In fact, this miracle was made possible primarily because of Dr. Akizuki's dietary recommendations and their extreme modification after the explosion. Two other factors also contributed to their survival. First, the hospital was built of bricks, which constituted for some patients and doctors relatively effective protection against the atomic bomb radiation. Secondly, torrential rains fell twice over Nagasaki after the bomb, on September 2 and September 16. The latter storm drenched Hiroshima. These rains, which ended each time with violent typhoons, were a difficult challenge for the bomb survivors. "It's hell on earth: torture by fire, and torture by water," Dr. Akizuki thought at the first rain. The flood was so intense that the meteorological observatory registered one foot of rain.

But the intensity of the storm turned out to be a gift from God, as did the typhoon "Makurazaki," which followed two weeks later. The abundant downpour could dissolve and drain away the radioactive fallout to the ground or wash it out to sea. After the typhoon, the number of deaths decreased at the hospital. The hospital attendants and Dr. Akizuki did not have any more nausea or bloody excrement. Their hair stopped falling out. It was forty days after the bomb had exploded. "It seemed that at last the number of victims in the city was going to decrease. Those who had to die were probably already dead. From the days of the typhoon the gradual approach toward inevitable death changed to the return of life," Dr. Akizuki said.

During this time, medical help from outside the city came very late and was unable to do anything for the new ailment. Perhaps it was fortunate, for as Dr. Akizuki wrote, "After all, there was nothing else to do than go back to brown rice and miso soup. . . . It was thanks to this food that all of us could work for people day after day, overcoming fatigue or symptoms of atomic disease and survive the disaster free from severe symptoms of radioactivity. I believe it although it is difficult to prove from a medical point of view."

Several years after the war, Dr. Akizuki and Chief Nurse Murai were married. Urakami First Hospital—now called St. Francis Hospital—had been rebuilt and Dr. Akizuki continued to serve as director for many years. Active in the peace movement, he also performed as director of the Nagasaki Association for Research into Hibakushas' (Atomic Bomb Survivors) Problems. Over the years, Dr. Akizuki became more religious but continued to attribute the miraculous survival of all his staff and patients to the diet. "We have a mission, to tell what happened here," he stated in the postscript to his autobiography. "That is why we feel God gave us life, to live until now."

Sources

Akizuki, Tatsuichiro. "How We Survived Nagasaki." Translated by Evelyn Harboun. *East West Journal* (Dec. 1980): 10–13.

Akizuki, Tatsuichiro. *Nagasaki 1945*, Edited by Gordon Honeycombe. London: Quartet Books, 1981.

2.

The Secret Melody of Peace

When I returned to Akita City and reached home, I was greeted by my parents' joyful, happy smiles. But I was saddened to discover that my elder brother, Toshio, was on his deathbed with tuberculosis. He had worked in a chemical company near Tokyo and the wartime conditions had aggravated his frail health. A few days later, I began to teach at the Catholic Holy Ghost Women's High School, filling in for my mother, who went to the hospital every day to care for Toshio. He was in bed awaiting his death. I visited him and was forced to wear a mask. The disease was believed to be transmitted through contamination by breathing. My brother gazed at me, and there was a weak smile on his pale, transparent face. We held each other's hand firmly. I pretended to be cheerful and encourage him, but his response was weak, though a smile stayed on his face. Several days later, we met once again, and of course Mother stayed with him constantly.

Several days later, while teaching at the high school, I received a call from my mother, saying, "Your brother passed away just now." Her voice trembled and she couldn't utter another sound. I said, "I'll come immediately."

With a trembling voice, Mother said, "Not now. After you finish your teachings in school."

I kept the news to myself, but as soon as school ended, I told several colleagues and dashed to the hospital. Mother was sitting at the side of the body, without saying anything, as lifeless as a ghost. As soon as Father's own school duties ended that evening, he came back from Honjo, where he was principal of the high school. For a few days, I helped my father with the cremation ceremonies at a Buddhist temple in Akita. About ten Catholic high school teachers and several neighbors gathered for the services, but due to chaotic social conditions at the end of the war, many of my brother's friends could not attend. When his ashes were carried to the temple in a small wooden case, I gazed at Mother, as if my gaze could protect her from collapsing. That evening, for the first time in my life, I saw my mother—that strong, disciplined educator—cry.

As Father consoled her, I pondered the meaning of death deeply in my soul. During the last few years, so many of my soldier friends had died. Hundreds of thousands of people in Hiroshima and Nagasaki had died. Millions had died in the Pacific, China, Manchuria, and Europe—all over the world—and now death by infectious disease, a perennial companion of war, had touched my family. I reflected on the truth that everyone is born and everyone passes away. I felt at the time that life is nothing but a dream, and that we pass through this world like travelers moving from one scene to another.

WORLD GOVERNMENT STUDIES

I continued to teach at the Catholic high school for another six weeks. When Mother had recovered from her sadness and could teach again, I returned to Tokyo University to continue my studies. My major interest was peace and the future of humanity. But these subjects as such were outside the formal curricula of the political science and law faculties. For the second time, I was selected as chairman of the dorm, and more and more I pursued my own course of study. As in high school, I began to visit nearby shrines and temples, meditating and praying whenever I had the time. My mind was searching for some practical and lasting way to realize world peace; it became clear that it would be meaningless for me to pursue an academic career. Though I had missed some of my studies because of the war, I decided to finish all requirements in three years.

Reconstruction began slowly in Tokyo in the winter of 1945 and during the following spring. Food was scarce everywhere, and the black market thrived. The Allied Occupation, under General MacArthur, took charge, and U.S. flags flew over the city. But hunger was widespread and the social situation remained tense. The Communist movement grew very active, and frequent labor strikes broke out. A general strike was planned, but stopped by order of the Allied Powers. Soon the Tokyo War Crimes Tribunal opened. Former Prime Minister Tojo and other leaders of the defeated Japanese military command were tried as war criminals. I visited the trial several times and observed the proceedings, wondering why this kind of drama was necessary to realize world peace. The court was convened in the name of justice and civilization, but after a worldwide tragedy of this magnitude, what really is justice and what is civilization?

One day I observed a huge demonstration of people, organized by the political left, in front of the Imperial Palace. I came not to participate, but to see why people gathered and what meaning or merit their assembly might have. I observed the excited faces and glittering eyes of thousands of people, but didn't share their excitement nor see how such agitation could bring lasting peace.

After graduating from Tokyo University, I wondered what to do. My best friend, Keichu Moriai, and most of my other classmates were planning to take the examinations leading to careers as lawyers, judges, government administrators, and diplomats. But these secure, officially prepared futures held no attraction for me. My uncle advised me to go into business and applied on my behalf to several business firms with which he was connected. But I could not tolerate the vision of spending my life on the staff of a company.

Returning to Tokyo University as a graduate student, I became interested in world federal government. Among various attempts to achieve peace and prevent a nuclear arms race, an international effort was being made to establish a world federal government, either through amending the newly adopted United Nations Charter or through the formation of worldwide conventions by people representing populations of different areas. On campus, I received valuable guidance in this direction from Professor Toyohiko Hori, a very decent, disciplined, sincere person; Professor Shigeru Nanbara, a devout Christian, political scientist, and chancellor of Tokyo University; and my other professors at the faculty of law and politics.

I started to visit people here and there who shared the same dream. I tried to find books and literature, past and present, related to this subject. I also began communicating through letters with world federalists in other countries, including the United States. I continued as chairman of the dorm and pursued regular studies, but for the most part, between prayers and meditation in front of nearby shrines, my mind was devoted to visions of realizing world peace through some form of world constitution. Among those I met in Japan were Reverend Toyohiko Kagawa, the Christian evangelist; Morikatsu Inagaki, the world federalist; and others seeking peace, including members of the Japanese Diet.

MEETING GEORGE OHSAWA

The person whose view of human society I was most deeply influenced by was neither a professor nor a scientist, a holy man nor a saint. I can only describe him as a free man. Our meeting came about in a curious way. One of the groups with which I was in touch after the war was the United World Federalists of North America. One day, a letter from New York came, informing me about the Student World Government Association in Japan. This small organization was located in Okurayama near Yokohama, just outside of Tokyo. It was headed by Yukikazu Sakurazawa, a poet, businessman, philosopher, and author of a few hundred books and articles, who had traveled abroad and lived in Europe during the late 1920s and early 1930s, synthesizing the teachings of East and West. For simplification, he used the pen name George Ohsawa in French and English. I decided to visit Okurayama one weekend. The address turned out to be a small part of a large building. There was practically no space, but I was cordially greeted by several students and invited to sit down at a low table. They offered me odd-looking tea, dark strange-tasting bread, and tekka, a root vegetable condiment that had been cooked down into a cinder-like black powder.

"Don't you think this is delicious?" they asked me. The bread was distasteful. The tea was bland. But having studied political science, I was diplomatic enough to reply, "Yes, so delicious." The students talked only about food. I asked them questions about world government and preventing the spread of nuclear weapons, but they couldn't answer well because they were not particularly knowledgeable in political science. So I asked who their leader was, and they said George Ohsawa. I asked to meet him, and they told me to come back the next weekend. The next week I returned to George Ohsawa's small house in Hiyoshi between Tokyo and Yokohama and noticed on the roof a big sign saying, "Student World Government Association." I thought he was either crazy or a genius.

Outside there were many shoes lined up, which I instinctively began to straighten out. Ohsawa's wife, Lima, came out and showed me in. Inside, there were about twenty young people eating dinner at a small table. In the room I saw a strange old man with a strange face. He looked something like a gangster and a poet, a complicated person with a combination of a very tough and tender mind. I bowed. As soon as he saw me, Ohsawa told everyone else to carry their bowls into the next room. They were very surprised. Then he told me to please sit down and have something to eat. Lima brought in some miso soup and closed the door.

"What are you doing?" George Ohsawa asked me.

"I'm studying world political problems—world government and world peace," I replied.

"Have you ever considered the dialectical application of dietary principles to the problem of world peace?" he asked. I was puzzled. I was a very diligent student, but had never thought about that. Political science, and even social science at large, except for some esoteric cultural and anthropological studies, never addressed the dietary practices of the human race. What possible relation could food and peace have?

"I never thought of that," I admitted.

"You have to study the relations between food and human destiny," he said, smiling. "Someday you will find that it is the key to world peace. Every week please come and eat with us."

I joined the evening meal. It was very distasteful to me. There was silence; no one spoke. I left.

Back in Tokyo, I discussed my visit to Ohsawa with some of my professors and elicited only disinterest. They were unanimous in their conviction that peace was an international problem. They told me that Ohsawa was just a health promoter and his ideas on peace were not worth serious attention. For the next eight months, I completely ignored my visit with Ohsawa. Then one day, I received a telegram from him: "Tonight we have a meeting on world government. Please come." I had no phone so I couldn't refuse the invitation. I felt I had to pay my respects. So once again, I set out for Yokohama. A group of students were gathered, and this time they were talking about world government, not about food, so I no longer felt so strange.

From then on, I visited the Student World Government Association every week or every other week. Whenever I went, they offered me a meal—strange food such as dark bread or brown rice balls. I still didn't understand the importance of food. But Ohsawa was drawing spirals on the blackboard and talking about the Order of the Universe, which governed everything from subatomic particles to star systems, from patterns of sickness and health to the rise and fall of civilizations, and this intrigued me. He didn't talk about food and sickness at all, just about yin and yang, the complementary opposites that make up all phenomena. While listening to his lectures, I started to think that his philosophy was really wonderful. It may cover the whole universe, but I still didn't see how to connect world government or one world with this approach. As a person born in the Far East, I knew from childhood about yin and yang, the two basic energies that give rise to day and night, summer and winter, man and woman, soft and hard, small and large, and other pairs of opposite qualities. But I did not know how to apply yin and yang to daily life. George Ohsawa didn't talk to me about food. He always talked about cosmology.

One day, he asked me to go to the movies with him. Although I was very modern in many respects, I never went to the cinema. I was very dedicated to my studies and felt this was a waste of time and could debilitate my self-discipline. I was surprised to find that Ohsawa slept through the entire movie. I thought, *Shall I wake him up?* He woke up just as the movie ended. His perfect timing impressed me.

Another time, a Sunday, we took a walk in a small forest. Ohsawa decided to test me on what I had learned from his lectures on yin and yang.

"Please try to divide everything into two," Ohsawa said, pointing to some flowers and leaves.

"That's very handy; I'll try," I said. But I couldn't do it. The words didn't come out.

"Michio, why are you hesitating?" Ohsawa said. "You know right and left, brightness and darkness, day and night. Try."

I said, "Oh, I see. It's so easy." But again, I was stuck. I couldn't do it.

For the first time, I realized how caught I was in the modern educational system. I was so shocked. My brain couldn't handle practical things. I couldn't use simple, ordinary words. I couldn't think in dynamic terms of smooth and rough, curved and straight, light and dark, up and down, back and front, inside and outside, center and periphery, and other elementary relations. Though it was so simple, I couldn't see yin and yang, the unifying principle, the Order of the Universe. It later took me ten years living in the United States to completely get out from beneath conceptual thinking and learn to express myself simply. Until then, I did not feel confident about life.

Ohsawa fascinated me, but I could not really grasp what he was saying during our meetings in Japan. I respected his courage and dedication to peace, but found some of his actions foolhardy. For example, in 1944, toward the end of the Second World War, he set out on a one-man peace mission through Manchuria with the goal of reaching Moscow and convincing Stalin to make peace between the United States and Japan. During the winter, he was arrested in Manchuria, which was probably just as well since the tundra to Siberia was frozen and it was forty degrees below zero. Moreover, he had never ridden a horse before.

For this action and his pamphlets against the Japanese militarists, Ohsawa was jailed, tortured, and sentenced to death. He survived only due to the valiant efforts of his wife, Lima, who brought him rice balls every day in jail and attended to his needs. Just before his scheduled execution, the war ended and he was freed by the Americans. Ohsawa never complained about his hardships. He had faith in the absolute justice of the Order of the Universe and always taught that by eating well, one would intuitively be in the right place at the right time. I was not so sure about this.

JOURNEY TO AMERICA

During this period, I continued to meet scholars in Japan who advocated world government and to correspond with world federalists in the United States and other countries. Norman Cousins, the editor of *Saturday Review* and vice president of the United World Federalists at the time, came to Japan to visit Hiroshima and the survivors of the atomic bomb. During his stay, he visited the Student World Government Association at George Ohsawa's house and also took a meal of miso soup and brown rice. At that time, I was very busy and couldn't attend, but later I met with him at the Imperial Hotel, where he was staying in Tokyo.

Through my communication with world federalists, I received an invitation to visit the United States. But at that period, it was very difficult for a Japanese person to travel abroad. It was the time of the Occupation, and Japan was very poor. Norman Cousins kindly endorsed my visit to America, so that I could obtain a passport and visa. Of course, George Ohsawa was very happy and encouraging and helped me very much. World federalists in Japan were also pleased and felt that I could represent their movement around the world.

In late autumn 1949, I arrived on the West Coast, but I didn't have much money and had to work in Los Angeles and San Francisco. After accumulating some funds, I set off for the East Coast, stopping in Salt Lake City, Denver, and Chicago to lecture about world government problems. In the summer, I attended a Quaker study center in New Hampshire. I went to Swarthmore College in Pennsylvania and visited the Peace Library, and to the Friends community at Pendle Hill, which is devoted to researching peace problems. I also visited the University of Chicago and talked with Robert M. Hutchins, the chancellor, as well as social scientists and atomic physicists who were peace promoters.

After making these preliminary contacts, I decided to settle in New York and continue my graduate work at Columbia University, encouraged by Reverend Toyohiko Kagawa and sponsored by the late Mr. Tsukada, a Japanese restaurant owner. As soon as I attended the first class, however, I became frustrated. I could not understand what the professor was saying because of my poor ability to understand spoken English. I could grasp some general ideas, but after several lectures I decided that I would not attend class and began studying myself. I bought a used typewriter and went to the political science section of the university library, which was located underground in a very dark place. I examined hundreds of papers and more than sixty drafts of proposed world constitutions published during the twentieth century, in addition to many debates, discussions, and reports related to the formation of the League of Nations, the United Nations, and a world federal government. Since my English was quite poor, I had to retype—with one finger, as I had never learned to type—many of the manuscripts before I could read them.

While comparing all this material, I discovered there were many conflicts within the international community: cultural differences, racial differences, religious differences, language differences, educational level differences, social and economic differences, ideological differences. How was the whole world to be united? How were representatives to be selected from different regions to participate in the world congress or parliament? Some proposed one representative for every one million people, but others opposed any system that would give equal representation to Africans, Chinese, and other less industrially developed people. I started to wonder. We definitely needed world government to prevent nuclear catastrophe. But the arrogance of each race or each country would still remain. People would still become sick. Families would still be unhappy. Crime would continue. I began to doubt whether the structural change of society alone could really realize world peace. It might exert some control over atomic bombs and other destructive measures. But it appeared difficult to alter hatred, fear, prejudice, and discrimination so deeply rooted in the human mind. Without recovering and developing our human quality, there was no way to establish effective world federation. Temporarily, agreements might be reached, but eventually they would collapse.

What was the solution? I decided to approach various ethical and social leaders. I went to see Albert Einstein, Harold Urey, Thomas Mann, Upton Sinclair, and other prominent scientists, authors, and statesmen. I wrote letters to Prime Minister Nehru of India and other leading figures devoted to the cause of world peace and world order. Everyone said, "Yes, Michio, we need world government, but it is not a lasting solution. We need something to make humanity really peace-ful. But we don't know what it is."

My contact with these men—moral and intellectual giants—further convinced me that, although the formation of a world federation was absolutely necessary for avoiding future warfare, it was not the ultimate answer for building a better world and enabling humanity to realize its physical, mental, and spiritual poten-tial. It became apparent to me that in order to realize universal peace and happi-ness, the human race needed to be elevated toward physical health, sound mind, and ever greater spiritual understanding. So long as the quality of the human species remained at the present level, disputes, arguments, crime, and conflict would constantly arise. They would again destroy world order, even if it were established through legal and political means.

In the course of my studies, I realized that the dream of world peace is not a new idea nor one born exclusively from the threat of nuclear war. Plato, ancient Oriental thinkers, Sir Thomas More, and many religious leaders have also envi-sioned a harmonious world order. Great military leaders such as Alexander, Cae-sar, and Napoleon also strove to create one world. Until now, however, all approaches had failed. Something was lacking. I asked myself: What is the prac-tical solution to this ultimate question? Religions? They have been offering solu-tions for the past several thousand years. Modern education? Judicial, economic, and political systems? They all appear to offer no lasting answer. Peace move-ments? They had usually ended up fighting among themselves. Science and tech-nology? I hoped studying medicine might provide a solution for healing human minds and conduct. But the great men I contacted all agreed there was no college, no university, no teacher, and no book on this subject. They told me that even the modern medical system could not fundamentally change the way people thought and behaved. I had to search and search.

One of my most memorable encounters was with Pitirim A. Sorokin, a won-derful thinker and the author of *Reconstruction of Humanity*. Born in Russia, he had come to the United States in the early 1920s and had taught sociology for many years at the University of Minnesota and at Harvard University. He even-tually came to the conclusion that international legal measures—such as strength-ening the United Nations—would not work. He decided that we must develop love for others in order to realize peace. He set up a research center for altruism and collected data on Catholic saints and other selfless persons. He wanted to find out why they became altruistic and whether there was some key to raising the consciousness and compassion of ordinary people.

One day, I telephoned him. The year was 1951. He was an elderly man of sixty-two nearing retirement, and I was a young man of twenty-five just starting out. I explained to him my search and asked him what his own quest for peace had brought.

"My life is too short," he told me over the phone. "My study so far is in vain.

I don't know why man is so violent. I don't know how we can develop altruistic love and attain peace. I'm getting old. There is no hope for my studies. I await my death." His voice was trembling.

As we talked, the words flashed on me: "The dialectical application of dietary principles to the problem of world peace." Maybe Ohsawa was right, I thought. Could daily food really be the single most important factor shaping our health and wellbeing? Was human destiny really a matter of what we ate?

I remembered a talk with Ohsawa before coming to America. He had smiled and wished me luck in finding what he called "the secret melody of peace." Clearly, what I was looking for could not be found in any classroom or book, in any house of worship or international forum. There was no one to teach me. I resolved to discover the secret melody of peace for myself.

PEACE PROMOTER

Susana Sarué and Miriam Nour, Lebanon and Israel

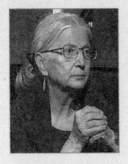

Miriam Nour

Modern macrobiotics came to the Middle East in 1975. Rema Cheblis, a young Lebanese girl, was suffering from a brain tumor. As the cancer had spread, she had become blind, deaf, and horribly disfigured. All the doctors had given up on her recovery and had prescribed heroin to deaden the pain. Susana Sarué, however, a student of mine completing her doctorate at the Sorbonne in Paris, heard of Rema's plight through mutual friends and went to Lebanon to help.

Susana took away all the candies, chocolate, and medications. She massaged Rema, slept with her, and went out with her every day to collect wild plants to make an especially nourishing soup. Along with brown rice and cooked vegetables, the soup gradually began to restore the little girl's vitality, which had been weakened by radiation treatments. For the first time in five years, Rema slept without interruption, and gradually she regained her hearing and sight in one eye.

One day she glimpsed herself in a mirror for the first time and saw that she had no hair and that the other eye socket was empty from where the tumor had pressed against it. Feeling she was no longer beautiful, Rema lost the will to live and stopped eating. Her death was very peaceful.

After Rema died, her parents, Brahim and Brigitte Cheblis, asked Susana to stay in Lebanon and do something so that her death would not have been in vain. Since the war began in 1975, the Cheblises had been working to restore peace between Christians and Moslems, as well as Palestinian refugees, who were also caught in the fighting. They had worked with many international relief agencies but had found nothing that really lasted. Perhaps macrobiotics could help bring peace to the Middle East.

Meanwhile, in March 1978, the first Israeli occupation took place in southern Lebanon. One day, the Cheblises woke up to find people fleeing from the fighting invading their house. Brahim, Brigitte, and Susana decided that they had to do something and, realizing the people had nothing to eat, decided to bake bread. There used to be a whole grain bread in Lebanon called Wise Bread because it gave wisdom and nourishment, but for many years the bread had been made entirely with white flour. In Lebanon, this flat bread composed up to 60 to 70 percent of the daily food.

With a little money donated by friends, they obtained five ovens, some fresh flour, and some equipment to prepare the dough naturally without artificial leavening. When the fighting eased, the ovens were brought into the homes of families who had a lot of children and who didn't have any work.

"Would you like to bake bread?" the mothers were asked.

"Of course," they answered, "there is no question. How can the children go without food?"

As soon as the ovens were installed, the people made the whole grain bread the same day and discovered they could make enough food for the entire week. They were mostly people from the mountains, so they ate this healthy bread and went to look for wild plants. Susana, Brigitte, and Brahim helped them find lentils, beans, and different things for each of the families to help them survive. They took the rest of the wild plants from the fields. Many families were able to save their lives thanks to the Wise Bread. The rest of the bread was given away to refugees from the south or sold to those who could afford it.

As the war continued, it became clear that everything in Lebanon was being destroyed by the implantation of modern culture. The demand for macrobiotic food was growing, to secure basic health and vitality as well as survival. To help people recover their own cultural roots, a food cooperative began in Brigitte and Brahim's kitchen. Soon it moved to an abandoned house next door and expanded into a store. The food center began by making organic fertilizer available, as well as providing information and books on traditional farming and food processing. The store sold locally made seitan (wheat gluten), bread, and jam, as well as miso, shoyu, and whole grain spaghetti imported from Italy. The store also carried sweets without sugar, sesame oil for cooking, and a wheat protein made from semolina. Recipes from traditional Lebanese cuisine that avoided exotic modern foods and styles of preparation were collected, such as *cabis*, a popular pickle. "If a mother does not recall, at least the grandmother remembers how to make a good meal with little or no meat, using fermentation and natural preserves," Susana noted. "Refined products have only been in existence here for fifty years." In the summer of 1978 a second corner shop was opened at Kaslik, on the coast to the north of Beirut, and in 1979 two other shops opened west of Beirut.

The macrobiotic approach to health and peace gradually attracted professional attention as well as local support. Stephen Malkonian, an agronomist who worked with a pesticide company for eight years, heard of Rema's case. Although very skeptical of macrobiotics at first, he decided to try the diet for himself. "I had had migraine headaches for years but after ten days, they stopped," he recalled. "I kept on that diet and started looking into the matter more deeply." After a year or two, Stephen felt he could no longer continue selling pesticides. He resigned from his job and began to bring in organic wheat from far-off villages. He started teaching macrobiotic courses in Beirut, which were attended by about fifty couples.

At the village of Kaa, Stephen helped set up an organic agricultural project on twenty-five hectares of land situated near the northern border with Syria. This land was practically a desert due to the erosion of soil in the region; but before World War I, the area of Kaa, like the neighboring regions, had been wooded. Wheat and barley were planted and harvested. An orchard was planted with a total of seventy varieties of fruit trees to see which trees would grow best in the soil. These included apricot, pear, pomegranate, cherry, almond, and peach trees. Artichoke, garlic, onions, and other vegetables were also cultivated. A small house in the desert was built for the family who helped in the work, using traditional methods of the region. The house also served as a training and information center for natural agriculture. "Our agricultural project is a green patch in the center of a vast desert," Stephen observed.

Back in Beirut, some Catholic priests who heard about the distribution of bread to the people gradually became macrobiotic. Père Maroun, who lived in a monastery ten minutes from the center of the city, joined the community and started bringing in brown rice and giving it to residents in the capital for half price. To schools and many others, he gave the rice for free. He said his hope was that if people would change their eating, they would see a difference not only in their health, but also in their attitude toward each other. He started preaching about food, telling his parishioners, "The church is not only for praying in this religion. Jesus said, 'Go and heal yourself.' So we must heal ourselves and our brothers and sisters."

In the east side of Beirut, a prominent broadcaster and journalist heard of macrobiotics and the priest's involvement. At the time, Miriam Nour had a two-hour radio program, discussing social news, arts, entertainment, and current events. It was very popular and broadcast throughout the Arab world. As Miriam learned about health and diet, she began talking about a macrobiotic approach to peace on her show and in her magazine stories. Her employers discouraged her new orientation. "If you want to stay in TV, on the radio, and in the magazines—and we want you to—don't speak about natural foods and love," she remembers being told. "Don't tell people not to go to war. Either you say what we want and we pay you a lot of money or you leave." She left.

At Père Maroun's monastery, Miriam was given space to open a center and begin giving cooking classes. Every day people came to pray, and many of them took her classes and began to change their eating style. Many came because of specific health problems—cancer, diabetes, obesity, epilepsy, migraines—and she worked with them. A doctor who knew the priest agreed to support the center medically. Other doctors were amazed to see how much better patients at the macrobiotic center were and started to lend their support as well.

At the monastery, Miriam and the others started growing vegetables with no chemicals, imported natural foods from Japan and Holland, and made available traditional Middle Eastern foods, such as lentils and wheat. Because the monastery was in a Christian area and people couldn't easily come from the Moslem side of Beirut, about 90 percent of those who came were Christians. As a journalist, however, Miriam could travel throughout the country; she began to take brown rice, miso, and literature to the Moslem areas and to give cooking classes in Arabic. She collected recipes and menus from the mothers and grandmothers. "The old people were very happy to be asked," she noted. "They believed in the traditional style, not in the modern hamburger and ice cream. They understood macrobiotics very well."

The macrobiotic center at the Catholic monastery was named Our Home, and the doors were never closed. It was open twenty-four hours a day and there was no key.

There was always an empty chair, an empty bed, a plate of food waiting for anyone who wanted to come. Prices were never put on anything. A box was kept at the door for donations. If anyone needed money, they could take some and no one would notice. The center was very poor but neat and clean and orderly.

The staff was surprised by the donations. One rainy night when there was nothing to eat, a man came to the door with snacks of rice and lentils. He said, "I felt that you needed this." Another time, a very rich man came with sacks of beans, saying "I know that you will use these." Once Miriam opened the box to take out some money and found only a diamond ring wrapped in a bit of paper that said, "This is all that I have" with no signature.

When Our Home first began, the monastery was a lovely, peaceful place. Bombarding of neighborhoods during the civil war continued, but it was in other areas. When she was not staying at the monastery, Miriam many times had to leave her house and go live in a shelter when the fighting broke out. People also moved from one area of the city to another as the pattern of rocket and artillery attacks changed. For a while, Miriam worked in one village where several thousand people had died. She was continuously impressed by how many Moslems and Christians helped shelter, feed, and clothe each other during the senseless attacks. "So many of these stories cannot be told through the mass media," Miriam later explained. "People around the world can only hear the voice of the bombs, and the reporters are only allowed to see one side."

Commenting on what she has learned applying macrobiotic principles to the situation in Lebanon, Miriam concluded, "Other countries—America, France—send us donations: canned food, sugar, white flour, margarine. And they send us free medication. It's a vicious circle—the food is eaten, the people get sick, they go to hospitals, they take the medications. The food is eaten, the people become more aggressive, angry, and warlike. And the people who send this junk food and medication, the synthetic clothing, also send the bombs. It is also they who say they want to make peace. But the war itself wants to fight because there is war in our hearts and minds. This is the lesson to learn through the experience of war—that it is inside each of us."

Sources

Naccour, Mary. "Sharing a Light in Lebanon." *East West Journal* (Dec. 1984): 32–37.

Stephan, Karin. "A Child's Gift of Courage to Susana Sarué." *East West Journal* (Dec. 1979): 52–55.

Stephan, Karin. "The Peaceful Revolution." *East West Journal* (Jan. 1980): 60–65.

Stephan, Karin. "Unity in a Lebanese Village." *East West Journal* (Feb. 1980): 60–63.

3.

Medicine for Humanity

My search for a way to realize peace had to begin somewhere, so I stopped all my library research and began to stand along Fifth Avenue and in Times Square in New York City. I sat on the stone staircase in front of St. Patrick's Cathedral near Rockefeller Center and watched thousands of people passing by, one by one. I watched their mannerisms and behavior, their postures and figures, their expressions and habits. Every day I watched them for signs of altruistic and peaceful behavior on the one hand or violent and aggressive behavior on the other hand, but soon I gave up. It was so confusing. Then I decided that one week I would observe only eyes. The next week I would watch only noses. So for a week, I would concentrate only on eyes—watching the eyes of thousands and thousands of people, going this way and that. The next week I would look at thousands of noses, then thousands of mouths, and thousands of ways of walking.

Days and weeks passed. At night, I would dream of thousands of eyes or noses. For nourishment, I ate rice balls made of brown rice wrapped in nori seaweed with a little umeboshi paste in the middle. About two months later I started to understand. Everyone was different. Everyone's eyes were different. Everyone's nose was different. Everyone's expression was different. These differences were to be respected, but why did they arise? I discovered that these differences resulted from two major factors: environmental conditions and food.

Environmental conditions included the changing climate, seasons, and weather, as well as the natural, social, and cultural environments in which individuals were brought up and were now living and the background of their parents and ancestors. Food conditions included everything that individuals have been eating during the present, during childhood, and in the womb, in addition to what their mother was eating, what their grandparents were eating, and what their ancestors were eating. I discovered that these influences shaped our present constitution and way of thinking. These factors were contributing to common qualities we share with all human beings, but they were also making everyone unique. At this time, there was no concept of DNA, though chromosomes and various hereditary factors were known. Hereditary factors are nothing but the

32

constitutional and genetic influence of the past and present environment and what previous generations ate.

From these discoveries, I could really understand for the first time the relation between food and world peace that Ohsawa had talked about. We create the future on the basis of our day-to-day way of life, including our way of eating. When the environment changes, we change. When eating changes, we change. I set aside my studies of political science and international law and began to study biology, chemistry, agriculture, history, religion, philosophy, culture, art, literature, music, and other subjects to understand more clearly the relationships between humanity, environment, and food. I did so not with the idea of becoming an expert or a specialist. I sought instead to find a comprehensive principle to unite our modern fragmented understanding.

I also continued to observe society around me, especially changing environmental and dietary patterns. To understand the day-to-day way people were eating, I would go to cafeterias and automats in Manhattan. I was very poor, so I usually didn't eat out myself. But I would watch others eat. Some people were eating very rapidly. Other people were eating very slowly. Some people gulped down their food. Others chewed it thoroughly. Some people were bright and cheerful. Others were depressed. Some people were energetic and healthy. Others were listless and sick. More and more, I understood their facial structures, their bodily constitutions, their mental and physical conditions, their human relations with other people. It became very clear how these were related to what they were eating. Thus began my true understanding of the Order of the Universe and the practical application of yin and yang.

BIOLOGICAL DEGENERATION

From my observations, I could see that degenerative physical, mental, and social disorders were rapidly increasing in modern society. Many people had heart disease. Others suffered from cancer. Among the old, arthritis was almost universal. Among the young, wild erratic behavior and mental illness were on the rise. I became more aware of environmental pollution and how water and air contamination were affecting our health and daily lives. Closely connected with chronic diseases was a deterioration of food quality. The food we were consuming was fundamentally different from that which our parents ate, and it was almost totally different from that of our grandparents and ancestors. Through refinement, mass production, chemicalization, artificialization, and other highly industrialized processes, a rapid change of food quality was taking place, and almost no one was aware of its effects on consciousness and behavior.

Realizing the basic cause of our modern ills, I felt sad at the prospects for humanity. Not only nuclear war but also biological disaster could lead to the decline and extinction of our species, *homo sapiens*. If biological degeneration continued unchecked, the end would probably come by the middle of the twenty-first century, even if we managed to avoid nuclear war. During this period, heart disease, cancer, diabetes, arthritis, sexual and reproductive disorders, allergies, and many other disorders would spread epidemically. Psychological disorders, including schizophrenia, paranoia, anxiety, and depression, would become common in daily life. Disputes, crimes, and conflicts within the family and community would mount. Religious and educational influences would be ignored. Economic and political systems would end in chaos. Poverty, disease, misery, and madness would spread through the entire modern world—with or without another world war.

The idea came to me then of a "medicine for humanity," which would seek to realize health, happiness, and peace. From my observations and studies, I found that all present-day medicine was devoted to the relief of pain and disappearance of outward symptoms. It did not, however, fundamentally concern itself with preventing disease, nor with the underlying environmental and dietary causes of good health. I looked up "medicine for humanity" and similar expressions in the catalogues of Columbia University Library and Widener Library at Harvard, but could find nothing.

To reverse the march toward biological degeneration and lay the foundation for a new era for the further development of human life on this planet, I realized that it was essential to recover genuine food, largely of natural, organic quality, and make it available to every family at a reasonable cost. Only then could consciousness be transformed and world peace achieved.

LIVING IN NEW YORK

Meanwhile, I had to improve my English, refine my way of expression, and support my life. I washed dishes at restaurants in New York and worked as a bellboy. In 1954, some friends and I started a small import-export company, R.H. Brothers (Resurrection of Humanity by Brothers) Trading Company, and set up small Japanese gift shops on West Ninth Street and then on West 44th Street. To help bridge Eastern and Western cultural understanding, I also took the initiative to bring a Japanese department store to New York's Fifth Avenue. But business was not my purpose. It just served as preparation for later teaching and helped me to experience the business world and to make a living. Slowly my command of English improved, and I was able to speak more fluently.

In November 1959, George Ohsawa came to visit New York. In the years since we first met, he and his wife had given up their center in Yokohama and left Japan to live and teach abroad. They journeyed first to India for a year and then to Africa to see Dr. Albert Schweitzer, who had been the only great world moral or intellectual leader to respond personally to Ohsawa's world government proposals. Eventually they reached Europe, where they attracted many students and inspired a pioneer natural foods company in Belgium called Lima Foods, named after Mrs. Ohsawa.

In the early 1950s, other students of George and Lima Ohsawa began to come to the United States. These included Tomoko Yokoyama, a young schoolteacher from a mountain village in central Japan. Ohsawa had been impressed with her dedication to world peace and arranged for her to attend a conference on world government in Paris. He gave her a new name, Aveline, and put her on a steamship sailing to San Francisco. I met her at the Greyhound Bus Station in New York in 1951, and we have been with each other ever since.

Herman and Cornellia Aihara also arrived during this period. They would later organize macrobiotic activities on the West Coast. During George Ohsawa's visits in the early 1960s, we made arrangements for him to give seminars and lectures. He came from France or Belgium every year or every other year and would stay for one week or one month. He often stayed at my and Aveline's home in Queens, New York (and later Cambridge, Massachusetts), and we would talk further about world peace—about developing a medicine for humanity. That is the beginning of our educational movement.

During this period, the Cold War between the United States and the Soviet Union was intensifying. Initial enthusiasm for world government in the late 1940s had waned following the Korean War, the Berlin Crisis, the Hungarian Revolt, the U-2 incident, the launching of Sputnik and the space race, the Cuban Revolution, and subsequent events. The United States and Russia became engaged in a deadly nuclear arms race, developing more and more destructive atomic and hydrogen weapons, bigger and more efficient intercontinental ballistic missiles, and ever more complex theories of deterrence and counterforce. Meanwhile, nuclear testing was at its height, releasing large quantities of radiation into the atmosphere that drifted across the world and fell on crops and harvests. In schoolrooms, children regularly held bomb drills, and some families built home fallout shelters, stocking them with food and weapons.

The peace movement at this time was small. In England, Bertrand Russell led the Ban-the-Bomb marches. In the United States, Einstein, Oppenheimer, Szilard, and some of the other original atomic scientists called for an end to the arms race. Citizens' groups such as the Committee for a Sane Nuclear Policy organized campaigns against nuclear weapons testing. *On the Beach*, a novel about the aftermath of World War III, had a tremendous impact on peoples' consciousness, and it was debated whether anyone could survive the next world war, and if so, where the ideal safe location might be.

At the time of the Berlin Crisis in spring 1961, tension and fear about a possible nuclear war reached a peak. George Ohsawa was in New York at the time and in his lectures, he advised people to evacuate larger cities to safer, rural areas. He made similar recommendations in Europe and Japan. A committee was formed in New York, and research indicated that the Sacramento Valley in northern California might be a safe place in the event of a nuclear war. Several hundred students of Ohsawa gathered to discuss the evacuation, and about twenty families decided to go. As chairman of the gathering, I indicated that I would continue to remain in New York until the international situation became more intense.

Those who decided to leave met many times at my home to discuss logistics of the move. On the day they left in a caravan of twenty cars, the *New York Times* published an article and quoted Ohsawa, who compared their move to the Exodus. Each night, the caravan stopped to camp out and dine on miso soup and brown rice prepared on kerosene stoves. In Chico, California, they found a warm welcome. Although they were surprised and relieved that war did not come, they set about starting new lives. Herman Aihara, Robert Kennedy, and other friends formed a rice cake manufacturing company, which later developed into one of the leading natural foods companies, Chico-San.

MACROBIOTICS

What should the way of life for the harmonious physical, mental, and spiritual development of modern humanity be called? In ancient Greece, Hippocrates followed a natural, commonsense approach to health and longevity, emphasizing environmental and dietary factors. His philosophy was summed up in the maxim, "Let food be thy medicine and thy medicine food." As the father of Western medicine, he introduced the term *makrobios,* or "macrobiotics," from the Greek words for "great life" or "long life." Since then, *macrobiotics* has come down through Western history to mean a natural way of life, including a simple, natural way of eating, leading to health, happiness, and longevity. The term was used by Herodotus, the historian of ancient cultures; Rabelais, the great French humanist of the Renaissance; and Christoph W. Hufeland, an eighteenth-century German philosopher, physician to Goethe, and professor of medicine who wrote a famous book, *Macrobiotics or the Art of Prolonging Life.* Until the early part of the twentieth century, Biblical patriarchs such as Abraham, long-lived people such as the ancient Ethiopians, and the Chinese sages were respectfully referred to as macrobiotic in popular works.

In the Far East, there were also cultural patterns, folk traditions, and wisdom schools based on a similar way of life. The traditional Oriental approach to health and longevity—based on the principles of yin and yang and the teachings of Confucius and Lao Tzu—was translated by Professor Joseph Needham in his 1959 multivolume history, *Science and Civilization in China,* as "macrobiotics."

In the early 1960s, during travels to France, Belgium, and the United States, George Ohsawa introduced the term "Zen Macrobiotics" to refer to his teachings. Zen Buddhists traditionally followed simple dietary practices, eating just a bowl of brown rice, miso soup, a few vegetables, pickles, and tea. Because Zen was popular in the West at this time, Ohsawa hoped to attract attention to his approach by linking it with Zen, though his own teachings were not limited to Buddhism. Needham's volumes, documenting the Far Eastern stream of macrobiotic thought, also began to appear about this time.

I adopted "macrobiotics" in its original meaning, as the universal way of health and longevity which encompasses the largest possible view not only of diet, but also of all dimensions of human life, natural order, and cosmic evolution. Macrobiotics embraces behavior, thought, breathing, exercise, relationships, customs, cultures, ideas, and consciousness, as well as individual and collective lifestyles found throughout the world.

In this sense, macrobiotics is not simply or mainly a diet. Macrobiotics is the universal way of life with which humanity has developed biologically, psychologically, and spiritually, and with which we will maintain our health, freedom, and happiness. Macrobiotics includes a dietary approach, but its purpose is to ensure the survival of the human race and its further evolution on this planet. In macrobiotics—the natural intuitive wisdom of East and West, North and South—I found the medicine for humanity that I had been seeking.

PEACE PROMOTER

Susana Sarué, Colombia

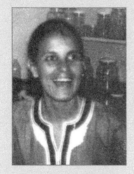

In the early 1970s, Susana Sarué (a student of mine who worked with Rema Cheblis in Lebanon) returned to Colombia to do field work for her thesis on malnutrition in the Third World. Half-Colombian and half-Chilean by birth, Susana had been studying macrobiotics in Paris and completing graduate work at the Sorbonne. She settled in a little village called Virareka. It had about 10,000 inhabitants and almost all of them, including small children, worked in a large sugarcane factory.

Over the years, the sugarcane plantation had displaced local farms and fields. Large amounts of chemicals were applied to the cane, which came to displace all other crops. Deserts replaced green fields of grains and vegetables. Almost all the food eaten locally was brought in from elsewhere.

`Susana Sarué

Arriving with no food or money of her own, Susana ate with the people and searched for a way to improve their diet. She studied the ingredients they cooked with, the materials the cookware was made of, the way they prepared their cooking fires, the odors they liked, the textures they liked, and the all-important symbols of prestige and social status that different articles of diet represented.

Visiting people's kitchens, Susana found that the rich used gas stoves and enjoyed steak, dairy food, and salads. The middle class cooked with paraffin and also ate a lot of highly processed modern foods. The lower class cooked with wood and emulated the upper classes in their food habits as much as possible. "The people ate white rice and beans, and they left room for meat, which they didn't have," Susana recalls. "They aspired to eat like that, so they would leave room. They lacked protein. They were very empty and hungry." Everyone consumed enormous amounts of sugar.

Susana also observed the local chickens. One day she realized that they naturally knew what to eat and were the healthiest and most energetic inhabitants of the village. She observed that the chickens were eating soy grits and sorghum, a tropical grain similar to millet. She realized that good-quality grains and beans were available, but that she would have to invent things for people to eat that also fit the terms of the idea they had of themselves. This insight led her to devise a whole range of foods made from natural ingredients, but which looked and tasted like the prestige foods the upper classes ate.

She made a variety of cutlets, burgers, and other "meats" with a soya base. She made soymilk instead of dairy milk and instead of sweetening it with refined sugar, she put a little syrup from the sugarcane and some cinnamon in it. Instead of yogurt, which the people wanted, she made "fromage du soja" (soy cheese). She even made an ice cream from sorghum and soya with molasses in it and cooked in such a way that it remained a cream.

The children's condition began to change quickly. They became more alert and intelligent in school and less famished. They no longer had large stomachs. They also became more active, which worried their mothers. "The mothers said to me, 'But the children are intolerable, they play all day.' I said, 'But those are normal children. That's how normal children behave.'"

With a girl from the village, Susana eventually opened a health food bar. They borrowed about $100 and rented a house. They put in a refrigerator, created a kitchen, and painted everything. They found a cook and started making soy burgers, ready to eat for mothers who did not have time to cook, and sold foods that were ready to cook. They made soy-milk yogurt with fruit. They even served an entire dinner plate with sorghum, soy meat, and local vegetables.

Susana noted how proud the people were of their health bar. "They began to plan out salaries, how much the rent should be, the gas, electricity, etc. They became their own administrators. They created a contest for the best recipe. Each person came with a plate, and the entire village would try it." For years, the villagers had been striking the sugar plantation but had never won. In her classes, Susana talked to the local women about yin and yang and the need to become free men and women. One day, Susana was invited to a meeting of married couples. She brought plates of already-prepared food. The men at the meeting asked if she were a communist and wanted to know what she had been telling their wives.

"Señores, I'm going to speak to you in your language," Susana replied. "You are earning 33 pesos per day, one dollar. You spend 25 pesos for your family, and you are still hungry. Your child has a bloated stomach and is always crying, and you have to see a doctor and spend money which you don't have, and you are always poisoned because you feel overwhelmed by life, and you don't want to think!. . . I'm going to show you how you can eat an enormous amount of food so you are no longer hungry. Look, this amount of soya will cost you this much; you can prepare food like this, like this, and this, which I will bring to you—the total cost for the family is 8 pesos."

The men said, "Tomorrow you begin [cooking], women. Tomorrow you begin." The women of the village said, "But you won't like it," and the men said, "No, we like it."

In this way, the families of Virareka were able to save money. One day, they went on strike. Their bosses at the sugar plantation said, "Well, the first day they won't come to work, but by the third day they will be starved and they will have to come." But the strike lasted two weeks, and in the end the workers' wages were finally raised.

Source

Stephan, Karin. "The Peaceful Revolution." *East West Journal* (Jan. 1980): 60–65.

4.

Erewhon Revisited

From my observations of people and lifestyles in New York, I began to see why people are different. I recognized why some were more altruistic than others, and some were more violent; why some were chronically sick and others remained well. Our day-to-day food changes and shapes us, giving us energy and vibrancy and changing the composition of our cells, including our brain cells. I was amazed that Albert Einstein, Pitirim Sorokin, Thomas Mann, and the other intellectual giants whom I contacted didn't notice this simple fact. Around the world, billions of other people didn't know either.

CHANGES IN DIET AND HEALTH

As my understanding and practice of macrobiotics deepened, my own health improved and I started to realize the influence that food had played in my own development. I was brought up on semi-polished brown rice, occasionally mixed with barley or beans, along with vegetables, bean products, sea vegetables, and occasional noodles, fish, and fruits. Of course, while I was growing up, the modern way of eating rapidly spread, penetrating our household as well as most others. Though our way of eating remained mostly traditional, from time to time we had white bread, brown sugar, milk, and butter, though these dairy foods were consumed only occasionally. Meat was eaten in our home very seldom, perhaps once a month in tiny volume, usually during special occasions. We had eggs once a week or every other week, and once Mother raised a couple of chickens, which produced nice organic eggs. Animal food usually consisted of fish or seafood, which was served a couple of times a week, and Father was especially fond of fish. I myself did not care much for animal food and did not eat it frequently. Instead, I was fond of noodles and sea vegetables; as I entered high school I developed a liking for fruits. Prior to this time, about age thirteen, my physical and mental condition had been very active and alert. Though physically slim, I engaged in many physical activities, including the martial arts, baseball, high jump, running, skiing, and bicycling, and I excelled in all these fields. After I began to consume more fruits, however, and started to like more refined white noodles, my physical vitality declined and I became more sedentary and introspective. Mentally, I started to isolate myself from my friends and classmates. I liked to be alone, reading books, writing poetry, and pursuing artistic and aesthetic subjects, as well as meditate and pray.

Upon entering college, I began to suffer early symptoms of tuberculosis, which I later associated with my excessive fruit consumption. I visited hospitals and received regular air injections to open my lungs, from a doctor who was a friend of the family. These periodic visits continued for about a year, and during this time I continued to write a lot of sentimental poetry. While still in college, I started to suffer spinal pain and was suspected to have some bone marrow deterioration, though medical exams were not extensively performed. Until the completion of college, over a period of a year and a half, the pain continued and I had to lean on piled cushions while reading. At school, I was excused from hard physical labor as the war intensified. However, in spite of my poor health, I was appointed dorm chairman and with the help of my closest friend and vice chairman, Keichu Moriai, actively coordinated the affairs of 600 students.

During World War II, dietary practice in Japan returned to a more traditional way of eating. Sweets, fruit, meat, dairy food, and other rich, luxurious foods were scarce. At my uncle's home in Tokyo, where I lived while studying at Tokyo University, our diet consisted of either half-polished brown rice or barley or dark-flour bread, miso soup with vegetables, sometimes wild grasses, occasional fruits, and fish. More frequently, we ate beans, tofu, and other bean products. My spinal condition disappeared during this time, but I did not know why or connect it with a change in diet. Later, when I was drafted, this more simple way of eating was also observed in the army, and my previous good health returned and stabilized.

Immediately after the war ended, in 1945, the food situation in Japan worsened, and even rice and other grains became difficult to obtain. Strict rationing was enforced throughout the country. In addition to basics, from time to time the Allied powers included a bucket of brown sugar, potato powder, or white flour in the rations. These foods were received by everyone partly with delight and partly with confusion. We could not use them as staples; however, they provided high caloric energy. During the rest of my university and postgraduate life, over the next four or five years, I continued to eat simply and maintained relatively good health.

Naturally, throughout this period of deprivation, I and everyone else was compelled to chew each bite very thoroughly to utilize its energy and nutrients to the maximum. It was considered a social sin to waste even a grain of rice or a piece of bread. It was during this time of scarcity that I met George Ohsawa. Although he was advocating and teaching dietary practice, my simple daily diet resembled his so much that it did not attract my attention or enthusiasm.

On the voyage to America in autumn 1949, I first encountered beef with mashed potatoes and pork chops with thick oily gravy, as well as buttered white bread and almost unlimited amounts of milk, dairy food, and sugar. On the SS *General Gordon*, I ate some of these foods, but I soon found that I preferred dark bread, oatmeal, and cooked vegetables, though they were often canned. I also preferred beans and fish to meat, though they were often deep-fried. In the beginning, I enjoyed sweet desserts and ice cream, but by the time the ship arrived on the West Coast I had come to dislike them.

After arriving in San Francisco on Thanksgiving Day, I began to partake of the ordinary American breakfast, lunch, and dinner while staying in church dormitories and friends' houses in San Francisco, Los Angeles, and New York. These foods included fried eggs, omelets, white bread, fried chicken, sometimes beef or pork, canned vegetables, canned and sometimes fresh fruit, milk, and butter. Although I sampled some of these rich foods, from taste and habit I enjoyed the simpler ones, always choosing darker bread, oatmeal, and more vegetables; more fish rather than beef or pork; the less-sweetened desserts; and fresh fruit rather than canned.

While in New York, I began to cook for myself, shopping at the local grocery store, and choosing these preferred items. I was especially delighted to find brown rice (though it was chemicalized), unrefined pasta, and dark bread. While working as a dishwasher in restaurants and as a bellboy in hotels and resorts, I could not eat what I really wanted. But intuitively, I tried to chew well. Moreover, I did not drink any alcohol, did not want soft drinks, and rarely ate heavily sugar-treated foods. While attending Columbia University, I had a small apartment in which I could cook. There, I prepared either brown rice or vegetable soup or unrefined pasta or noodles, though occasionally I would eat at a coffee shop nearby.

I continued to cook for myself for about a year in New York until Aveline came and joined me. Although intellectually and spiritually, I was coming to understand George Ohsawa's teachings about food and destiny, it was Aveline who really secured my health and consciousness. She began to cook brown rice. She also baked whole rye or whole wheat bread, made unrefined pasta and salted biscuits, and obtained fresh vegetables from Chinatown. When I went out to binge on ice cream, she would accompany me but not order anything for herself. She would just watch meditatively and, without saying a word, influenced me to stop. Thanks to her wonderful cooking and high spirit, I was able once again—after so many years—to become one with the natural environment and begin to realize my eternal dream.

In New York, my physical health improved, and I had boundless energy to pursue my work, studies, and responsibilities as a father to a growing family. However, it took about ten years to recover a simple, clear way of thinking and expression. I began to study what kind of food people were eating when the Old and New Testaments were written. By eating that food, I could understand their world view, and whole sections of the Bible that had long puzzled me suddenly became clear. The same thing with the traditional Hindu, Buddhist, Confucian, and Taoist teachings. By eating the food that Krishna, Buddha, Confucius, or Lao Tzu ate, we can understand the minds that gave rise to the great cosmological teachings of the East. I began to see universal order operating in people, mountains, stars, and galaxies.

The same principles that governed the movement of subatomic particles and the growth of trees and flowers shaped our personal and social destinies. One by one, the solutions to the problems of modern society emerged as my own health strengthened and my consciousness broadened and deepened.

TEACHING IN BOSTON

After changing myself, I wanted to apply my understanding of food principles immediately to the problem of war and peace. There was, however, virtually no natural, organic food available in the United States. Good-quality grains, vegetables, beans, bean products, sea vegetables, fresh fruits, and many other traditional products, including miso, shoyu, and unrefined sea salt, were not available at all at this time. Chemically contaminated food made up 99 percent of what was sold in the grocery stores and supermarkets. It was clear that I could not depend on the food industry to begin developing food for human development, or what I called "medicine for humanity." They were oriented totally in the other direction: speeding up the processes of nature through artificial methods in order to maximize profit. There was a small health food movement at this time, but it was based largely around vitamins and supplements, not whole foods. It became apparent that we must begin to change society ourselves through public education and then through natural foods production.

In 1965, our family moved to Boston. I had given some seminars in Massachusetts and found there were many young people in New England who would be receptive to macrobiotics. It was also the spiritual and intellectual energy center of the continent. Many social and philosophical movements, such as the Pilgrims, the American Revolution, the Abolitionist movement, the Transcendentalists, women's suffrage, Mormonism, Seventh Day Adventism, Christian Science, and others, originated in New England and spread across the rest of the country. This corresponded with traditional Oriental philosophy, in which the northeast direction or region governs thought and consciousness.

Along with Aveline and our children, I settled in Cambridge and began to teach a handful of friends who had been studying with me when I came up from New York occasionally to lecture. At the same time, I started giving workshops in Oriental philosophy at Harvard University, but I soon found that I had made a great mistake. The students and faculty there were not interested in the Order of the Universe at all; they wanted only knowledge, conceptualizations, and data. I felt as if I were in a department store, offering God, spirit, and infinity. They had come to buy underwear, socks, or cheap shirts, but not life itself. So I began to lecture at home and receive whoever would come.

One day during a lecture at my home about traditional Oriental medicine, I exhibited some acupuncture needles. Shortly afterward, I was visited by the Cambridge police. They warned me that I was practicing medicine without a license and said unless I left town, I would be prosecuted. I explained to them the long history of acupuncture in the Far East. Actually, I was not practicing acupuncture, just introducing the subject in discussion, as an example of a symptomatic approach to the relief of disease compared to changing our daily way of eating.

This was at the height of the Cold War, before the thaw in relations between China and the United States. Merely showing acupuncture needles was considered illegal. I could have taken legal action and probably would have won in court, but I knew that this would have only increased polarity and misunderstanding. I told the authorities that my family and I would leave.

From Cambridge, we moved our educational activities to Wellesley, which also had a sizable college population. We didn't know that it was also very conventional, and soon problems with the town arose. Under the name of the East West Institute, we had rented a space from an educational institute to lecture, demonstrate macrobiotic cooking, and practice Aikido. But we attracted so many students—including some with long hair and beards from Boston—that the town fathers asked us to stop. The neighbors complained of too much traffic and congestion.

From Wellesley we moved to Brookline. We continued to invite students to live and study with us for short periods in our home. It soon became clear that we would need a larger and more formal teaching and cooking facility. In 1966, I began lecturing two evenings a week in downtown Boston in the back room of the Arlington Street Church, a Unitarian-Universalist church that was very active in the peace movement during the Vietnam War. In the beginning, only a few students came, but gradually the numbers increased. Every year since our days in New York, Aveline and I had imported a small quantity of the best natural, organic-quality miso, shoyu, sea vegetables, and other traditional foods from Japan for our personal use, as well as for our friends and students. We spent many evenings transferring these foods from bulk containers into smaller bottles, bags, or boxes.

During some of my lectures, Aveline would distribute rice balls that she had prepared in the kitchen at home. The demand for good-quality, ready-made foods such as these, as well as the imported goods, increased, and it no longer became practical to stock them at home. A small basement food store was opened, followed by two small restaurants: Sanae, which means "sprouting rice" in Japanese, and the Seventh Inn. We stocked brown rice and other grains, beans, seeds, nuts, fresh vegetables, miso, shoyu, and a few other items. We selected the term "natural foods" to distinguish our approach from modern refined, chemicalized, and highly processed foods, as well as "health foods" that consisted primarily of vitamins, juices, flakes, bran, and other partial or processed foods.

Aveline named our little shop Erewhon, after the Utopian romance written by Samuel Butler in 1872. In his novel, Butler satirized modern civilization's turning away from nature. In the world of the Erewhonians, disease is viewed as a crime, while crime is viewed as a disease. Sick people are put in jail because they have violated natural order by not taking care of themselves, while lawbreakers are hospitalized and given healthy foods to change their immoral behavior. The inhabitants of Erewhon observe a simple, orderly way of life. They possess machines but do not use them because the machines end up possessing their time and creative energy. Instead, the machines are kept in the museum as artifacts of past cultural disharmony. Butler's book, like Lewis Carroll's novels *Alice's Adventures in Wonderland* and *Through the Looking Glass,* held up a mirror to the topsy-turvy world of Victorian society and, by extension, modern society as a whole.

Unlike previous Utopian communities that were established in a distinct geographical area, we hoped to create a healthy, peaceful community of people in the midst of modern society. Unlike past Utopias that had ideological belief systems and philosopher-kings, we had no dogma or creed, no formal membership or governing elite. Everyone was in charge of his or her own destiny.

THE SPREAD OF MACROBIOTICS

Soon, Erewhon Trading Company moved into a larger store on Newbury Street, a few blocks down from Sanae and the Arlington Street Church. Within two years, the wholesale operation moved to a warehouse on the Boston Wharf, distributing constantly to an ever-increasing number of natural foods stores in New England and the mid-Atlantic states. In the beginning, there was very little organic food available in the country, and most of our energy was devoted to visiting farmers and convincing them to try our methods. At first, they were very skeptical. The mid-1960s was still a time of cheap energy, and the disastrous effects of chemical spraying had not yet become widely apparent. By appealing to ancestral traditions, common sense, and in some cases guaranteeing to purchase the entire crop, we talked farmers in California, Texas, and Arkansas into growing rice and other foods organically. Until this time, to our knowledge, the only commercial brown rice in the United States was produced with pesticides in Texas and marketed under the label River Rice. We were grateful for this rice; however, until an organic quality of brown rice was readily available, we could not truly begin to secure the health of modern society.

We also talked to many food processors, manufacturers, exporters, distributors, retailers, and consumers. From the start we realized that it was not economical or ecologically sound to continuously import macrobiotic specialty foods from Japan. But we had to rely on these Japanese imports, with which we were most familiar, until good-quality natural foods were produced in this country and a whole foods cuisine native to North America was reestablished.

MACROBIOTIC EDUCATION

From this small seed, the natural foods movement developed. Spearheaded by Erewhon, high-quality natural food distributors in North America serviced thousands of retailers and co-ops and hundreds of restaurants by the mid-1970s. Though not all of them were managed directly by macrobiotic principles, they were obviously serving for the betterment of the public health. Millions of people started to eat brown rice, millet, barley, whole oats, whole wheat bread, grain burgers, tofu, miso, tempeh, shoyu, tahini, organic vegetables and fruits, unfiltered juices, seaweed, naturally sweetened desserts, sea salt, unrefined vegetable oil, spring water, and other foods that our movement introduced and popularized. Meanwhile, public education expanded. We began constant lectures, seminars, and study sessions for the education of the food industry, government and social leaders, the medical profession, and the general public. Natural food industries began to spread, not only in North America, but also in Central and South America, Europe, Australia, and the Far East.

Along with securing the best possible natural quality of food, it was necessary to guide individuals and families in the direction of more healthy dietary patterns and cooking methods using these foods. In the Boston area, several study houses were opened for the convenience of students who came from other states and abroad. These study houses offer experience in the macrobiotic way of life, teaching philosophy and practical applications in daily life. By the early 1970s, several hundred teaching centers were established in this country and all around the world by our associates, friends, students, and people who shared the same dream. These centers offered macrobiotic cooking instruction, in addition to classes in East-West philosophy, traditional medicine, shiatsu massage, palm healing, meditation, natural birth and family care, yoga and martial arts, along with a spirit of respect and love for parents, ancestors, and all people in society.

The *East West Journal*, a monthly newspaper, was established in 1971 to introduce macrobiotics and a new vision of the present and future world to a wider audience. Books, magazines, and pamphlets were published and continue to be published in many languages through a network of centers, associations, and publishers. In 1973, the East West Foundation was set up in Boston to coordinate and administer macrobiotic educational activities in the United States. The following year, under the auspices of Kushi International Seminars, Aveline and I began lecturing every year to students, physicians, and health professionals in Europe, Latin America, and occasionally the Far East. In 1977, the Kushi Institute was founded in Boston to train and certify macrobiotic teachers, counselors, and cooks. Affiliate institutes subsequently opened in London, Amsterdam, Antwerp, Barcelona, Florence, Switzerland, Lisbon, and Tokyo, with hundreds of graduates fanning out each year to teach cooking and give way-of-life consultations in their local areas; start small, natural food processing industries; work in schools, restaurants, businesses, and hospitals; and perform other community service. The Kushi Foundation was established in 1980 to further scientific and medical research, as well as oversee our educational activities. In 1983, we opened a teaching facility at a former Franciscan retreat in the Berkshire Mountains of western Massachusetts and began advanced instruction in spiritual training, as well as in cooking, culture, and the art of living.

Through these activities, millions of people around the world turned to proper dietary practices using better-quality natural food, moving toward a healthier way of life. By the late 1960s and into the 1970s, the way modern society looked at food had altered radically, and entire dietary patterns began to change. Meanwhile, once basic natural, organic-quality food was available, we could turn our attention directly to the modern biological and psychological crisis. We began to focus on the problems of cancer, heart disease, diabetes, arthritis, and other degenerative diseases.

Over the years, the success of macrobiotics in preventing diseases that had baffled modern medicine began to attract the attention of researchers. In the mid-1970s, doctors at Harvard Medical School and the Framingham Heart Study began a series of studies on people in the macrobiotic community in Boston. They found that macrobiotic people had the lowest cholesterol levels and the most ideal blood pressure levels ever recorded by any group in modern society. These blood values were similar to those in traditional societies around the world, where heart disease, cancer, arthritis, and other degenerative disorders were unknown. These promising findings and other research on macrobiotics were published in the *New England Journal of Medicine, Journal of the American Medical Association, American Journal of Epidemiology,* and other professional journals and had a major impact, educating society to the dangers of the modern diet high in saturated fat, dietary cholesterol, and refined sugar. The medical researchers cited the macrobiotic community as providing an almost utopian model for the rest of society, because it was drawn from all walks of life and required no special family, religious, racial, or ethnic ties or background. For example, J. P. Deslypere, M.D., head of a Flemish medical team investigating macrobiotic blood values, body weight, hormone levels, and nutrient levels, concluded: "In the field of cardiovascular and cancer risk factors this kind of blood is very favorable. It's ideal, we couldn't do better, that's what we're dreaming of. It's really fantastic, like children, whose blood vessels are still completely open and whole. This is a very important matter, deserving our full attention."[1]

From 1974, regular medical seminars were held in Boston, attracting hundreds of doctors, nurses, and other health care professionals. The East West Foundation also convened an annual conference on a dietary approach to cancer, in which scores of individuals and family members who had relieved existing tumors and malignancies with macrobiotics presented their experiences. These accounts were published regularly in the *East West Journal* and *Case History Reports* (a series of personal accounts published by East West Foundation), and often included the results of X-rays, CAT scans, blood tests, and other medical diagnostic techniques.

By the end of its first decade, the impact of the natural foods and natural health movements penetrated the highest levels of society. In Washington, D.C., my associates and I met with leaders at the White House and Congress to discuss our work and present recommendations for public health and national food and agricultural policy. In 1977, the Senate Select Committee on Nutrition and Human Needs issued a report titled *Dietary Goals for the United States.* This landmark report connected meat, sugar, and other articles in the modern diet with six of the ten leading causes of death in modern society and called upon the public to begin eating substantially more whole cereal grains, fresh vegetables, and fruit.

By the early 1980s, our preventive dietary approach to cancer had begun to be accepted by the medical profession, and various medical schools began research- ing the effectiveness of the macrobiotic dietary approach in relieving existing tumors. In 1981, the Lemuel Shattuck Hospital in Boston began a macrobiotic and natural foods lunch program in its cafeteria. A double-blind experiment with long-term psychiatric and geriatric patients demonstrated significant reductions in psychosis and agitation in patients on the macrobiotic diet. At the Tidewater Detention Center in Virginia, antisocial and aggressive behavior among juvenile offenders was reduced by 45 percent by restricting certain foods in a macrobiotic project. In 1985, a group of inmates in the 1,800-man Pohawtan State Prison in Virginia started eating macrobiotically in a state-sponsored program. In the mid-1980s, we began working with people with AIDS in New York; medical researchers have begun to report on the success of the macrobiotic dietary approach in stabilizing this often fatal disorder.[2]

Though our work with the scientific and medical professions, as well as correc- tions and educational facilities, continued to expand, in the late 1970s I began to focus once more on the problems of international conflict, arms control, and world peace. In 1979, the first North American Macrobiotic Congress convened—with delegates from many states and provinces—to discuss applying our understanding of natural order to the problems of modern society, especially the peace issue. The Congress organized five working committees—agriculture, food processing, and food distribution; family and community affairs; education; medical, scientific, and governmental affairs; and publications—which over the years have initiated a vari- ety of activities, including the adoption of the motto "World Health—World Peace"; the observance of World Peace Day (August 6) at macrobiotic centers around the country; and the drafting of dietary and environmental guidelines to help minimize the effects of radioactivity in the event of a nuclear accident, such as those that occurred at Three Mile Island in 1979, Chernobyl in 1986, and Fukushima in 2011. Similar macrobiotic congresses have assembled annually in Europe, the Middle East, and the Caribbean, drawing representatives from many states and nations. In the future, we plan to convene the first World Macrobiotic Congress for One Peaceful World. One of its aims will be to draft a preliminary constitution for the new world order that will emerge in the mid- to late-twenty-first century.

Several governors, ambassadors, and heads of states who have come to see me and started to eat macrobiotically have expressed an interest in these propos- als, and our associates have organized an International Macrobiotics Society at the United Nations headquarters in New York, with branch chapters at U.N. offices in Geneva. In 1986, we started a One Peaceful World educational mem- bership organization. If a nuclear exchange can be prevented in the next several decades, these societies and assemblies will become the basis for the future world government that will finally mark the end to the threat of global war.

In the early 2000s, we worked closely with Congressman Dennis Kucinich, who proposed creating a Department of Peace. This Cabinet-level office would serve as a presidential counterweight to the Defense Department and Joint Chiefs of Staff, mediate major international and domestic crises, and promote peace education in schools, hospitals, and the workplace, including the introduction of healthy, mostly plant foods. Further achievements of ours can be found in the Peace Promoters sections of this book.

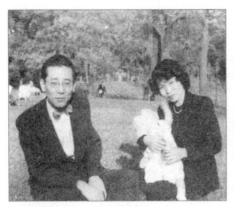

Michio and Aveline Kushi with daughter Lily in New York in the early 1950s.

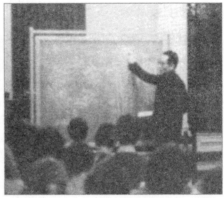

Michio Kushi lecturing at Boston's Arlington Street Church in the mid-1960s.

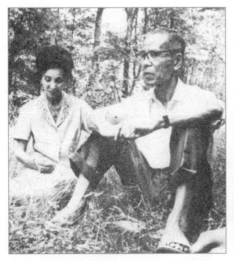

Lima and George Ohsawa relax on a visit to New York's Central Park.

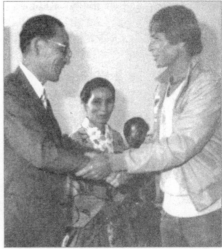

John Denver visits the Kushis in Boston and performs a benefit concert for macrobiotic education and global harmony.

PEACE PROMOTER

Chico Varatojo and Tó Zé Aréal, Portugal

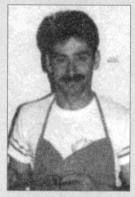

Antonio "Tó Zé" Aréal

José Joaquim, at age thirty-five, was considered one of the worst prisoners in Portugal. Nicknamed "Al Capone," he had a spare, handsome face, high cheekbones, dark eyes, and hair combed straight back that fit the classic image of the gangster. From stealing cars as a teenager, José graduated to safecracking. For his last robbery, José was sentenced to twenty years (later reduced to ten years) at Lisbon's Linho prison. Linho is one of the most heavily guarded of Portugal's prisons. Most of its inmates are doing time for robbery or assault.

José suffered from asthma and had heard from a fellow inmate at Linho that macrobiotics could heal sicknesses. He decided to try it. Prison officials gave him permission to cook for himself on a small camping stove in his cell. Since he was not allowed to use knives, he had to cut all his vegetables by hand, and in the beginning he had to pay for his own food. After experimenting for a year on his own, he called Unimave—the macrobiotic center in Lisbon—and immediately received some meals prepared from the outside, as well as supplies and books. By this time (spring 1979), several other inmates decided to eat macrobiotically, and the prison agreed to pay for their food.

Soon after, Chico Varatojo, a director of Unimave, started to teach regularly at Linho. Every week he lectured on Oriental philosophy and medicine, as well as traditional Portuguese cooking and diet. He also demonstrated shiatsu massage, visual diagnosis, and other practical techniques that he had learned at the Kushi Institute in Boston and the East West Center in Middletown, Connecticut. Soon, thirty prisoners had become macrobiotic. Linho officials allowed them to use a large kitchen, and they began to cook and eat together once or twice a week.

Reflecting on his past, José says that his criminal activity was primarily the result of his unbalanced diet, which consisted mostly of animal foods, especially meat. He says, in retrospect, that these foods caused him to be excessively aggressive, violent, and hyperactive. In the younger inmates, he noted a "big change after a week in most men who start macrobiotics; they become much more calm and have a more spiritual feeling." José no longer suffered from asthma, except when he strayed from the diet.

Like José, Antonio José (Tó Zé) Aréal was regarded as one of Portugal's most dangerous criminals. Tó Zé became famous for masterminding the payday holdup of the Standard Electric Company in Cascais, a town between Lisbon and the castle city of Sintra. Brandishing submachine guns and wearing stockings over their heads, Tó Zé and four other gang members entered the payroll office through a hole in the wall. To ensure their escape, Tó Zé shot out the wires with his machine gun, cutting off the electric power and phones for miles around. The gang made off with the equivalent of $120,000 and three hostages. Later they commandeered a getaway car and were the subject of a vast manhunt by police, dogs, and helicopters in the mountains of Sintra. Eluding their captors, they were eventually caught in Lisbon trying to get false papers to flee the country. Tó Zé was sentenced to three consecutive terms, the first one for ten years. At Linho, Tó Zé was put in solitary confinement for the first week and later kept under constant watch.

In Linho, Tó Zé met José Joaquim, who interested him in macrobiotics. At first, Tó Zé made many mistakes. Someone told him to avoid meat and sugar, and soon he went to the opposite extreme, eating only brown rice and hiziki seaweed. After two weeks, he was back on drugs, which he had begun using at age sixteen. He continued to make mistakes, adding two tablespoons of salt for every cup of rice, and burning the rice. Soon he became very sick from the combination of drugs and salt and was sent to the hospital with typhoid. In the prison hospital, he was given sugar water and nineteen pills to swallow each day. After two weeks, Tó Zé was sent back to his cell. Eating rice and soybeans, he reflected on his life. He decided not to take any more drugs and resolved to get some outside help with his food.

After Chico Varatojo came to the prison and started giving lectures and consultations, Tó Zé felt much better. "After I began to read Michio Kushi's *The Book of Macrobiotics,* my understanding of the macrobiotic way of life grew," Tó Zé recalled. "My cooking got a lot better. I began to have discharges—physically, I went from 146 pounds to 104; I had diarrhea, headaches, kidney pain; mentally, I was often irritated, confused, and depressed. The spiritual transformation is more difficult to describe but it was powerful. About one year after I began eating this way I started to feel much better. I could understand people better and many things about my past, how food, family, and environment had interacted and affected me. This new way of life also gave me motivation, and a larger, cosmological view as well as changing me physically. The food changed me."

Looking back, Tó Zé recalled that his childhood in the Portuguese countryside had been very peaceful and happy. The family's diet consisted mostly of cornbread, poultry, fish, vegetables, and fruit. But at age eight, his parents separated, and he moved to the city, where he was exposed more to dairy food, sugar, and meat. At age sixteen, he started to smoke hashish and marijuana and to take amphetamines, LSD, cocaine, and then heroin, which he was using regularly by the time he was eighteen. Joining the army at eighteen, he rose to sergeant and taught hand-to-hand combat, how to handle guns, and deployment of bombs. Toward the end of his two-and-a-half year tour, he started to take drugs again, which played a large part in his criminal career.

After four-and-a-half years of confinement in Linho, Tó Zé's sentence was commuted early, partially because of the changes in his attitude and behavior. Assis Teixeira, the director of Linho, remarked, "I keep in touch with Tó Zé—I feel that he is permanently changed." Commenting on the influence of macrobiotics in general, Senhor Afonso, another prison official, noted, "Yes, there is a great difference in them [the macrobiotic prisoners], especially in those who have left the prison. It is not easy to describe—for one thing I can say that now they take more initiative. Actually, there is no problem here with anyone who is macrobiotic; this way of life enjoys a very good reputation. I believe the food and the outside stimulus both helped. The food can change people."

In the spring of 1982, my wife, Aveline, and I visited Portugal. We drove out to Linho to say hello to the macrobiotic inmates, intending to stay only ten minutes because of a busy schedule. But everyone was so eager to study and talk that we stayed over three hours. We were impressed and touched by the men's enthusiasm, energy, and spirit. We were used to being asked questions about personal health and were refreshed by the prisoners' challenging questions of a spiritual and philosophical nature. We discovered that prisoners are often much healthier physically than people who have degenerative disease; they have an excess, rather than a lack, of vitality. They may have committed a violent or illegal action, but many have a spirit of adventure and inventiveness and express positive and creative ideas. Many prisoners are also far superior morally than some people in society, especially some in the fields of politics and finance. Their minds are often simpler, sometimes to the extent of naiveté, compared with highly intellectual manipulators. All they lack is a balanced dietary foundation and proper guidance.

After leaving Linho, Tó Zé went to work with Unimave in Lisbon. He cooked in a macrobiotic restaurant, made seitan and tofu five days a week, and attended classes and lectures. In 1983, Tó Zé came to the United States to study at the Kushi Institute. While in Boston he lived at our home in Brookline, often cooking traditional Portuguese dinners for our whole household. Everyone was deeply moved by his humility and hard work. No one could ever have imagined his violent past. In New Bedford, a large Portuguese-speaking community on Cape Cod, Tó Zé helped start a macrobiotic center and gave many lectures and consultations. After his return to Portugal, he worked at a macrobiotic company, helping countless people—including many prisoners—realize a more healthy, peaceful way of life. Eventually, he married, had a family, and started a successful natural foods business making tofu, tempeh, and other natural foods. Fellow prisoner José Joaquim also worked at a natural foods company, producing rice cakes and attending macrobiotic classes in Lisbon. Their instructor, Chico Varatojo, went on to become a leading macrobiotic teacher, counselor, and eventually a lecturer at medical schools and hospitals in Portugal and around the world.

The experience at Linho is one example of what macrobiotic practice can accomplish. From it we can envision the possibility of reforming the entire correctional system, of changing the practice of restriction and punishment to one of love and understanding—a giant step in the direction of One Peaceful World.

Sources

Chico Varatojo, personal letter, April 16, 1986.

Seaker, Meg. "Fighting Crime with Diet: Report from a Portuguese Prison." *East West Journal* (July 1982): 26–34.

5.

We Are Eternally One

While I am optimistic about the future, there is nothing automatic about averting war or biological degeneration. In fact, while our movement and the parallel holistic and environmental movements are gaining momentum and helping to spread health and peace all around the world, the dominant trend toward the modern diet, terrorism and war, and unsustainability still continues. If biological degeneration—and therefore social decline—proceed at the present rate, humankind may collapse before our movement is strong enough to secure the world's health and safety. This collapse would include economic systems overburdened by rising expenditures for physical and mental health, disabled workers, and a decline in productivity and efficiency of the remaining workforce. Paralysis of political systems would arise from physical, mental, or emotional disorders—with which a deluded majority or a fanatical minority constantly suffers—while uncontrollable social chaos may result from increasing environmental destruction, accelerated industrialization, and a sense of futurelessness (living without hope of a worthwhile future) living in the age of global warming and climate change. The family and social systems would further deteriorate through the inability of humans to produce healthy offspring by natural means.

WE ARE WHAT WE EAT

While society as a whole is beginning to turn toward a more healthy way of life, there is still a long way to go. Irradiation of food has begun on a large scale, threatening to accelerate the spread of degenerative diseases, deformed babies, and mutations. Also, many people are confused about alternatives. For example, instead of beef, many people are now eating poultry, especially chicken. In my experience, eating too much chicken is a leading cause of arthritis, or the hardening of joints and bones. In addition, factory-farmed chicken is very poor in quality compared to natural, organic chicken.

Every year, thousands of people come to me for dietary and way-of-life consultations. One day, an older man who was suffering from a form of muscular dystrophy came to me. The muscles in his hands and legs had progressively thinned, and he could grip things and walk only with great difficulty. Because muscle is composed primarily of protein, doctors had advised him to eat substantially more meat, poultry, dairy food, and other animal products. But he only got worse. Eventually, he would be crippled and might even require surgery or transplants to stay alive.

After observing the man's condition for a few minutes, I turned to his wife and said, "Your husband has turned into a chicken."

She looked at him in astonishment and gasped, "My husband is a chicken." It turned out that almost every day for many years she had been giving him chicken and eggs.

I explained to them that modern nutrition is good for analyzing the amount of nutrients in food, but as yet, knows nothing about the *energy* of food. Vegetable-quality protein is very different from animal-quality protein, even though under the microscope their chemical composition is the same. The energy of different foods is very easy to measure with the mind, if you are eating well and can think in terms of yin and yang. However, most modern people's way of eating is so chaotic, they cannot think in this simple, basic way.

In this man's case, too much animal protein was the underlying cause of his illness. His limbs had become spindly like chicken feet, and his shoulders had become tight as if he were beginning to sprout wings. The way he continually shook his head up and down and other mannerisms he displayed were those of a chicken. After just a few months of eating whole, natural vegetable-quality foods, he could pick up things with his hands, and he had a half-human way of walking again.

Chicken is just one of many foods abused today. Too much pork and ham produces swinish behavior—very stubborn and egocentric. Too much fish leads to short tempers, arguments, and fishy actions. Also, there is too much beef and dairy food being consumed. This makes for strong, cow-like bodies—big in structure, but low in intelligence. Beef eating makes for violent and aggressive tendencies, while dairy food dulls the emotions and creates a passive, docile mentality that is content to follow the herd. Myself, I am very fond of nuts, and someday may turn into a squirrel.

THE PEACEFUL REVOLUTION

We are presently entering the period of bionization (the use of artificial body parts); many people have already experienced synthetic replacement of bodily organs or functions to one degree or another. If this is "logically" extended beyond physical manipulation into the realms of thinking, emotion, and spirituality, it will become increasingly difficult, if not impossible, to live as a naturally free human being.

Whether we go in this direction or not largely depends on what happens during the upcoming years. If instead of going toward increasing artificiality, people begin to choose more natural methods for recovery from cancer, heart disease, infertility, AIDS, and other degenerative and immunological disorders, as well as family problems, crime, and international conflict, then there is a good possibility that the course of history can be changed. We have been encouraged by the trend toward alternative and complementary medicine, as well as integrative medicine (in which both traditional and conventional best practices are offered). If modern civilization reorients its direction toward the elimination of disease, war, and unsustainability at their origins, and not (as is presently the case) merely dealing with symptoms of conflict and climate change, we can prevent our species' decline.

What we now refer to as "macrobiotics" is actually the most natural method for achieving this change. By improving the quality of our daily foods, we begin to improve the quality of our blood and body fluids. We can achieve sound physical and psychological health without having to depend on drugs, operations, or other artificial treatments. This improvement in quality begins with one's own physical condition and extends to all aspects of life, including judgment, mental qualities, and spirituality. When we return to eating food for human development, our facial features improve and return to normal. Our eggs and sperm become very good quality, and our children and grandchildren will develop stronger constitutions and conditions than we have.

When applied socially, macrobiotics can bring about a future based on the continuous development of individual and social health, with all people working toward the goal of a genuinely healthy, productive, and peaceful world culture. The people who practice this way of life will naturally begin to feel a sense of family unity with each other as a result of eating whole, unprocessed foods, which tends to create similar physical and mental qualities. This family feeling can then naturally develop into a worldwide planetary family commonwealth based on mutual love and respect.

PURSUING OUR DREAM

At the end of the Second World War, I began to experience one-world consciousness as the need for world federal government became apparent and as the scarcity of food in Japan made us chew well and appreciate the little that we had. Until economic conditions improved, and refined, processed food again became available, this vision was widespread.

When I graduated from Tokyo University, there was the option to take many examinations to enter the legal profession, government service, and academic life. My friends had passed these and were preparing for official careers. I knew, however, that I could not become a judge, diplomat, or professor. Although I did not know yet how to realize my dream, I knew that this was not my life and that I would go to another country.

Just before graduating, we had a party and one by one, each of us discussed his dream. One classmate said he would become an official and change the present government; all were planning great things. When my turn came, I said, "I do not know about my future, but it seems that my dream of world peace and world government is the biggest and maybe even an impossible dream, but I will pursue it wherever it leads me." My classmates wished me good luck and then went on to become very respectable leaders of society. I came to America, and while they were in secure positions, I was earning my bread from day to day as a hotel bellboy and dishwasher. While they were moving in the highest circles of society and art, I was observing people in churches, cafeterias, and subways, and drawing spirals in my notebook.

After ten or twenty years, my former classmates became chiefs of their sections and departments and prominent lawyers, government officials, and diplomats. Along with others of our postwar generation, they were responsible for Japan's rapid economic recovery and unparalleled technological development. During business trips to the United States, they would often visit me.

Almost all of them said, "Michio, you really chose the right way. I did not know how my job would spoil and weaken me and make me lose my dream." We had all discussed our dreams to change the world with passion then, but now they said, "I know that the end of my life is coming. I will become an executive, or a minister, and retire and finish. By comparison, you are different. You have no occupation and do not worry about the future. You kept your health and are happy. Even when you die, your dream will go on forever."

I said, "See? That is why I said that my dream is the biggest and most universal."

By the early eighties, many of my former classmates suffered from high blood pressure, stroke, stomach cancer, or other degenerative disorders now common in Japan and the whole modern world. Others have retired and await their deaths. Just a few remained active. One of these was my best friend, Keichu Moriai. We were just like brothers. On a visit to Washington, D.C. for a conference, he looked me up. Although we had not seen each other in thirty-five years, we embraced warmly.

We were amazed at the course each other's lives had taken. Keichu told me that Japan had assumed the lead in bionization. For the last seven years, he had been chairman of the Japan artificial organ manufacturers association, while I had been involved in educational activity to prevent it. He told me that it was now theoretically and technically possible to replace all human bodily organs and systems, including the head. However, his industry had not yet begun manufacturing computerized heads because they had not received any "purchase orders."

From talking with him, I could see that investment and banking circles, government and industry, medicine and law, and other segments of society in Japan, the United States, Europe, and elsewhere were supporting bionization, robotics, and psychonization for humanitarian purposes. In the face of biological and psychological degeneration, they could not envision any natural alternative to easing human suffering and unhappiness.

I described to Keichu the principles of macrobiotics and our natural way to restore humanity's health, happiness, and peace without technological intervention in basic life processes. Lest he be concerned that I would be angry or upset with him or that macrobiotics would organize protests against his industry, I reassured him that our approach was entirely peaceful.

Our meeting was symbolic of the end of modern civilization as we know it. The choice before humanity now is clearly the one envisioned by *Erewhon, Brave New World,* and *1984*—government by artificial manipulation and control of basic life processes, or government by natural education and self-reliance. In a way, our talk was like a summit conference between representatives of the two possible futures opening up to humanity. The human race will either restore its health and consciousness by returning to a more natural way of life and put an end to disease and war, or follow an artificial way of life and be succeeded by an artificial species.

Before long, it was time for our reunion to end. There was that feeling between Keichu and myself that we were going in opposite directions. However, from the point of view of the infinite Order of the Universe, we are always in harmony with one another. According to the logarithmic spiral—the universal form—we were both going in the same direction. I told Keichu that eventually people would become unhappy from organ transplants and turn to macrobiotics. There was no need to worry. Though we appeared to be diametrically opposed, we are always eternally one. Let's love and help one another in the brief time we are here on this beautiful planet.

In parting, Keichu and I shook hands and agreed, "Let's cooperate and build One Peaceful World."

THE TWENTY-FIRST CENTURY AND BEYOND

Since the 1980s, the trend toward biological and spiritual degeneration and the artificialization of society has dramatically increased. AIDS, avian (bird) flu, swine flu, Legionnaires' disease, Ebola, and other new viral epidemics have spread around the world. With rising living standards and a more affluent way of eating, cancer, heart disease, diabetes, and other chronic illnesses have become the leading causes of death in developing societies, eclipsing malaria, tuberculosis, and other infectious conditions. The digital and electronics revolution has seen tremendous advances in communication, education, research, business, trade, and other domains. At the same time, it has resulted in the spread of artificial electromagnetic radiation and potentially harmful energy fields that are contributing to reduced natural immunity in humans. The effects include an increase in leukemia, lymphomas, and other malignancies; the decline of bees and other insects, plants, and animals; and the voracious need for raw materials, especially conflict metals and rare earth metals that are used to manufacture cell phones and computers. Along with continued reliance on coal, oil, natural gas, and other fossil fuels, globalization fuels global warming, climate change, and economic disparity that threatens to destroy the natural environment and create an oppressive global order dominated by multinationals and wealthy elites.

On the positive side, the last generation has witnessed a sea change in the modern way of eating. From an animal-centered diet, society has turned toward a plant-centered way of eating. The U.S. government's change from a recommended dietary pattern based on the "basic four food groups" (half of which were made up of meat and dairy products) to the "food guide pyramid" in 1992 (with a foundation of whole grains and grain products and plenty of vegetables and fruits, and only small amounts of animal products) reversed humanity's trend over the last 10,000 years of eating increasingly more animal food. In 2011, the U.S. Department of Agriculture (USDA) replaced the food pyramid with MyPlate. In this guide, 75 percent of the suggested plate consists of grains, vegetables, and fruits, while the remaining 25 percent consists of protein from either plant or animal sources. A small "glass" of low-fat dairy sits next to the plate. This is major progress and we support this guideline strongly.

Macrobiotics led the way in this historic reversal. Organic gardening and farming, the primacy of whole foods, and alternative and complementary healing have all gone mainstream in the United States and spread around the world. Scientific and medical studies inspired by the macrobiotic community have been conducted by the National Institutes of Health (NIH), the Centers for Disease Control and Prevention (CDC), and other health agencies, medical schools, and universities. The *New England Journal of Medicine, Journal of the American Medical Association, Lancet,* and other leading journals have documented the benefits of a macrobiotic approach to heart disease, cancer, diabetes, and other chronic diseases. In 1998, the Smithsonian opened a permanent Michio Kushi Collection at the National Museum of American History, acknowledging the contribution of macrobiotics to the health and well-being of the country, as well as to world peace.

As the twenty-first century began, macrobiotic principles and practices had been widely recognized and adopted at every level of society. Though our own organizations—including the Kushi Foundation, East West Foundation, and other educational centers—remained small and modest in scope, the direction we long pioneered started to prevail. In coming decades, it will only strengthen, along with rising consciousness of balance, proportionality, and sustainability in other domains. New careers and lifestyles, including an explosion of online businesses and services, home and community-based arts and crafts, decentralized energy networks in which people can sell back their excess energy to the grid, and other appropriate and renewable advances, promise to create a new, more just and peaceful society.

The momentum toward gender equality, women's rights, gay liberation and marriage, and multicultural identity have also started to reverse centuries of injustice and contribute to a planet in which human diversity and tolerance, like biodiversity in the plant and animal kingdoms, ensures optimal fulfillment and realization of our potential as a species.

As a result of changes like this, humanity is beginning to see life with fresh eyes. Both age-old religious dogmas and modern scientific myths are no longer reliable compasses to living free, healthy lives. They are in sharp decline and will be displaced in the near future with new paradigms. In biology, modern evolutionary theory is giving way to new schools of thought emphasizing cooperation, rather than competition, among species. The study of classic genetics, which holds our destiny is fixed or determined by our genes, is being replaced by epigenetics, the view that diet, lifestyle, and consciousness predominantly influence and shape our destiny and can even affect our germ line and be passed on to future generations. In the nature vs. nurture controversy, nurture now has the upper hand—a conclusion we teach in our classes on diagnosis when we say condition (or day-to-day eating and way of life) trumps constitution (or what we are born with).

In the medical field, Darwinian medicine and other holistic approaches are showing that new viral and other microbial diseases emerge because of fundamental changes in the agricultural and food system. Monocultures, artificial chemicals and fertilizers, and mechanical harvesting methods disrupt ecosystems and interfere with the delicate checks and balances in the soil. The end result is the emergence of novel strains of viruses that have few, if any, natural enemies. Meanwhile, poor-quality modern foods have compromised human immune function. When exposed to these virulent new microbes, the blood, lymph, and other bodily fluids and protective factors are not strong enough to produce antibodies or discharge them from the body. Instead, they gather, accumulate, and eventually destroy cells and tissues, organs and functions from within. This is the pattern for AIDS, Ebola, and similar contemporary scourges. The return to a more natural way of farming, eating, and healing will render these new epidemics a dim memory.

On the social front, modern industrial society is now collapsing as fossil fuels run out and contribute to global warming. Less well-recognized is the metals crisis. By about 2035, most of the metals on which civilization has been founded, including gold, silver, copper, bronze, and iron, will disappear, as well as new industrial metals and rare earth metals used in making computers and cell phones. Present-day technology has no solution for this impending crisis. However, from a macrobiotic view, the answer lies in transmutation, the creation of comparatively rare, valuable elements from common, inexpensive ones. Since the 2000s, Quantum Rabbit, a small macrobiotic research company started by my students, has created about twenty elements in the laboratory, including titanium, palladium, scandium, and others. Because the theory behind this process is dismissed as alchemy, modern science refuses to confirm the results. Like the cardinals that refused to peer through Galileo's telescope because their dogma didn't allow for the moons of Jupiter, today's biochemists and astrophysicists have stuck their heads in the sand in the face of a simple, practical solution to the energy and materials crisis. In coming years, transmutation (also known as quantum conversion and cool fusion) will move from proof of concept (testing in parts per million) to production and practical use. Mining, competition for scarce resources, and territorial wars for oil, uranium, and other valuable resources will become obsolete.

Finally, as these changes are implemented, the guiding paradigm of modern cosmology—the Big Bang—will itself be replaced. The Big Bang is a violent model of the universe that coincided with the discovery and development of nuclear energy and is the creation myth of the Atomic Age. It posits the birth of the cosmos in a primordial explosion in which time and space themselves, as well as all the elements, were created. Modern physics describes the sun in similar terms. As one research paper has concluded: "The sun is not commonly considered a star and few would think of stars as nuclear reactors. Yet, that is the way it is, and even our own world is made out of the 'fallout' from stars that blew up and spewed radioactive debris into the nascent solar system." Like a bomb blast, modern science regards life as random, chaotic, and without purpose. Genetic mutation, rather than design, governs evolution.

Meanwhile, age-old religious superstitions still abound. Sickness, violence, and war are attributed to sinfulness or divine punishment. In actuality, they are the natural consequence of our unnatural diet, lifestyle, and way of thinking. The coming new era of humanity will witness the emergence of peaceful, harmonious new myths, theories, and paradigms. The cosmos, life and death, and our own lives will be seen as part of an eternal spiritual journey. The Big Life—*makrobios*—will replace the Big Bang as the guiding myth. Rather than the mother and father of all violent explosions, the universe will be seen as a beautiful flower with trillions of spiral metals that unfold naturally and peacefully in perfect harmony with universal law.

I am more hopeful than ever that common sense and universal consciousness will spread across our planet. As I embark on the next stage of my own endless voyage, I am confident the earth will become a shining, radiant manifestation of one healthy, peaceful world. By understanding the various spirals of creation, we come to know our eternal origin and destiny and become one with life as a whole.

PART II

Understanding Our Origin and Destiny

The destiny of nations depends upon what and how they eat.

—JEAN ANTHELME BRILLAT-SAVARIN

6.

The Order of the Universe

In yin and yang—the complementary opposite energies that make up all things—I found the compass to manage my own health and destiny, as well as contribute to well-being and peace at a social and planetary level. George Ohsawa helped orient me in this direction, as did my wife Aveline (through her wonderful cooking) and my meetings with remarkable men like Einstein and Thomas Mann, as described in Part I. However, as my macrobiotic practice deepened, I gradually discovered my own personal dream in life and its connection with humanity's universal dream of a healthy, peaceful world.

In essence, our planet, our lives, and our food are the terminus of a long, unfolding spiral of materialization and the genesis of a complementary opposite spiral of spiritualization leading to enlightened awareness. These great twin spirals, glanced at in the pictographs, cooking vessels, pottery, and the monumental architecture of ancient cultures and civilizations, are referred to broadly as the Order of the Universe. In this chapter, I shall summarize this process and its manifestations in different regions of the world.

THE SPIRALLIC UNIVERSE

The infinite universe is a paradise full of joy and peace. It is without beginning and without end. It is spaceless and timeless. However, because it is moving in all dimensions at infinite speed, it creates phenomena that are infinitesimal and ephemeral. These manifestations have a beginning and an end, a front and a back, measure and duration, and may be viewed as forms appearing and disappearing in an ocean of cosmic energy.

Many concepts mentioned in this book tie back to the idea of "complementary antagonisms." This refers to two thoughts that are opposites but which complete each other. Each needs the other to carry out its purpose. The infinite universe, though itself invisible and beyond the apprehension of the senses, differentiates into two antagonistic and complementary tendencies of centrifugality and centripetality—expansion and contraction, space and time, beginning and end, yin and yang. At the intersection of these two forces, numerous spirals are produced in every dimension.

All phenomena are *spirallic* in nature, regardless of whether they are visible or invisible, spiritual or physical, energetic or material. Many of the spirals arising in the infinite ocean of existence appear manifest to our eyes. The physical universe, stretching over ten billion light years in every direction and itself spiral in structure, contains billions of spiral galaxies, some hundreds of thousands of light years in diameter, which periodically appear and disappear. In turn, these galaxies contain hundreds of millions of spirallic solar systems.

In each spirallic solar system, various planets, together with millions of comets, are spiraling around the spirallic center called the sun. Each planet receives a charge of incoming, centripetal force towards its center—a spirallic energy we call gravity. Meanwhile, as a result of turning on its axis, an outgoing, centrifugal force is generated toward the periphery. Together these two forces combine to keep the planet in orbit about the sun.

On Earth, a small planet within a solar system belonging to the spiral galaxy called the Milky Way, centripetal force and centrifugal force produce unaccountable phenomena that appear and disappear, changing constantly. These planetary phenomena include invisibly minute spirals such as electrons, protons, and other subatomic particles; various kinds of elements that combine to form organic and inorganic compounds; and numerous kinds of botanical and zoological life, including human beings, which appeared during the most recent era of biological evolution on the planet.

As all life exists within worlds of multiple spirals, human life is also spirally constituted and governed. Not only individual human lives, but also human history as a whole, are subject to the laws of spirallic motion and change. The two antagonistic and complementary forces govern the development of human affairs, underlying patterns of growth and decay, health and sickness, peace and war.

In the Far East, the natural dynamics of change—the ceaseless interplay of yin and yang—was traditionally called the Tao. A free, healthy, happy, peaceful human being was someone who understood and could intuitively harmonize with this order. In Japan, the word for Tao is Do. The terms for many Japanese arts contain this word. For example, the way to harmonize yin and yang by serving tea is called *sado*, or tea ceremony. The application of yin and yang to brush writing, or calligraphy, is called *shodo*. Together, the martial arts are known as *budo*, while the art of swordsmanship is *kendo*. The art of physical adaptation to the opponent is *judo*; the art of harmonizing ki, or natural electromagnetic energy, is *aikido*; and the art of archery—achieving union between the self and the target—is *kyudo*. Far Eastern medicine is known as *ido*, the art of harmonizing yin and yang in daily life with food and the environment.

In ancient India, a similar orientation prevailed. In the Bhagavad Gita, the holiest scripture of Hinduism, Krishna teaches Arjuna, a despondent warrior who has thrown down his weapons before the decisive battle, that the secret of life is learning to balance opposites: "For, Arjuna, he who has transcended the pairs of opposites is easily freed from bondage."[1] Everything in the universe, Krishna explains, is the product of two complementary principles, spirit and matter, which he names in various Sanskrit terms such as Purusha and Prakriti. In turn, the relative world is divided into three *gunas,* or "qualities": (1) *tamas,* the force of ignorance, delusion, and inaction; (2) *rajas,* the force of enterprise, passion, and action; and (3) *sattva,* the force of clarity, joy, and knowledge. Tamas and rajas are akin to yin and yang in Far Eastern philosophy, while sattva is the balance between the two. In the Bhagavad Gita, Krishna teaches Arjuna the central importance of a balanced diet and shows him how to balance foods, especially whole grains, according to these principles to win the inner war and attain lasting peace.

In the ancient Middle East, the teaching of Jesus was also based on a dynamic understanding of the complementary relationship of opposites. The New Testament relates many examples of this teaching, as when Jesus fed the multitude with two small fish and several loaves of bread. The two fish may be interpreted to represent yin and yang, or the principles of "movement" and "rest" as he referred to these tendencies in the *Gospel According to Thomas.* It is clear that Jesus is not just feeding the people physically. He is also teaching them the Order of the Infinite Universe, or what he referred to as the Justice of the Kingdom of Heaven.

The universal principle of yang and yin—or rajas and tamas, movement and rest—is the intuitive common understanding of all the world's great religions, including Confucianism, Taoism, Shintoism, Hinduism, Buddhism, Zoroastrianism, Judaism, Christianity, and Islam. Together with these religious adaptations, we are able to see the same understanding embodied in ancient astronomical and calendrical observations, in architecture and public construction, and in many traditional arts and crafts. From megalithic times through the farming revolution, from the rise of civilization until the eve of modern times in about the seventeenth century, the Order of the Universe was intuitively known and expressed—sometimes to a greater degree, such as during eras of peace and prosperity, and sometimes to a lesser degree, such as during eras of war and decline—guiding the day-to-day lives of countless families and individuals, tribes and societies, cultures and civilizations. Historically, however, consciousness of the Order of the Universe has steadily waned over the last several thousand years, reaching near total eclipse during the last 400 years. In our era, the laws of harmony have been rediscovered in partial or fragmented form. For example, modern science deals with opposite pairs of forces, such as centripetal and centrifugal energy, positive and negative electromagnetic force, anabolic and catabolic reactions, acid and alkaline, waves and particles—but as yet has no unifying principle to connect them with each other and understand life as a whole. In the same way, history, literature, and the social sciences make partial use of categories such as soft and hard, static and dynamic, sensate and spiritual, Dionysian and Apollonion, aristocratic and plebian, and individualistic and collective to analyze and interpret events.

One modern thinker who began to apply this principle systematically to history was Arnold Toynbee, who based his life's work on a dynamic understanding of the alternating movement of two complementary opposites, which he termed "challenge and response." In the introduction to his twenty-volume *Study of History,* he explains that these concepts originated from a study of yin and yang and that they are indispensible to understanding the movement of human affairs:

> Of the various symbols in which different observers in different societies have expressed the alternation between a static condition and a dynamic activity in the rhythm of the Universe, Yin and Yang are the most apt, because they convey the measure of the rhythm directly and not through some metaphor derived from psychology or mechanics of mathematics. We will therefore use these Sinic symbols in this study henceforward.[2]

THE SPIRAL OF CREATION

From God or One Infinity, all life has proceeded through seven spirallic stages of increasing consciousness and complexity (see Figure 6.1 on page 67):

1. The absolute, undifferentiated world

2. The world of polarization

3. The world of energy or vibration (light)

4. The pre-atomic world

5. The world of elements

6. The vegetable and animal kingdoms

7. The human race

The universal process of materialization (physicalization) reaches the center of the spiral with the creation of human beings, the most highly evolved species of biological life. The inward course of physicalization, however, starts to turn at its center to the reverse course, returning again through the preceding levels and ultimately merging into God or One Infinity, the origin of all. This return process is one of spiritualization, in which our human development, understanding, and spirit become increasingly refined until we reach universal consciousness.

One of the principal laws of nature is the law of harmony. According to this law, yin and yang are always balancing in different dimensions to maintain harmony at all times during every step of the changing process. Thus, each being is constantly realizing a harmony within itself as well as harmony with external conditions. Harmony is continuously being made between past and present, and the future. Each being is continuously achieving harmony with other beings, with groups of beings, with the environment, and with the universe itself. The two antagonistic and complementary forces do not act as destructive forces against

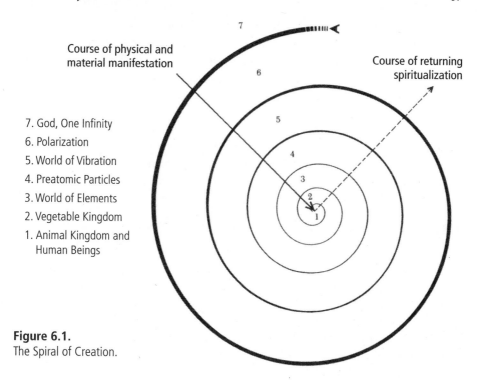

Course of physical and
material manifestation

Course of returning
spiritualization

7. God, One Infinity
6. Polarization
5. World of Vibration
4. Preatomic Particles
3. World of Elements
2. Vegetable Kingdom
1. Animal Kingdom and
   Human Beings

Figure 6.1.
The Spiral of Creation.

each other, but they act as opposite factors to maintain balance. Opposite energies attract each other and similar energies repel each other in order to achieve harmony always as a whole.

Another law summarizes the principles of cause and effect. In the process of endless change, yin and yang intersect in serial motion. Upward motion, for example, causes downward motion as a subsequence; downward motion causes upward motion in the succeeding phase. Faster motion causes slower motion as the next step; the slower motion is succeeded by faster motion. The rate of change varies, furthermore, according to whether the spiral is predominantly centripetal or centrifugal and whether we are at the beginning, middle, or end of the spiral. Meanwhile, there are no independent manifestations arising separately out of time—unconnected with the past—or out of space, unconnected with the environment in which we live. Therefore, there are no mutations and accidents (in the modern sense) occurring in the universe. Everything has its cause, and everything becomes the cause for the next process in its change. Therefore, all phenomena are related to each other, and all are connected to each other in the process of change, in time and in space.

Isolation, separation, randomness, and meaninglessness exist only in deluded imagination. In reality, there are no separate and autonomous manifestations. The infinite universe is always in perfect harmony. Though we live in the relative world, we are governed by the absolute world. Human destiny is subject to the universal destiny of the cosmos, though the dimensions of time and space differ from each other. According to the law of unity, all phenomena appear differently, yet all phenomena arise from the same origin and return to the same source. All beings move differently, yet all beings are governed by the same universal laws of change. The other laws and principles of spirallic motion and change are summarized in Appendix B. (See page 322.)

The Order of the Universe is really very simple. Most children readily understand it, and it is apprehended by the adult mind through more intuitive natural and aesthetic comprehension. This capacity is nothing but primary common sense, the birthright of everyone who is living in harmony with nature and their environment.

THE LAWS OF CHANGE AND HUMAN DESTINY

Modem theories, assumptions, hypotheses, and laws of the physical and social sciences are usually partial in nature or at variance with the traditional understanding of the natural order, including the proper selection and preparation of daily food. For example, modern anatomy is based on an analytical understanding of the human body, which sees life as a chemical process governed chiefly by the DNA in the nucleus of the cell, rather than as a biological process influenced by the whole and all the parts of the larger environment. Similarly, modern nutrition has a static understanding and looks at food exclusively in terms of caloric measurement and chemical composition, completely ignoring its energetic quality and effects. Because they are not based on a comprehensive view of universal order, modern technologies—including those responsible for securing health and human services, medical care, and freedom from violence and war—are unable to safeguard humanity's health and happiness. On the contrary, through an unnatural food and agricultural system and an uncontrollable nuclear armaments race, an unsustainable modern civilization is threatening to destroy human life altogether on this planet.

From an evolutionary point of view, if these trends continue, biological degeneration, nuclear war, and global warming and climate change can be seen as the consequences of our failure as a species to adapt to our natural environment. However, such a tragic destiny is not inevitable. We have a choice. Applying the universal principles of change described above to problems of human life and its development, we can make the following judgments:

1. Humanity as a whole is constantly changing, as is every individual.

2. All of the facets of human life are constantly changing and evolving, including the physical, psychological, spiritual, and social dimensions, as well as the relationship between human beings and their environment.

3. All physical and psychological changes that human beings experience, in addition to all other aspects of life, change according to orderly laws and principles.

Yin and yang—the laws of harmony and relativity—govern all bodily and mental functions, including digestion and elimination; inhalation and exhalation; extension and constriction in muscular motion; expansion and contraction of internal organs; antagonistic and complementary functions between the orthosympathetic and parasympathetic nerves; harmonious balance between hormones; balance between red and white blood cells in the circulatory system; smooth coordination between right and left hemispheres of the brain; balance between salt and water retention in the kidneys; and many other similar relationships.

4. All human functions and movements are proceeding in relative harmony between the internal environment (body, organs, thoughts, emotions) and the external environment (natural and social conditions).

5. All physical and psychological manifestations arising in human beings, including symptoms of disease, do not occur accidentally, but arise as the result of certain causes.

6. Human behavior and consciousness, including symptoms of disease, are conditioned by outward causes. Humanity's internal condition mirrors the external environment and, in turn, influences that environment. The primary factors absorbed from the environment are: (a) the food we eat and the liquids we drink; (b) the air we breathe; (c) the sound waves we hear and the light waves we see; (d) the atmospheric impulses and other external stimulants we sense; and (e) cosmic rays, waves, and invisible forces that we may not sense, but that nevertheless influence thought and consciousness.

7. Each of these causative forces is composed of antagonistic and complementary factors (see Table 6.1 on page 70).

8. Different combinations of these causative factors produce different effects in the physical and psychological constitution. These physical and psychological differences give rise to different manifestations in daily thought, action, and behavior, as well as in various conditions including orderliness and disorderliness, health and sickness, peace and war, and life and death.

9. When these causative factors are observed in proper harmony, the individual realizes and maintains physical health and psychological well-being and society realizes peace and prosperity. When they are observed chaotically, the individual experiences physical and psychological disorder and society experiences crime, war, and social chaos.

10. Among the causative factors, food and drink are the two primary factors that the individual and society can control and manage, while other factors—such as air quality; atmospheric conditions; external vibrations, stimulations, and impulses; cosmic rays and waves—are less manageable or practically impossible to control.

TABLE 6.1 EXAMPLES OF YIN AND YANG		
	MORE YANG	**MORE YIN**
Food and Liquids	Animal-quality complex carbohydrates	Vegetable-quality simple carbohydrates
	Animal protein	Vegetable protein
	Saturated fat	Unsaturated fat
	Sodium	Potassium
	Low fiber	High fiber
	Oil-soluble vitamins	Water-soluble vitamins
Air	Carbon dioxide	Oxygen
	Hydrogen	Nitrogen
	Lower humidity	Higher humidity
	Higher pressure	Lower pressure
	Higher temperature	Lower temperature
	Positive ions	Negative ions
Vibrations	Lower frequency	Higher frequency
	Higher speed	Lower speed
	Longer waves	Shorter waves
	Infrared light	Ultraviolet light
	Electromagnetic waves	Nonelectromagnetic waves
Stimuli and Impulses	Heavy pressure	Light pressure
	Sharp pain	Dull pain
	Hot sensation	Cold sensation
	Strong sensation	Weak sensation
	Stimulants that create downward energy	Stimulants that create upward energy

11. Food and liquid, as part of the organic and inorganic life of this planet, synthesize the fundamental forces and energies of the universe and are themselves the culmination of all preceding stages of biological evolution. By observing food and liquid intake in proper balance, the individual is able to maximize his or her adaptation to the environment and realize physical health, psychological well-being, and continued mental and spiritual development. Similarly, social health and well-being, including global peace and security, depend upon the proper balance of these factors. We are able to classify, from yin to yang or yang to yin, the entire scope of food and drink. We can then classify further within each category. In the beginning, the simplest division is made between foods that are excessively yang or excessively yin and should be avoided or reduced whenever possible (with some exceptions for non-temperate zones), and foods of more central balance that are suitable for regular consumption. Table 6.2 summarizes these categories.

TABLE 6.2 CLASSIFICATION OF FOODS AND SUBSTANCES

STRONG YANG FOODS AND SUBSTANCES (FROM MORE TO LESS YANG)

Refined table salt

Eggs

Meat

Hard salted cheese

Poultry

Fish and seafood

Tobacco

Insulin, steroids, and some other drugs and medications

BALANCED FOODS (FROM MORE TO LESS BALANCED)

Whole cereal grains (brown rice, millet, whole wheat, oats, rye, corn, quinoa, buckwheat)

Beans and bean products (lentils, chickpeas, azuki beans, etc.)

Root, round, and leafy green vegetables

Sea vegetables

Unrefined sea salt, vegetable oil, and other seasonings (if moderately used)

Spring and well water

Nonaromatic, nonstimulant teas and beverages

Seeds and nuts

Fruits (apples, cherries, berries, melons, etc.)

Moderate sweeteners (rice syrup, barley malt, and other grain-based natural sweeteners, if moderately used)

STRONG YIN FOODS AND SUBSTANCES (FROM MORE TO LESS YIN)

Tranquilizers, antibiotics, and some other medications

Drugs (marijuana, cocaine, etc., with some exceptions)

Foods containing chemicals, preservatives, dyes, pesticides, GMOs

Alcohol (whiskey, gin, beer, etc.)

Strong sweeteners (sugar, honey, molasses, etc.)

Aromatic and stimulant beverages (coffee, black tea, mint tea, cola and soft drinks, etc.)

Spices (pepper, curry, nutmeg, etc.)

Refined oils

Soft dairy foods (milk, cream, yogurt, ice cream)

Large, watery fruits and vegetables (tomatoes, potatoes, eggplants, mangoes, coconuts, etc.)

White rice, white flour

12. By observing a proper diet, the individual maintains a healthy and orderly condition in harmony with the natural and social environment. Food and drink largely determine the quality of the individual's blood and lymph; the quality of cells, tissues, and organs; the quality of the digestive, circulatory, nervous, and reproductive systems; the quality of thought and consciousness; the quality of behavior; the quality of human relations; the quality of society; the quality of human interaction with the natural environment; and the quality of the human spirit to be passed on to future generations. Diet guides and shapes all human activity, including the lives of individuals, families, communities, cultures, societies, and civilizations, and is the primary means by which the human race as a whole controls its destiny on this planet.

PEACE: THE ART OF BALANCING OPPOSITES

Among wholesome foods, whole cereal grains, either wild or domesticated, are the most balanced form of nourishment. In various forms, they have constituted humanity's staple food for millennia and, until modern times, were eaten as the main food throughout the world. Every civilization prior to modern times recognized whole grains as the Staff of Life, and the different types of grain, farming methods, cooking, and other ways of preparing foods gave rise to the wonderful diversity and richness of human culture and society. Rice and millet were principal foods in the Far East; wheat, oats, and rye in Europe; buckwheat in Russia and Central Asia; rice, teff, sorghum, and millet in Africa; barley and wheat in the Middle East; and maize in the Americas.

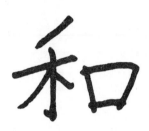

The connection between whole grains and peace was central to traditional understanding. In the Far East, the word for "peace"—*wa*—is formed from the ideograms (written characters) for "grain" and "mouth" (see Figure 6.2). Ancient people intuitively knew that a diet based predominantly on grains and vegetables created a peaceful mind and society. The Tao Te Ching, the Confucian classics, the Upanishads, and other Eastern classics embody this wisdom.

Figure 6.2. "Wa," a Character for "Peace" or "Harmony."

A similar way of thinking prevailed in the West. Dietary commonsense is a central theme in the story of Odysseus, the greatest warrior in the ancient Greek

Agriculture and Peace in the *Odyssey*

In the *Odyssey*, the pivotal episode occurs nearly twenty years later when Odysseus, after the loss of nearly all his men and still far from home, seeks guidance from his ancestors and fallen comrades at the entrance to the Underworld. There, he meets the ghost of Tiresias, the blind seer and wisest man in antiquity. The spirit of Tiresias tells Odysseus that his trials and tribulations will end when he reaches home and travels far inland to a place where the people eat simple food and do not know about modern warfare. Odysseus is told to carry an oar on his shoulder and when a passerby comes up and mistakes it for a shovel to winnow barley and wheat, he is to plant it firmly in the ground. Odysseus takes this advice to heart. When he reaches Ithaca and finally rescues his wife (Penelope), his son, and his father, he tells them that he has one more task to accomplish and sets out to the fields of ripening grain with his battle oar. In this way, the long-separated family—symbolically the human family—returns to its agricultural roots and, in the words of Homer, attains "blessed peace."

world. In ancient Greek myth, he feigns madness to remain at home when the Trojan War begins. However, Odysseus is eventually exposed when his young son Telemachus is put in front of the plow. Uprooted from his grain fields and his family, he is forced to join the expedition.

In the Bible, Isaiah's prophetic injunction to beat swords into plowshares invokes a similar image of an implement of war being turned into a tranquil farming tool. In its search for peace, humanity is encouraged in both cases to return to the traditional Staff of Life—whole grains—and literally center itself in the earth.

In modern usage, we usually refer to peace as meaning a truce between belligerents. Originally, however, the word had a much larger meaning. The English word "peace" comes from the Latin *pax* and means the act of making, or coming to, an agreement between two opposites. The principle of peace is balance. The words "pact" and "compact" derive from this same root and also mean agreement. Peace is the dynamic balance between two seemingly opposite forces.

True peace is a harmonious union of opposites, not simply a cessation of conflict. It is an active, creative state in which individual differences are unified as part of a larger whole.

In the Far East, a dynamic understanding of peace existed until comparatively recent times. Peace was viewed as the balance of yin and yang—the two complementary and antagonistic qualities that make up all phenomena. For example, in the I Ching, or Book of Changes, there is a hexagram (figure) for "peace" (*T'ai*), combining yin and yang lines in perfect harmony (see Figure 6.3 right). Confucius' commentary states:

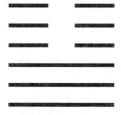

Figure 6.3. Yin and Yang Lines Forming Peace.

> Peace. "The small departs, the great approaches. Good fortune. Success."
> In this way heaven and earth unite, and all beings come into union.
> Upper and lower unite, and they are of one will.
> The light principle [yang] is within, the shadowy [yin] without; strength is within and devotion without; the superior man is within, the inferior without.[3]

Describing the meaning of *peace* (shalom) in the Judeo-Christian tradition, *The Interpreters' Dictionary of the Bible* defines it as: "The state of wholeness possessed by persons or groups, which may be health, prosperity, security, or the spiritual completeness of covenant. In the [Hebrew Bible] no particular distinction is made among these categories; military or economic peace is similar to the bodily and spiritual health of the individual."[4]

In the broadest, most universal sense, peace and health are the same. Peace and happiness are inseparable. Individual peace and social peace are one. In practice, peace refers not just to achieving balance between the nuclear powers, but also between the Arabs and the Jews, the Hindus and the Moslems, Protestants and Catholics, Shiites and Sunnis, and other pairs of opposing parties.

Peace refers to balancing all aspects of our daily lives. It includes balancing the cold of winter and the heat of summer, balancing the hours of wakefulness during the day and the hours of sleep at night, and balancing the amount and quality of the foods we eat and drink every day with those we consume on holidays, at parties, and other special occasions. In fact, the more we reflect on existence, we realize that nature—of which we are a small part—is made up of countless opposites. Not only are we constantly balancing myriad factors, consciously or unconsciously, but also these factors are constantly changing. Thus, everything eventually turns into its opposite. Summer changes into winter; youth changes into old age; action changes into rest; the mountain changes into the valley; land changes into ocean; day changes into night; hate changes to love; the rich and powerful decline; the poor and meek prosper; war turns into peace; former enemies become friends; civilizations rise and fall; species come and go; life changes into death and new life is reborn; matter changes into energy; space changes into time; galaxies appear and disappear.

Arising out of God or One Infinity, yin and yang are the eternal forces and tendencies governing all phenomena, visible and invisible, individual and group, part and whole, past and future. To know the principles and laws of change is to attain the Tree of Life, to enter the Kingdom of Heaven, to achieve Perfect Peace. When we know these principles and laws, all spiritual and religious concepts, all scientific and philosophical ideas, and all individual and social efforts are unified and understood to be complementary aspects of a larger whole. These forces and tendencies are a compass enabling us to realize order and harmony at all levels. By knowing them, we can turn sickness into health, sadness into joy, and war into peace.

PEACE PROMOTER

William and Joan Spear, Connecticut

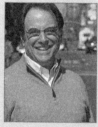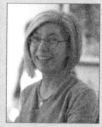

Bill Spear and Joan Spear

Since the late 1970s, William Spear, with the support of his wife Joan, had been offering a variety of international seminars, workshops, conferences and individual services in the field of macrobiotic education, natural alternative health approaches, sustainable ecological design practices, personal transformation, and end-of-life counseling.

Bill's own journey to health and well-being began while living in Denmark in the early 1970s, where he was diagnosed with kidney disease and was advised to begin dialysis treatments immediately. Within hours (and against medical advice) he left the hospital, began to practice macrobiotics in earnest, and never looked back. He's never been a patient in a hospital since.

In 1974, together with Michael and Jeanne Rossoff in Washington, D.C., Bill was among a group of friends who cooked weekly lunches at St. John's Church, directly across the street from the White House. Motivated to change government policies concerning food, he and Bill Tara testified in front of the Senate Select Committee on Human Needs and Nutrition during their investigation of the relationship between diet and health.

After accepting a position to work with the Center for Living with Illness and Dying at Yale University, Bill Spear moved to Connecticut and opened the East West Center (later called the Macrobiotic Association of Connecticut, and currently Fortunate Blessings Foundation, Inc.) in Middletown, Connecticut. Continuing in his efforts as a community organizer and activist, he and his wife expanded the center to include the Nutrition Information Center and Women's Resource Center, which focused on home-birth, women's issues, and childcare. To alleviate a need for better access to good-quality organic macrobiotic ingredients and specialty items, in 1979, Bill and Joan opened the Bridge, a cauldron-style traditional food company that distributed throughout the state and into wider regions.

Throughout the later 1970s and early 1980s, Bill traveled globally with my family, offering courses on the macrobiotic approach, diet and health, and the unifying principle applied to social issues. The East West Center also sponsored numerous seminars with me and my wife Aveline, Shizuko Yamamoto, and many other teachers, leading to Bill's selection as an original member of the Kushi Institute faculty in 1979. He further became a regular lecturer and counselor at the Macrobiotic Center of New York, working closely with Annemarie Colbin, Kezia Snyder, and Shizuko Yamamoto.

During this time, when the AIDS crisis emerged, Bill was instrumental in helping to organize frequent support groups for men with AIDS. He also contributed to research on the efficacy of macrobiotics in minimizing the side effects of autoimmune diseases. It was at that time—as a result of numerous end-of-life encounters with clients—that Bill reached out to Elisabeth Kübler-Ross, author of *On Death and Dying*, with whom (along with Tibetan lama Sogyal Rinpoche) he began years of in-depth training. Together, they represented lifetimes of vast experience with people in transition.

After moving to northwest Connecticut in the mid-1980s, Bill started to offer small workshops for hospice volunteers and caregivers throughout the United States., eventually developing the Gentle Passage (also known as the Passage), a five-day intensive residential retreat program first offered in Kiental, Switzerland, at the International Macrobiotic Center. The retreat provided a path of personal transformation, supplying a safe space in which participants could face and release past and present issues that prevented them from experiencing life fully in the present through developing personal and spiritual practices of heart-centered unconditional presence.

In the early 1990s—following talks in Moscow, Leningrad (now St. Petersburg), and Chelyabinsk near Siberia—war broke out in Yugoslavia, and Bill began to offer workshops throughout the Balkan area. Moved by these conflicts and determined to prepare himself for work with survivors of torture and war, Bill sought out traditional Buddhist teachers—including His Holiness the Dalai Lama—with whom he began what would remain a life-long study. Over the course of the next five years, he collaborated with Zlatko and Jadranka Pejíc of the Center for the Improvement of the Quality of Life in Zagreb, Croatia.

During the same time, teaching courses on *feng shui* (harmonization with the surrounding environment) throughout Europe and the United Kingdom, Bill founded the International Feng Shui Society and published *Feng Shui Made Easy*, which became a bestseller. The revised edition, released in 2010, was translated into sixteen different languages. As a result of the success of the book, he started lecturing and giving consultations all over the world on the art of placement for individuals and businesses.

In 1995, Bill developed Open Heart, Deep Spirit as a follow-up to the Passage. OHDS is a three-day residential retreat focusing on discerning the path of destiny, creating the future, and embarking on the next step in self-development, namely, freeing one's energies to be of unconditional service to our fellow human beings and the planet.

In 1998, Bill established the Silent Oceans Trust, a five-year effort intended to bring attention to the dangerous presence in the world's oceans of low-frequency sonar, which was seriously damaging to marine mammals. Taking the message to the U.K., Sweden, Japan, and Australia, Silent Oceans sought to prevent proponents of this ill-advised technology—as diverse as oil companies and defense departments—from continuing the practice. Silent Oceans and other environmental groups joined forces and sued the U.S. Navy, winning their case and gaining an injunction against the Department of Defense. As a result, the National Resources Defense Council took up the issue and, backed by famous faces such as James Taylor, Robert Redford, and Pierce Brosnan, published a widely circulated white paper on the subject.

As a result of the events of September 11, 2001, and the massive tsunami in the South Indian Ocean on December 26, 2004, Fortunate Blessings Foundation launched Second Response, an initiative that began as an international relief program to assist children who had been traumatized by natural disasters, war, torture, and other misfortunes. After the initial emergency phase of a disaster, Second Response trauma teams traveled to impacted areas to offer support to children and training to caregivers by using the carefully crafted methodology of mind-body exercises, called PLAYshops.

During PLAYshops, participants directly engage in an experiential session on methodologies that employ body or somatic exercises to release repressed emotions. The learning objective is to introduce the phenomenology of trauma and PTS (Post-Traumatic Stress) to participants through specific exercises designed to prevent PTSD (Post-Traumatic Stress Disorder).

In recent years, Second Response's trauma teams have assisted children in Indonesia, Samoa, Japan (following the 2011 nuclear accident at Fukushima), and the Philippines, as well as victims of the Nepalese earthquake and various weather-related and man-made disasters in the U.S. Second Response's PLAYshops—now with the additional component of Strategies for Self-Regulation—facilitate a natural release of fears, grief, anger, and other emotions. They effectively demonstrate to caregivers ways to understand the nature of PTSD and identify special cases and the needs of children who are severely traumatized.

Bill and Joan are a bright, shining example of the macrobiotic spirit of One Grain, Ten Thousand Grains—expressing endless gratitude to nature and society and dedicating themselves to creating a world of enduring health, happiness, and peace. The parents of three sons who exemplify the Spears' commitment to One Peaceful World, they live in Litchfield, Connecticut and have continued to teach and counsel around the world.

7.

Lost Paradise

O ur study of human destiny is based on a view of life that encompasses the entire universe while revealing the order that operates at every level within it. At the foundation of this understanding is the logarithmic spiral. This basic form, which appears throughout nature, reveals the mechanism of creation and the fundamental unity and interconnectedness of life. Knowledge of this simple but comprehensive form permits us to unify all of the seeming contradictions in our modern science and history, as well as to understand the origin of war and the way to peace. In this chapter, I will explore the basic cycles and rhythms that shape and influence our life, from the largest galactic cycle to the cycles of biological evolution, from the precession of the equinoxes to the spiral of history.

THE GALACTIC CYCLE

Modern science has enabled us to measure some of the celestial events that are shaping human destiny. We know that life started on our planet more than 3 billion years ago and that our solar system is revolving in an approximately 200-million-year cycle around the center of the galaxy. We may refer to this cycle of the solar system around the Milky Way as the "galactic year." More than ten revolutions ago, bacteria emerged and slowly developed into primitive sea life and fish; only two revolutions ago, in the late Paleozoic Era, the first amphibians were formed. Less than one revolution ago, giant ferns and dinosaurs covered the earth.

The galactic year may be divided into seasons (see Figure 7.1 on page 79) in a similar way to the ordinary 365-day solar year. Of course, the sun's orbit around the galactic center is not perfectly uniform—nothing is! At various times during this cycle, the solar system is nearer the center of the galaxy; at other times, it is farther away. When the solar system is farther away, it becomes larger—a yin state of expansion. When it is nearer to the galactic center, the solar system becomes smaller—a yang state of contraction. When the solar system expands, naturally, the distance between the sun and the earth becomes greater. As a result, the earth then receives less solar radiation and becomes colder—a yin condition. At the opposite time, when the solar system becomes contracted, the distance

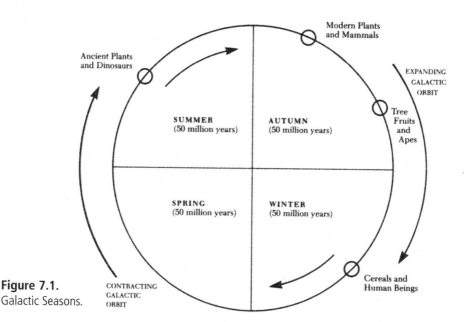

Figure 7.1.
Galactic Seasons.

between the sun and the earth shortens, and the earth receives more solar radiation. The earth becomes hotter and its surface becomes muddy and swamp-like. A yang condition arises. The atmosphere becomes more humid and plants become bigger.

Thus, when the solar system is farthest from the center of the galaxy, that time is the middle of the galactic winter season. The middle of galactic summer comes when the solar system is closest to the galactic center. In between are galactic spring and autumn. Actually, the solar system's journey around the galactic center is gradually shortening over the eons, but practically speaking, at the present time each galactic season lasts about 50 million years.

Diverse Species Emerge

Through the course of an estimated sixteen galactic revolutions over 3.2 billion years, many evolutionary changes have taken place. Warm, hot, cool, and cold galactic seasons have alternated to create different geological and climatic conditions, giving rise to new, diverse species of plant and animal life. Ferns, for example, developed in a season of galactic winter; they contracted in the intense cold and their leaves split into many sections. Then, in the following galactic spring, ferns began to expand and cover the earth. About this time, too, reptiles and birds prospered, eventually developing into giant reptiles and dinosaurs under the expansive influence of the warm weather during galactic summer.

About 64 to 68 million years ago, as our solar system moved into galactic autumn, the huge trees began to die, along with the large animals. The cooler weather brought different forms of life; the plants became less juicy and smaller, and herbs, grasses, and grains came out. In the animal kingdom, corresponding changes caused mammals to develop. Animal life is dependent, directly or indirectly, upon plant life. Animals evolved, or changed, by eating the changing vegetation that was available to them during this colder epoch. The early primates that ate principally seeds, nuts, and fruits evolved into apes, chimpanzees, and baboons.

The ancestors of human beings developed possibly more than 10 million years ago by incorporating the most recent form of plant life—whole cereal grains—into their diet (see Figure 7.2 below). Wild cereal grasses, combining the seed and the fruit together, represented a unique evolutionary adaptation to the increasingly cold climate brought about by late galactic autumn and early galactic winter. Moreover, compared to earlier plants, cereal grasses grew more vertically,

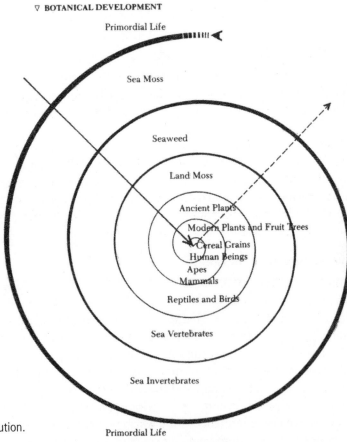

Figure 7.2.
The Spiral of Evolution.

thereby absorbing a greater portion of the natural electromagnetic energies streaming in from the heavenly bodies above and the turning of the earth on its axis below. By eating wild grains as their principal food, early hominids assumed a more upright posture, and their consciousness, nourished by the energies of sky and earth, greatly expanded.

Humankind, then, is a product of late galactic autumn to early galactic winter. We can understand this cycle by seeing how our own activity changes during the calendar year. Our sexuality reaches a peak in the spring, our physical nature is dominant during the summer, while late autumn to early winter is the time we think best and devote more time to school or study. The influences of the galactic season are similar: Spring saw the differentiation of many species, summer the physical development of orders and phyla, while late autumn and early winter produced a thinking being—homo sapiens.

The Evolution of Humanity's Diet

The traditional diet of humanity consisted primarily of whole cereal grains, vegetables, and other foods of plant origin, especially in the savannahs of Africa, our species' ancient homeland. Only a small supplemental part of the daily diet over the last several million years was made up of foods of animal origin. However, during periods of extreme cold, extreme heat, or other unusual environmental conditions, the proportion of animal food varied considerably. As part of an active, outdoors way of life, a small volume of animal food (especially fish and seafood) has traditionally been eaten by human beings in relatively good health. The exact amount has depended on geography, climate, the weather, personal level of activity, and other factors. According to the most recent genetic findings, our species originally left Africa about 65,000 years ago. The exodus took the first wave south to South Asia, the Andaman Islands, Melanesia, and Australia—all warm, tropical regions where a plant-based diet was natural. A second wave about 40,000 years ago saw our species leaving Africa and spreading in more northerly and easterly directions, including Europe, Central Asia, East Asia, and Siberia, where a diet higher in animal food was appropriate in the colder environment and climate.

With the rise of the Darwinian theory of survival of the fittest in the late 1800s came the modern notion that homo sapiens and their ancestors were primarily carnivores and that meat, poultry, and other animal foods higher up on the evolutionary ladder were superior foods for human development and constituted the most important part of the diet. This approach was popularized by Justus von Liebig, the German chemist and father of modern nutrition, as well as Herbert Spencer, the British sociologist who coined the term "the survival of the fittest." Until recently, most conventional scientists have not been eating the same kind of food that ancient people ate. As a result, they can collect data about ancient cultures, including spiral designs and inscriptions, but they cannot understand the cosmology and the mind that formed them. To understand the mentality of ancient people, it is necessary to have the same quality of food and thereby develop the same wavelength of consciousness. This can be done only by researchers and others who are eating grains as main food.

As modern society has turned toward more natural foods in the last generation, scientists are beginning to reevaluate their assumptions of humanity's remote past, assumptions based on the fragmented and incomplete nutritional theories of the last century. Studies of Paleolithic cultures, as well as dietary investigation of the modern hunter-gatherer tribes, have shown that they consumed primarily vegetable-quality food, including undomesticated grains, wild plants and grasses, tubers, seeds and nuts, berries, and roots. Fish and animal life was taken only when necessary and consumed in small amounts. Archaeologists are discovering that many stone-age tools, such as those found at Olduvai Gorge in Tanzania and other noted archaeological sites, are implements for vegetable processing rather than animal processing.[1] A reexamination of the bones and tools of early humans going back two million years has even led some scientists to conclude that early humans were scavengers and not hunters at all, eating only occasional animal food that had been killed by some other species.[2] An anthropological study of fifty-eight hunter-gatherer societies that existed in the late 1980s revealed that 50 to 70 percent of their diets consisted of complex carbohydrates from plant sources.[3]

Summarizing the new view of early humanity's original diet, *The New York Times* reported:

> Recent investigations into the dietary habits of prehistoric peoples and their primate predecessors suggest that heavy meat-eating by modern affluent societies may be exceeding the biological capacities evolution built into the human body. The result may be a host of diet-related health problems, such as diabetes, obesity, high blood pressure, coronary heart disease, and some cancers.
>
> The studies challenge the notion that human beings evolved as aggressive hunting animals who depended primarily upon meat for survival. The new view—coming from findings in such fields as archaeology, anthropology, primatology, and comparative anatomy—instead portrays early humans and their forebears more as herbivores than carnivores. According to these studies, the prehistoric table for at least the last million and a half years was probably set with three times more plant than animal foods, the reverse of what the average American currently eats.[4]

Stone tools found in Mozambique dating to 100,000 years ago showed that Paleolithic cultures were processing sorghum and other wild grains and baking grain products. Similar pre-agricultural sites have been found in ancient Palestine in the Middle East, Moravia in the Czech Republic, Italy, and Russia dating to about 25,000 years ago or more. These findings contradict claims put forward by present-day advocates of the "Paleo diet" that our ancestors ate predominantly meat and other animal products and little, if any, grains. The original Paleolithic way of eating, as a consensus of food historians and other researchers are now finding, was plant-centered. In his audio course *Food: A Cultural Culinary History*, Ken Albala of the University of the Pacific refers to ancient hominids as "gatherer-hunters," not "hunter-gatherers," because they ate predominantly wild plants, seeds, nuts, tubers, and roots and only marginally animal foods.[5]

The most important breakthrough occurred in 2013, when archeologists found that the entire hominid line of evolution branched off from chimpanzees and developed 3.5 million years ago, when primates started to eat wild grasses and sedges. According to the study published in the *Proceedings of the National Academy of Sciences* and led by researchers at the University of Colorado Boulder, "A new look at the diets of ancient African hominids shows a 'game change' occurred about 3.5 million years ago when some members added grasses or sedges to their menus."[6] This study confirms the longtime macrobiotic teaching that our human form and structure originated when ancient hominids began eating wild cereal grasses and discovered the art of cooking.

THE CYCLE OF THE NORTHERN SKY

There have been, and will be again, many destructions of mankind arising out of many causes; the greatest have been brought about by the agencies of fire and water.

—PLATO, *TIMAEUS*

In addition to the galactic revolutions, human destiny is also strongly influenced by the cycle of northern celestial motion, the approximately 26,000-year cycle of the precession of the equinoxes. As the sun and planets journey around the galactic center, their orbit traces a gentle wavelike motion. From a point removed from the earth, our planet would be seen to wobble slowly like a child's top, with its north-south axis pointing first in one direction, then in the other, making one complete "wobble" about every 26,000 years. That wobbling motion of the earth's axis traces a circle across the night sky, with a series of stars in the northern constellations serving successively as pole star (see Figure 7.3 on page 84). In the lifetime of any individual or culture, the movement is imperceptible—only one degree every seventy-two years. But over millennia, there is a slow, steady, perceptible energetic shift.

This precession was first described in writing by the Greek philosopher Hipparchus in 127 B.C.E. In astrology, the 26,000-year cycle was divided into twelve houses and gave rise to the Ages of Aries, Pisces, Aquarius, and so on. In that cycle—depending on how the earth's axis is aligned relative to the plane of our galaxy—we receive varying amounts of stellar and solar radiation, electromagnetic energy, and other impulses and waves originating from the center of the Milky Way as well as the billions of other galaxies in the infinite universe.

As a whole, the earth is surrounded by a vast protective belt of electromagnetic fields, but the area over the poles is relatively open. The shower of energy from the pole stars therefore exerts a strong influence on the earth; as a new star or constellation moves into ascendancy, it produces a regular change of electromagnetic charge on the earth. In comparison to the South Pole, which faces more toward the center of the galaxy, the North Pole faces more toward the periphery, receiving energy from billions of other galaxies. As a result, the North is more highly charged than the South.

The 26,000-year cycle (also known as the Platonic or Great Year) falls into two halves, each lasting about 13,000 years, which have been traditionally described as the Golden Age and the Age of Darkness; the Time of Paradise and the Time of Wilderness; Spiritual Civilization and Material Civilization; or other complementary opposites. The precessional cycle can further be divided into four seasons: First, summer, or the peak of light; next, fall; then, winter, or the depth of darkness; and finally, spring. Transitional stages of four more constellations between these four points make a total of eight constellations in the Great Year.

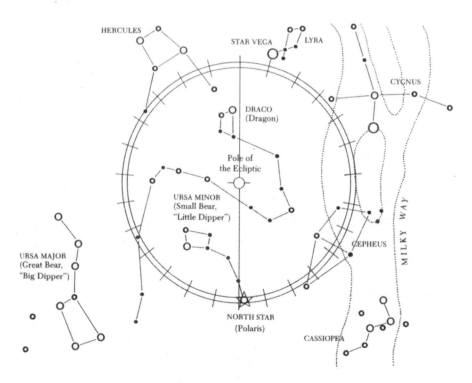

Figure 7.3. Constellations of the Northern Sky.

The Golden Age

About 20,000 years ago, during the peak of precessional summer, the earth's north-south axis was oriented toward the Milky Way, aligned with the plane of the galaxy, and the northern sky was illuminated with millions of brilliant stars. The great mass of stars clustered in that plane shed their influence directly down from overhead, highly charging the earth and all forms of life growing upon it. Our ancestors were constantly bathed in a shower of light and radiation, pouring in through their spines, meridians, electromagnetic energy centers, organs, tissues, and trillions of cells. They became very highly energized, and their consciousness developed heightened awareness and capacities. In contrast, humans around the globe today are unable to see the stars or experience their energies because of the growing incidence of light pollution. This has negatively affected our ability to maintain our health and sleep soundly, and also impacts animals and plants with which we interact (see "Creating a Naturally Bright New Era" on page 86).

Not only was the human brain much more activated during that period, but all the botanical sources of food became much more vigorous, requiring hardly any cultivation. This is the Golden Age of which ancient poets speak. For example, Ovid writes:

> Golden was that first age which, with no one to compel, without a law, of its own will, kept faith and did the right. There was no fear of punishment, no threatening words were to be read on brazen tablets; no suppliant throng gazed fearfully upon its judge's face; but without judges lived secure. Not yet had the pine-tree, felled on its native mountains, descended thence into the watery plain to visit other lands; men knew no shores except their own. Not yet were cities begirt with steep moats; there were no trumpets of straight, no horns of curving brass, no swords or helmets. There was no need at all of armed men, for nations, secure from war's alarms, passed the years in gentle ease. The earth herself, without compulsion, untouched by hoe or plowshare, of herself gave all things needful. And men, content with food which came with no one's seeking, gathered the arbute fruit, strawberries from the mountain-sides, cornel-cherries, berries hanging thick upon the prickly bramble, and acorns fallen from the spreading tree of Jove. Then spring was everlasting, and gentle zephyrs with warm breath played with the flowers that sprang unplanted. Anon the earth, untilled, brought forth her stores of grain, and the fields, though unfallowed, grew white with the heavy, bearded wheat.[7]

In Roman mythology, the Golden Age is associated with Saturn, the god of the harvest, whose color is yellow and whose symbol is the scythe for reaping grains. In China, the Golden Age is symbolized by the Yellow Emperor, who is associated with the same planet.

While we cannot be sure of how life was organized in that era, the world's

Creating a Naturally Bright New Era

**Light pollution across North America adversely impacts animal
and plant life, as well as dims human consciousness.**

A new world atlas of artificial night sky brightness shows that more than 80 percent
of the world population and more than 99 percent of Americans and Europeans live
under light-polluted skies. According to the online journal *Science Advances,* the
Milky Way is not visible to 80 percent of Americans and 60 percent of Europeans.
Nearly half of the United States, 88 percent of Europe, and 23 percent of the planet
as a whole experience light polluted nights.[8] This includes Iraq, Syria, and other
parts of the Middle East, where warfare has artificially lit up the sky.

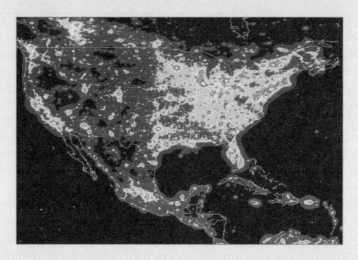

Principal sources of light pollution are residential lights, streetlights, highway lights,
motor vehicle headlights, sport stadium lights, electronic advertising billboards,
shopping mall lights, park lights, airport lights, and offshore oil platforms. These
create such a hazy glow that they block out the light of the heavens above, including our home galaxy, the constellations of the Zodiac, and even the North Star.

Like other modern technologies, gas, electric, and digital lighting have improved
our safety, comfort, efficiency, and material well-being (think illuminated freeways
and smartphones). At the same time, they have threatened ecological diversity and
adversely affected our health and consciousness.

The artificial light around cities and extending into many rural areas has interfered
with the migration of nocturnal birds because they cannot follow the moon and
stars. Over 450 species of birds, including many endangered varieties, are apt to
collide with night-lit towers. In the Gulf of Mexico, female sea turtles are more likely

to avoid coming to shore and nesting because of changes in the reflectivity of the water. Light pollution also disorients bats, moths, and other animals that come out at night, and millions are killed each year by flying into streetlights. The metabolism of snakes, salamanders, and frogs has also been altered.[9]

The synthetic glow affects the growth and flowering of plants as well. A recent British study found that low-intensity amber light inhibited the flowering of a wild relative of peas and beans that is a key source of food for the pea aphid insect in grasslands and road verges.[10] Multiplied many times over, tiny changes like this could cascade and have a profound impact on delicate ecosystems.

Light pollution also affects humans, disrupting sleep, causing headaches, affecting sensory nerves, and contributing to depression. Alteration of circadian rhythms is further believed to increase the risk of obesity and diabetes. Some medical researchers suggest that artificial light, especially the blue component in white light at night, is carcinogenic. Exposure to artificial light at night, or LAN, increases cancer risk, especially for breast, prostate, and other hormonal cancers. Women who work night shifts have shown higher rates of breast cancer. Reduced melatonin—a protective hormone produced at night during sleep—is believed to be a key factor in this increase in cancer in people who work or stay up at night and are exposed to artificial light.[11]

As we see in this chapter on Lost Paradise, the Milky Way and other stars and constellations in the night sky influence and shape biological and spiritual evolution. They constantly charge our mid and forebrains, eyes, chakras, meridians, and other systems, organs, and functions, especially if we eat whole cereal grains that have small antennae that receive and concentrate this cosmic energy and vibration. This current of incoming spiral energy orients us to beauty, truth, peace, justice, freedom, and other universal ideals.

As the 25,800-year Vega/Polaris cycle and Spiral of History come to an end, it is imperative for humanity to develop broad, comprehensive thinking, stay focused, and not lose its direction or bearings. The Ki energy streaming from the heavens is indispensible for developing a calm, clear mind; envisioning a healthy, peaceful future; and realizing our common dream.

With the eclipse of night, the consciousness of modern society is rapidly dimming. Like the birds and the turtles, we are disoriented and have lost our way. Fortunately, the Kushi Institute, situated in a remote region of the Berkshires in western Massachusetts, is one of the few places on the Eastern Seaboard that has a clear, unobstructed view of the Milky Way. We are hopeful that macrobiotic education will continue to provide inspiration and guidance as the world artificially brightens. By respecting the natural rhythms and cycles of nature, including day and night, humanity can pass safely through this time. We can recover the compass of yin and yang, apply it to problems of society, and create a naturally bright new era.

myths and scriptures almost universally tell of a time when humanity reached advanced cultural, spiritual, and scientific levels and maintained a worldwide peaceful, unified civilization. This ancient civilization then apparently collapsed through a series of natural catastrophes that ushered in the next half-cycle, the Time of Wilderness.

The Draconian Age

About 13,000 years ago, halfway back on the 26,000-year cycle, we moved out of the galactic plane as the star Vega of the constellation Lyra came overhead (see Figure 7.4 below). *Vega* is a word of Arabic origin, meaning "fall." However, *Vega* is not a "falling" or shooting star. *Vega* refers to the Fall from Paradise—the end of the Golden Age or the preceding precessional summer, when celestial energy was at its peak. Lyra, the Harp, further is linked with the musician Orpheus in Greek mythology, who descended to the dark Underworld searching for his bride Eurydice. The tale of their separation symbolizes humanity's looking back to a lost Golden Age.

During the end of the Golden Age, the earth's position relative to the plane of the galaxy began to tilt—offering less of an opening for the energies that flow from the Milky Way—and the energy of plants and animals dimmed, while human consciousness lowered and became more materially oriented. This period marks the time roughly 13,000 years ago when the world appears to have been

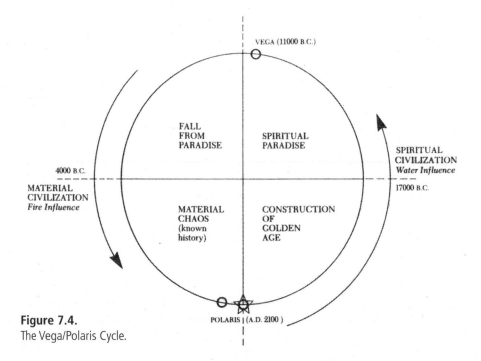

Figure 7.4.
The Vega/Polaris Cycle.

engulfed in a tremendous flood or series of floods, as recounted in mythologies around the world (best known to us as the Gilgamesh legend and the biblical story of Noah). The water catastrophe may have been due to a partial geological axis shift of about thirty degrees. Scientists tell us that the earth's axis has shifted approximately once every 25,000 years. For example, the earth's last south magnetic pole was possibly in Australia. There is also evidence that a giant comet entered the solar system at this time and broke into fragments. Some of these hit the northern polar region, generating enormous amounts of heat that vaporized ice caps, destabilized the earth's crust, and sparked a deluge.

The entire dark side of the cycle covering the period from 13,000 years ago to the present is dominated by the constellation of Draco, the Dragon. In Sumerian tradition, this constellation is associated with Tiamat, the monster of primordial chaos. In Christian tradition, it is associated with the serpent that tempted Adam and Eve and led to the exile from the Garden of Eden. A star in the tail of Draco, one-quarter of the way around the circle, was the pole star during precessional winter and the point on the cycle farthest removed from the Milky Way. Draco ruled the Ice Ages and the deepest darkness in which humanity was submerged preceding the dawn of recorded history. The Great Pyramid at Giza is oriented to Thuban, the star in the tail of Draco that served as the pole star during this time.

Next on the cycle, after Draco, comes Ursa Major. The "Great Bear" or Great Dipper is associated with many myths, including the *Iliad* and the *Odyssey*. The Greek epics describing the story of humanity's journey through this precessional epoch are rooted in an ancient myth referring to a great celestial bear hibernating in the winter and then reemerging in the spring. In the *Iliad*, Achilles, the Greeks' chieftain, holes up in his tent like a bear for a long period before emerging and leading the victory over the Trojans. Achilles' shield is emblazoned with the symbols of the Great Bear and other polar constellations, surrounded by concentric circles depicting the ages of humanity.

After Ursa Major comes Ursa Minor—the "Little Bear" or Little Dipper—which rules precessional spring and which points to Polaris, the current pole or North Star. During this epoch, which saw the rise of agricultural civilization, metallurgy, and the nation-state, humanity has faced the Promethean challenge of mastering the use of fire. With each succeeding minor age, the challenge of using fire properly has intensified. What we may call the Fire Civilization is now ending, just as the deluge ended the Water Civilization opposite us on the circle that occurred when Vega was the North Star. However, the "destruction by fire" universally prophesied by ancient cultures need not be sudden in the form of nuclear, chemical, or biological warfare, though that is certainly possible. Other modern fire phenomena include global warming and climate change; the rapid spread of industrialization, chemicalization, and urbanization; the loss of biodiversity; artificial electromagnetic radiation; and new viral epidemics. The destruction by fire may be more gradual and already upon us in the form of improper dietary practice (e.g., synthetic foods, chemical farming, and GMOs) and catastrophic misuse of technology (e.g., highly artificial energy), resulting in the pollution of our internal and external environment.

According to astronomers, in about C.E. 2100, the earth's north-south axis will point almost directly at Polaris in the Little Dipper. This will signal the end of the preceding 13,000-year-half-cycle, dominated by the darkness of Draco, and the beginning of a new 13,000-year-half-cycle dominated by the light of the Milky Way. This date need not be taken literally as the turning point. The momentous changes that humanity is currently experiencing have been forming over the last several centuries and will take possibly several more centuries to solidify. Practically speaking, however, the events of the first third of the twenty-first century—especially the spread of artificial food, the accelerated destruction of our environment, the proliferation of weapons of mass destruction, and the drive toward genetic manipulation—are the most critical humanity has ever faced.

The events of the years preceding C.E. 2100 will determine whether our species survives the challenge of fire and passes safely into the next phase of the cycle: the Era of Humanity and the beginning of planetary family consciousness.

THE SPIRAL OF HISTORY

World history moves in a spiral. There is as marvelous an order and unity to human affairs, including the rise and fall of civilizations, as there is to the helical development of galaxies, solar systems, plants and animals, DNA, and subatomic particles (see Figure 7.5 on page 91). To understand the momentous changes that are converging at this time—including the development of atomic energy, the exploration of space, and the invention of personal computers and smartphones—we need to reflect on the spirallic order of which our lives on this planet are a small part.

The Stages of the Spiral

The Spiral of History can be divided into twelve sections, like a clock. They are not actually equal but, because the spiral is logarithmic, become increasingly smaller in size and shorter in time. The first sections span over a thousand years in duration, while the last section extends less than fifty years. Because of the spirallic nature of historical development, history actually does repeat itself to a degree. For instance, the time of intense war activity marked by the Crusades and the Mongol invasions occurs during the same period of its era as do the World Wars in our era. In the same way, the age of discovery, which saw contact established between East and West and between the Old World and the New World, falls in the same section as the modern space age, which saw the launching of the first earth satellites, the landing on the moon, and probes of the solar system. The impetus, or character, of each section is the same; the main difference is that the earlier periods took a longer span of time.

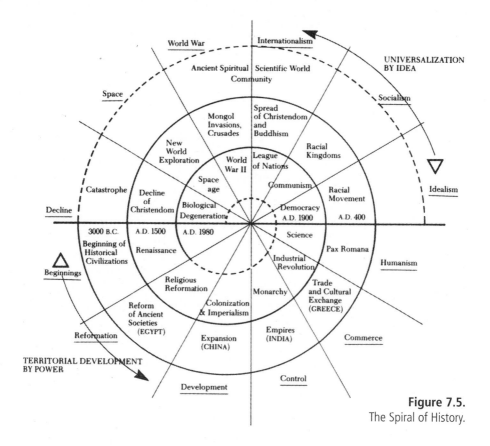

Figure 7.5.
The Spiral of History.

The Spiral of History alternates between periods of territorial expansion and conquest by power and periods of universalization by idea, or what can be called the spread of global or international ideologies. Each half-orbit of the spiral encompasses six sections and represents one of our historical ages. The stages of the spiral unfold in an orderly sequence. An initial period of territorial expansion comprises the more yang, or material, phase of the cycle. It includes the first six stages:

1. A new society, culture, or civilization begins;

2. Reform of the original system is instituted;

3. Development proceeds;

4. Power is consolidated;

5. Trade, commerce, and culture flourish; and

6. Material and cultural exchange stimulates new ideas.

At this point, the period of universalization by idea begins, which comprises the more yin, or spiritual, phase of the cycle. It includes the last six stages:

7. Idealism takes root and develops;

8. Socialization occurs with the spread of the ideas or doctrine to new territories;

9. Internationalization results;

10. Conflicts arise among competing ideas or ideologies, leading to world war;

11. Warfare stimulates technological development, leading to exploration and discovery, especially in a spatial dimension; and

12. Expansion in space leads to decomposition of systems and ideas, and the old order declines and falls.

At the end of the cycle, the process is renewed, and a new community, culture, or civilization begins. As you can see from Figure 7.6 below, there are seven half-orbits in the Spiral of History. These seven half-orbits make up seven ages, or epochs. Like the seasons of the year that are not exactly equal in length, the boundaries between these ages are approximate and, to a certain extent, overlap. The essential thing is to glimpse the underlying order to history and its accelerating speed.

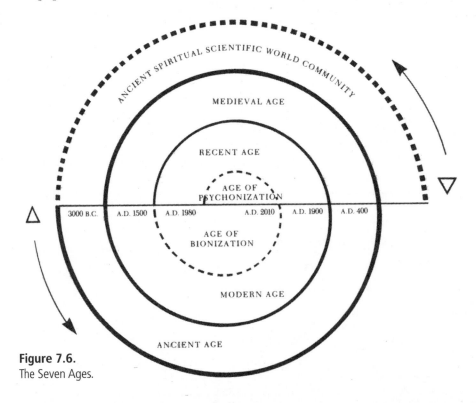

Figure 7.6.
The Seven Ages.

Historically, the change of society—as well as the development of technology and consciousness—has accelerated logarithmically. For example, within historical times, the use of fire has increased at an exponential ratio as the source of cooking fuel, home heating fuel, and metallurgical energy; other technological energy changed from wood to charcoal (about 3,000 years), from charcoal to coal (about 1,000 years), from coal to petroleum (about 300 years), from petroleum to electricity (about 100 years), and from electricity to nuclear power (about thirty years).

Foretelling the Future

Because of the logarithmic nature of the spiral, modes of life remained relatively unchanging over many generations in ancient civilizations, such as those of China and Egypt. By contrast, we know that life today is far different than it was even ten or twenty years ago. The years leading up to the mid-2030s will be the time of greatest yang-condensed force, the center part of the historical spiral. High pressure governs this era. High pressure is manifested as:

1. High speed (rapid advances in transportation and communication);

2. High production (increased mechanization);

3. High efficiency (introduction of computers, robotics, and smartphones);

4. High consumption (e.g., high-calorie, high-fat, high-protein, and high-salt diets); and

5. Great movement (fast circulation of people and money and rapid movement in general).

Under this pressure, many things are exceeding their levels of tolerance and are beginning to disintegrate. These include the institutions of society; the family structure; books and the printed word; brick and mortar businesses; the church, temple, and mosque; the nation-state; the mental stability of people; and the cellular stability of bodies.

Social changes cannot be separated from the changes in the physical environment, which are also progressing at an ever-increasing rate. Pollution of the water and air from industrialization, chemical farming, and genetic engineering are resulting in corresponding increases in atmospheric heat and pressure. The heaviness of the atmosphere is a very important effect accompanying the contraction of the historical spiral. It is contributing to global warming and significant climatic changes that could, in a relatively short span, produce profound effects on the natural environment, on which all life—including human life—depends. Upsetting the delicate ecological balance around us that has taken eons to develop could result in rising temperatures, melting ice, and massive die-offs of plants and animals. Other tumultuous earth changes may occur, such as those in myth and legend that are associated with the natural catastrophes that may have coincided with the ancient world community's collapse at the end of an earlier epoch. Our disregard of nature's subtle rhythms and cycles is also leading to further derangement of natural electromagnetic balances and an isolation from celestial forces, dimming our consciousness and judgment and making world war, biological decline, and social economic collapse more likely.

In the short period ahead, leading up to the 2030s, all aspects of human affairs—religious and ideological, political and economic, social and cultural, national and international, individual and universal, material and spiritual, and all other factors—will converge. This age will be the most confused, complicated, and condensed period that humanity has experienced in its history, as even age-old boundaries between species, sexes, and genders dissolve.

During the last 12,000 to 13,000 years, the earth's energy has steadily continued to decrease as we moved farther and farther away from the plane of the Milky Way. A period of milder climate about 6,000 years ago prompted Sumer, Egypt, China, the Indus Valley, and other centers of civilizations to build again toward a unified world civilization, but this movement was only temporary. The overall course of history continued with civilizations struggling in the darkness, fighting nature by inventing ever bigger and more powerful, destructive technologies. We are now reaching the climax of that darkness, the most fragmented and destructive era of human history.

This is the celestial and historical background of our present evolutionary challenge; our more conventional recorded histories all chronicle events within this age of decreasing electromagnetic influence, and this period of our history—the unbroken line of the spiral representing a fraction of our life on this planet—is now drawing to a close.

THE ERA OF HUMANITY

As the current Spiral of History ends in the early mid-twenty-first century, a new spiral will form that will last for about the next 12,000 to 13,000 years. This new era has already begun to unfold as the old era draws to a close. The relationship of these two spirals is similar to an Olympic relay race, in which two runners run in parallel for a brief distance until the baton is safely passed (see Figure 7.7 on page 95). When a secure hold is established, the new runner accelerates and takes off on his or her lap while the old runner fades away. In the human race— the contest to preserve and develop our natural biological quality and spirit— this period of overlap extends from roughly 1980 to 2100, when the Pole Star in Ursa Minor (Poseidon) arrives directly overhead. The Spiral of History and the coming new Era of Humanity will proceed in parallel for a while until the new orientation is strong enough to lead and the old orientation decays. Realistically, it may take the momentum of the past disharmonious factors two or three generations to fade away.

Thus, although worldwide modern civilization will continue to decline and fall over the next several decades, humanity need not necessarily disappear. At the same time that biotechnology is developing, a new orientation of civilization will arise among those people who have individually reoriented their way of life according to the laws of nature and the Order of the Universe. Through their understanding and efforts, the construction of a new healthy and peaceful world will begin, by the unification of all antagonistic factors in human affairs.

As the new orientation spreads, existing political, economic, ideological, and cultural systems will be seen as complementary to one another and will be allowed to evolve naturally as civilization as a whole develops in a more peaceful direction. The safe start of this new spirallic age will be signaled by the

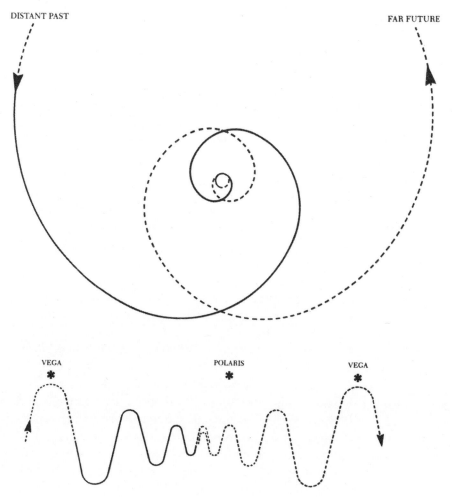

Figure 7.7. The Meeting of Ancient and Future Worlds.

establishment of a world federal government, or planetary commonwealth, to oversee the final abolition of nuclear weapons and other weapons of mass destruction, to preserve the earth's natural resources and wildlife, and to facilitate the biological, psychological, and spiritual health and happiness of humanity. Around the year 2100, the North Star (Polaris) will move directly overhead. This will hopefully mark the safe entry into the new Era of Humanity and the beginning of a new cycle of peace and unity that can be expected to last for many thousands of years, as the celestial influence of the Milky Way increases.

HUMANITY AT THE CROSSROADS

In the course of its development, human society has passed or will pass through three types of civilization:

1. A more spiritually oriented civilization, focusing on artistic, intellectual, and religious pursuits;

2. A more materially oriented civilization, focusing on health and well-being, productivity, and technological pursuits;

3. A more comprehensive civilization synthesizing the spiritual and the material.

For the past five or six thousand years, the more materialistic orientation has dominated. Before that, the more spiritual orientation was dominant. In the next era, the more comprehensive orientation will prevail.

During the remainder of this century and the early part of the next century, there will be a shift from material leadership (a reliance on power, economic wealth, territory, and autonomous nation-states) to more intuitive and ethical leadership (a reliance on balance, human rights, environmental sustainability, and collective world government). In fact, from the late nineteenth century, we can see the unifying principle beginning to emerge again at the forefront of human thought—for example, the shift in modern physics from viewing matter as substance to an understanding of particles as energy—and in general, leadership that emphasizes material superiority is losing its credibility and rapidly decaying. That decay will continue as social and economic chaos continues to spread. National economies around the world have already begun to encounter very serious difficulties. Meanwhile, the familiar cultural and religious teachings expressed through institutions such as the schools and churches, temples, and mosques are losing their authority or influence over people, especially those that emphasize hierarchial organization, dogmatic creeds, and an exclusively otherworldly orientation and minimize the importance of the body, food, and the material world. The whole of modern society, which has been oriented in a one-sided materialist direction or in a one-sided spiritualist direction, has started to disintegrate. This disintegration will reach a peak and turn into its opposite tendency: unification. Even science has been losing its authority.

Unless it is synthesized with a more balanced, intuitive understanding, it too will die out.

Because the spiral is balanced between opposite tendencies—power and ideological development—the point we now occupy is a time of decomposition, yet it occurs during the period of ideological development. Two possible futures are opening before us. One way we can go, as we have seen, is total destruction with all systems collapsing. This destruction, we may say, will be by fire—modern civilization's technology is based on fire. Energy is produced by burning coal and oil, by natural gas and hydraulic fracturing ("fracking"), and now, by splitting the atomic nucleus, which produces an incredible amount of heat. The center of the centripetal spiral is very condensed and active, and as we approach it, our use of energy is becoming greater and greater. If we collapse, by improper cooking, by abuse of energy, by war, by viral pandemics, by global warming and climate change—by fire—we must return toward the peripheral orbits of the spiral and return to a primitive way of life, or else be succeeded by some other species.

On the other hand, if we pass through the center without total collapse, we will begin spiraling centrifugally (away from the center). At this juncture, the twelve major tendencies of the historical spiral would continue, but in a totally different orientation. Many changes would take place. Most importantly, our values would change into their opposites. Our present-day valuables would become worthless. These present-day values are material ones: gold and diamonds, stocks and bonds, cars and clothing, fame and recognition. In the future, however, spiritual understanding, philosophical understanding, and mental development will become valuable. People will start to measure a person's worth or a person's happiness by these more comprehensive standards. Now, we judge each other largely by material worth and status. Although the coming age will be a spiritually oriented one, technology would still be developed and assimilated into the new orientation. The difference will be that technology will follow a sustainable orientation, rather than be used in military applications and threaten the environment.

Thus, the choice before us as a species is still open. There is nothing inevitable about the future ending of humanity. On one hand, human society and culture may end violently (see Figure 7.8 on page 98). We may "drop the baton" and eliminate ourselves from further evolutionary development. The apocalyptic outcome would stem from a resistance to the Order of the Universe, with people continuing to destroy their world through acquisition, fear, and indifference. On the other hand, the tightening spiral could be peacefully reversed (see Figure 7.9 on page 99). For this to happen, the community of people who harmonize with the natural order would need to grow and prevail. Through cooperation, reconciliation, and creativity, they will take the initiative to develop strong, healthy families, sustainable businesses and communities, and create a more peaceful world by radiating peace in their personal lives.

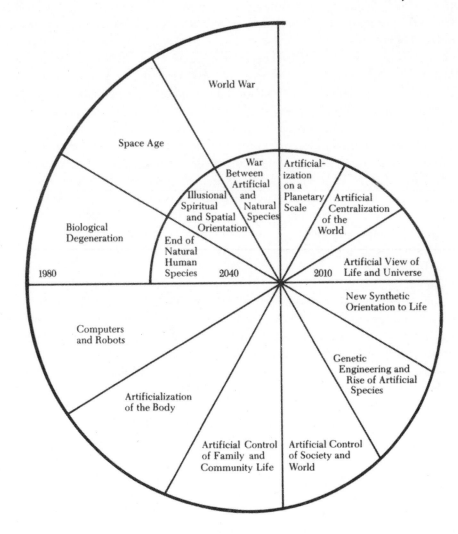

Figure 7.8. Choice of Futures: 1. Biotechnology.

THE ROOTS OF ANCIENT PROPHECY

Tens of thousands of years ago, the whole world was unified as one. In most parts of the globe, ancient peoples were eating in a macrobiotic way (mostly grains and vegetables), building temples and observatories, studying the principles of yin and yang (under various names), and generally leading healthy, peaceful lives. After the earth's atmosphere and energy field began to change, the knowledge and understanding of ancient cosmology and wisdom declined and remained in fragmental form for thousands of years. As great changes (including large floods, a possible partial axis shift, and the retreat of the glaciers) obliterated most traces of the past, memory of a united world community was all but fcrgotten except

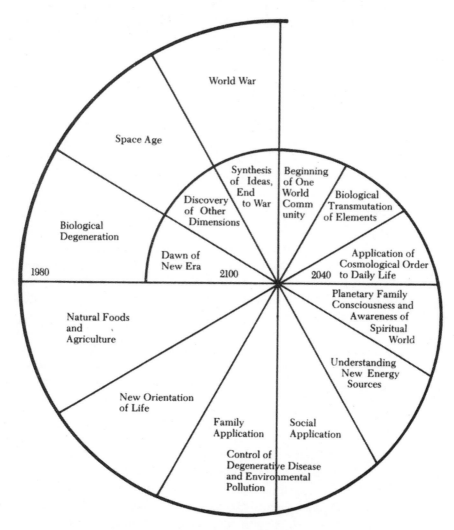

Figure 7.9. Choice of Futures: 2. Planetary Family Consciousness.

in myth, legend, and standing stones. Though scattered across the earth, a small remnant of people with some comprehensive understanding remained and developed communities and countries with an aspiration toward oneness and unity. These included Sumeria, upper Egypt, the Taklamakan Desert region of China, regions in the Himalaya mountains, the Pyrenees mountains in Spain and France, the Andes mountains in South America, and elsewhere. Wild cereal grains were domesticated and civilization again began to flourish. But soon God—the image of One—became idolized. At the same time, power, in the political sense, soon took over. Animal food consumption increased, wars broke out, and a spiral of violence developed that has accelerated ever since.

Intermittently, during the last month of the precessional year (a period of about 2,150 years, or one-twelfth of the cycle of the Northern skies (also known as the Zodiac cycle), prophets and spiritual leaders such as Homer, Moses, Buddha, Confucius, Lao Tzu, Jesus, and Muhammad arose, warning people to abandon their childish ways and habits—especially improper diet and war—and prepare for the coming One World. These prophets and teachers were considered, by future generations, to be the originators of new religions, such as Judaism, Christianity, Confucianism, Taoism, Buddhism, and Islam. However, they were really teaching timeless, spirallic truths, encouraging people to return to the Order of the Universe. The peaceful world they envisioned was not some otherworldly heaven, but a return of Lost Paradise (for example, the anticipated Second Coming among early Christians) that would commence with a change in the Pole Star and the start of the illuminated half of the cycle of northern celestial energy. Although 2,000 years is a relatively short span in the historical spiral, people could no longer think dynamically in terms of yin and yang and see human evolution and history as a long wavelike motion extending from the infinite past into the infinite future. The teachings became mystified and turned into very limited predictions pertaining to a minor era or single nation rather than universal prophecies spanning an entire epoch and the world as a whole. Dogmas developed and a big church or mythology was built around each prophet or teacher. The teachings became mysterious and no one could understand them. Worship replaced understanding. Science replaced worship. Under whatever form of prevailing ideology, exclusivity, intolerance, and fanaticism spread.

SUMMARY

The light has continued to diminish for the last 2,000 years as humanity approaches the center of the Spiral of History. For us now living, the important thing is to pass through this time, experiencing all the opposing tendencies but not becoming engulfed by them. Who today can really be like Noah and his family and survive? The people who understand each individual tendency, as part of the whole, will endure. Those who can embrace all conflicting ideas and synthesize all antagonistic ideas as complementary factors in one harmonious whole will lead humanity through this crisis, the culmination of millions of years of biological evolution. Men and women, boys and girls, who have the unifying principle—*makro bios* (the original Greek term for macrobiotics), the longest and largest possible view of life—will pass through the center of the spiral safely. They will carry the baton or flame of health, happiness, and peace to untold future generations and enable the human race to continue. For 99 percent of the time, humanity has eaten primarily whole, unprocessed foods. People today who eat, think, and dream like their ancestors will pass through safely. They will create the foundation for a peaceful world civilization that will continue for the next 10,000 years, culminating in a new Golden Age leading to the stars.

PEACE PROMOTER

Alex Jack, Vietnam and China

During the 1960s, the world was moved to reflection by the self-immolation of Buddhist monks and nuns in Vietnam. The Buddhist peace movement, which sought a neutral Southeast Asia independent of both the communist and Western blocs, gathered widespread popular support and brought down several military governments in Saigon. In 1966, the South Vietnamese Army (with U.S. helicopter support) crushed the nonviolent demonstrations in Hue, the old imperial capital. Thich Tri Quang, the charismatic Zen priest who led the peace movement, took sanctuary in the An Quang Pagoda near Saigon.

Heavily armed police and military forces ringed the pagoda, but even they dared not enter and arrest Tri Quang because of his undisputed moral authority. In the spring of 1967, Alex Jack, then a young journalist in Vietnam reporting for a syndicate of American university, college, and small-town publications, arranged to interview Tri Quang. "He was slight and soft-spoken, but radiated a commanding spiritual presence," Alex recalls. "His eyes were positively aglow with compassion and understanding, and it was easy to see why he was considered the Gandhi of his country."

Alex asked him many questions about war and peace, and the Buddhist leader patiently explained the goals of the Third Force movement and delved into many areas of Far Eastern history and philosophy. Tri Quang said he was profoundly moved by the sorrow of Vietnam, but not in the least fearful about the effects of warfare on his country or even the threat of nuclear weapons.

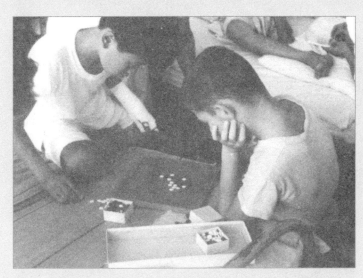

Figure 7.10.
Alex Jack, at age twelve, visiting Hiroshima Hospital in 1957 and playing with children still suffering from the effects of the atomic bombing.

"Vietnam has been fighting for two thousand years," Tri Quang observed. "The religious faith and common sense of the people will survive, whichever side prevails. But what disturbs me most is the quality of rice."

"Rice?" Alex asked. "What does rice have to do with war and peace in Southeast Asia?"

"Rice is foundation of civilization in the Far East," the Zen master explained. "It nourishes personal health and family life, culture and art, philosophy and religion. During the war, most of the rice fields here have been destroyed by bombs and chemicals. The rice in our country now comes primarily from Texas. It is a polished white rice—completely devoid of life and energy. If Vietnam adopts this way of eating, it will be the true end of our civilization and culture."

At the time, Alex did not fully understand Tri Quang's concern. The year before, while studying philosophy and religion in India, Alex had become a vegetarian. Hindu and Buddhist texts, as well as the Gandhians he talked to for a field-work project on attitudes toward war and peace, emphasized the importance of food for health and spiritual development, but this was the first time someone had presented to him a social analysis of the effect of food on society and human destiny.

The interview with Tri Quang was an important step in Alex's development. His interest in the Far East had originated in 1957 when, during the eve of his twelfth birthday, he accompanied his father to a peace conference in Japan. In Hiroshima and Nagasaki, he visited boys and girls his own age who had been injured in the atomic bombings and had spent most of their lives hospitalized and suffering from the effects of atomic radiation. Several years later, his father, Reverend Homer A. Jack, a Unitarian minister, became director of the National Committee for a Sane Nuclear Policy in New York City. In the early 1960s, Alex's whole family was active in peace activities, including public education on the effects of nuclear fallout on milk and other items in the food chain.

Back in Boston, where he entered theological school, Alex became active in the peace movement, speaking and writing about his experiences in Vietnam and Cambodia. In the fall of 1967, he and several associates organized a peace rally on the Boston Common and the Arlington Street Church. The rally drew thousands of people and resulted in the conspiracy trial of Rev. William Sloane Coffin, Dr. Benjamin Spock, and several others for encouraging draft resistance to the war in Vietnam.

In 1975, after taking macrobiotic courses in shiatsu massage and palm healing, he started working at the *East West Journal* and began attending my lectures and seminars regularly. At the *Journal,* he eventually became editor-in-chief. Later he began writing books with Aveline and myself and served as director of the Kushi Institute in Becket on several occasions.

Regular confrontations broke out between the peace groups and police, federal marshals, army recruiters, and religious and university authorities. Alex began to notice that it was very difficult for people who ate meat, sugar, and other articles in the modern diet to remain calm and nonviolent. "The peace movement was much more angry and violent than the early civil-rights movement. A few years earlier, I had been a civil-rights volunteer in Mississippi and Alabama, and there was a genuine feeling of community and devotion to nonviolence. Meals were a major social occasion, and everyone would eat together in a spirit of gratitude. The traditional Southern diet of cornbread, black-eyed peas, grits, collard greens, and other mostly grains and vegetables was much healthier than the diet we usually ate up North." In Boston, Alex began to shop at Erewhon and eat at the Seventh Inn and Sanae, two macrobiotic restaurants started by my students in the Back Bay. The food was very wholesome and he felt at home in these settings, though he said, "the macrobiotic persona at that time—short hair, three-piece suits, and a dogmatic mentality—didn't appeal."

At the Boston University School of Theology, Alex and his associates organized a sanctuary in the university's chapel for GIs who didn't want to fight in Vietnam. This action paralyzed the seminary and Alex was dismissed from the school. As the war continued, the peace movement turned into an antiwar movement, and Alex became more and more uncomfortable with its violent tendencies. He eventually quit organizing protests, served as editor of an underground newspaper, and moved into a commune in Cambridge, Massachusetts. In the early 1970s, he spent several years traveling and hitchhiking around the United States and Europe on a spiritual odyssey. "I found that gurus expanded the consciousness but didn't nourish it," he recollects. "During my quest, I kept cooking whole foods and found myself attracted to macrobiotic environments. Finally, I realized that enlightenment begins at home, and we are all responsible for our own health and happiness."

Returning to Boston, Alex started a small press and began to publish his own material, including a play about his experience in Southeast Asia. In 1975, after taking macrobiotic courses in shiatsu massage and palm healing, he started working at the *East West Journal* and began attending my lectures and seminars regularly. At the *Journal*, he advanced from typesetting to the editorial department and eventually became editor-in-chief.

During the late 1970s and early 1980s, Alex worked to develop macrobiotics in a more social direction, editing special issues of the *East West Journal* that focused on the impact of cancer and heart disease on society, the dilemma of nuclear war and energy, and the relation between the modern diet and world poverty and hunger. "This material was very valuable in helping people understand the underlying connections between diet, consciousness, and behavior," he says. "But it was generally negative rather than positive. We needed to move from analysis to synthesis, from pessimism to optimism, especially on the peace issue."

Following the tragic death of John Lennon in 1980, a reader suggested that the magazine sponsor an event in honor of the slain singer. John and Yoko Lennon had begun eating macrobiotically and met with my wife and me on several occasions. His music, especially songs like "Imagine," had a strong influence, helping people to envision a more peaceful future. At the *Journal*, Alex organized the John Lennon Memorial Peace Contest, which asked readers to write a short essay looking backward from some future time and describing how all the bombs were dismantled and how peace was realized on the earth. Scores of entries were received, from mothers, fathers, children, grandparents, teachers, writers, scientists, and many others. "It was a wonderful exercise and created so much positive energy," Alex recalls. "By projecting into the future, it became clear to everyone that criticism and protest would not be enough to change the world. We had to develop a healthy, peaceful community offering a bright, hopeful alternative. In addition to the nuclear freeze, a woman president, and other ideas that later became popular, our readers came up with dozens of other practical suggestions for what the ordinary person or family could do."

In 1980, Alex had an opportunity to realize one of his own dreams, bringing macrobiotics to China, where white rice, sugar, chemicalized food, and other articles of modern diet had almost entirely supplanted the traditional way of eating. His father, who was now Secretary-General of the World Conference on Religion and Peace and head of the association of Non-Governmental Organization Committee on Peace and Disarmament at the United Nations, invited Alex to accompany him on a visit to Peking. In the Chinese capital, Alex arranged to hold a macrobiotic banquet for religious and civic leaders at the Fayuan Temple, a Zen temple west of the Forbidden City, which dated to the seventh century. The sole surviving Buddhist vegetarian restaurant in Peking

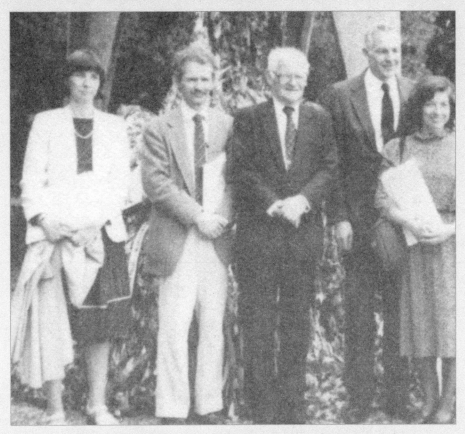

Alex Jack with his father and friends on a visit to Hiroshima Peace Park.

arranged to cater the affair, and Alex supervised the cooking of organic brown rice that he had brought with him from America. He also cooked miso soup made from the first batch of fermented soybean paste commercially made in the United States.

"I felt the winds of destiny blowing me to the eastern shore of the Silk Road, where rice cultivation and miso making began thousands of years ago," Alex wrote afterwards in *East West Journal*. "The appointed hour [for the banquet] duly arrived, and under a crystalline sky we set off for a short visit beforehand to the Temple of Heaven. Each year at this site the Emperor would spend a night fasting and meditating in the Hall of Prayer for Good Harvests. Opposite this famous structure, with its three conical roofs of glazed blue tiles, stands a smaller Temple of the Gods. A single canopy adorns this shrine and a circular wall encloses its courtyard. If you stand close to the inside of the round wall and say something, your words will travel around the circumference and come back from the other direction. It struck me as a sudden reminder of the long East-West journey which the ancestors of the rice grains in my knapsack had traveled over many centuries."

At the banquet, Alex gave a short talk on macrobiotic activity in the West and expressed the gratitude of macrobiotic families around the world for the rich heritage of Chinese philosophy and culture. Several of the Chinese guests said this was the first time they had ever eaten unpolished rice and found it surprisingly tasty. A government official confided that he did not even eat white rice but mostly meat and other animal foods, and had not previously considered the dialectical value of foods to personal and social health. The Roman Catholic bishop remembered that in Chinese, the Lord's Prayer is translated as, "Give us this day our daily rice." The head of the Taoist Association smiled broadly and presented Alex with a stone rubbing of the *Tao Te Ching* from a Sung Dynasty inscription. The leader of the Chinese Buddhist Association said that the banquet marked the rebirth of the Great Life movement in China.

Since then, several other macrobiotic friends have visited and taught in China, and several books that Alex co-authored with my wife and myself were translated into Chinese. On the way back from China, Alex visited settlements for refugees on the Thai-Cambodian border and talked to international relief officials about the importance of providing whole grains and other nourishing foods instead of polished grains, infant formula, and other unhealthy fare. Back in the United States Alex, Karin Stephan (a macrobiotic yoga teacher), and their associates started the Staff of Life, a small macrobiotic food-relief organization which raised thousands of dollars for whole foods projects in the Third World. "Through educational and service activities of this kind," Alex concludes, "we are best able to remain peaceful ourselves, further global harmony, and keep alive the dream of endless generations of our ancestors from all over the world."

Sources

Jack, Alex. "Beyond the Gun-sights: Traditional Medicine and Buddhism Resurface in Cambodia." *East West Journal* (Oct. 1980): 26–37.

Jack, Alex. "Bringing Brown Rice Back to Chinsi." *East West Journal* (Feb. 1981): 48–53.

Jack, Alex. "The John Lennon Memorial Peace Award." *East West Journal* (Dec. 1981): 40–43.

8.

The Origin and Causes
of War

*"There are a thousand hacking at the branches of evil
to one who is striking at the root."*

—HENRY DAVID THOREAU

As you have learned from previous chapters, there are periods of heightened
conflict as well as eras of harmony within the Spiral of History. In the *Iliad*,
this was depicted as the Cities of War and Peace on Achilles' Shield. In this chapter, we look at the nature of war and its root causes.

WAR AND HUMAN NATURE

Is fighting basic to human nature? Some psychologists believe that human beings
are innately aggressive and have a "killer instinct." According to this argument,
there will always be wars. Pacifists and members of certain religious groups, on
the other hand, say that human beings are innately peaceful and war is not
inevitable. In between these two theories is the view that individual human
beings are generally tranquil, harmonious, and gentle, but that in groups or larger
social units, human beings easily grow aggressive.

To understand the origin and basic causes of war, we need to look at human
history. Within the 26,000-year cycle of the precession of the equinoxes, there have
been eras of peace and harmony and eras of war and disorder. In the early
twenty-first century, we are now living following the end of a long era of global
violence and disorder, including World War I, World War II, the Korean War, the
Vietnam War, and the wars in the Persian Gulf and Afghanistan, in which tens of
millions of people were killed, injured, or uprooted from their homes. In conjunction with advances in technology, communications, and transportation, the rise
and spread of terrorism throughout the world has made violence appear more
ubiquitous; however, as a whole, the spread of democracy, human rights, and
trade actually has made daily life more peaceful.

During precessional summer, as we discussed in the last chapter, when the
earth was milder and more of the radiation of the Milky Way showered down
from overhead, humanity experienced an era of peace and prosperity. During

this Golden Age or Garden of Eden, natural agriculture prevailed, requiring little (if any) labor in the fields. New findings have begun to confirm that this was an era of material abundance, rather than competition and fighting over scarce food resources (as was earlier believed).

In the Middle East, using a small stone-age sickle, an anthropologist found that he could harvest about one kilogram of edible grain for each hour's labor in a stand of wild wheat. From this, he calculated that in prehistoric times, a family could easily have harvested enough grain to feed itself for an entire year with only three weeks' labor. Producing a comparable amount of cultivated grain today would take many times as much work because the soil today is depleted, the seeds are less viable, and the ancient strains were hardier.[1]

Archaeology is also beginning to find direct confirmation that this earlier era was peaceful. A study of megalithic culture, including cave drawings and stone tools, shows no evidence of weapons of war or organized social aggression by one group against another. War also seems to be unknown in the earliest civilizations. For example, the pre-dynastic Egyptians made maces, but there is no indication that they were used as weapons rather than as ceremonial implements.[2]

In northeastern Thailand, archaeologists have recently found evidence of a bronze-age culture much older than that of the Tigris and Euphrates valley in ancient Mesopotamia, which (until recently) has been believed to be the cradle of civilization. By 3600 B.C.E., the Ban Chiang people, as they are called, lived in permanent villages, grew rice, wove silk for clothing, and wore bronze jewelry. According to scientists, they learned and perfected bronze-making much earlier than metalworkers in the Middle East. However, unlike later cultures in Mesopotamia, they appear to have been entirely peaceful and did not use their advanced technology for destructive purposes. Analysis of more than one hundred skeletons found no deaths by violence, and no weapons of war have been unearthed.[3]

In the American Midwest, the 1970s excavations at Koster (seventy miles north of St. Louis) revealed the outlines of a prehistoric Native American culture that occupied the site peacefully for 9,500 years. The inhabitants of Koster lived on wild cereal-like seeds, water lotus, hickory nuts, deer, fish, and other wild plants and animals. They had tools for grain and vegetable processing, as well as baskets and leatherwork. By 5000 B.C.E., they were living in permanent wooden houses and establishing long-term villages. Until about C.E. 800, when they came into contact with highly complex Mississippian cultures, there is no sign of invasion or violent death. The Inuit, the Western Shoshone, and other traditional peoples in North America also evolved complex social organizations that endured for centuries without warfare.[4]

In addition to war, the infectious and degenerative diseases of early and modern civilizations were also virtually nonexistent among the first human societies. "The diet of our remote ancestors may be a reference standard for modern human nutrition and a model for defense against certain 'diseases of civiliza-tion,'" medical researchers concluded in a recent study on the paleolithic diet in the *New England Journal of Medicine*.[5] With the passing of Vega and the coming of the constellation Draco as the North Star, however, the galactic stream of energy overhead started to decline, natural catastrophes multiplied, and the sick-nesses and conflicts characteristic of recorded history set in. During this time, as the most recent ice age intensified, the atmosphere as a whole was much colder, heavier, and denser. As the lush vegetation of the preceding Golden Age receded, humanity's traditional diet of wild cereal grasses gave way to pro-portionately more animal food, more cooked food, and more salt, which con-tributed to increased vitality as well as aided in preserving other food. The principal way of life at this time was scavenging and hunting, and large game such as reindeer, bison, horses, sloths, and mastodons were consumed as a sup-plement to foraged plants.

During the era of advancing ice, humanity faced many difficulties as the envi-ronment became harsher and as consciousness naturally declined with the shift of the Milky Way's plane relative to earth. As the former ancient world com-munity broke up, memory of past principles of peace, harmony, and balanced cooking and food selection began to fade. The story in Genesis of how the serpent tempted Adam and Eve to eat previously forbidden food may refer to the arrival of a star in the constellation of the Dragon (Draco) as the new North Star. Primi-tive war, as reflected in the story of Cain and Abel, appears to have developed at this time.

THEORIES OF WAR

In addition to innate aggressiveness, various theories have been advanced about the historical causes of war. Many people, especially sociologists and political sci-entists, tend to divide the causes into various individual components. The first cause, they say, is imperialism. Secondly, there is economics, as in the case of over-whelming poverty or gross lack of raw materials, which motivates a war or inva-sion to redress the imbalance. Alternately, there is the case of secondary economic systems which need to expand and exploit in order to survive, as seen in mer-cantilism, modern capitalism, or communism. A third cause of war is overpopu-lation, which requires annexing additional land for expansion and development. A fourth cause is generally categorized as militarism. This category includes aggressiveness in a nation's mentality and its consequent acquisitions and bene-fits. This, of course, is closely connected to imperialism. The fifth category of social causes that analysts have isolated is religious dispute. People have fre-quently waged war as a matter of religious belief. These wars have occurred either to spread religious doctrine or to suppress other faiths.

These explanations are fine as far as they go, but we have to keep in mind that they are simply surface effects, manifestations of deeper underlying causes. The real causes of war are far more fundamental. Let's take imperialism as an example. Modern imperialism was common among Western countries from the seventeenth to the twentieth centuries and was characterized by a high degree of war, military occupation, and state brutality. The Chinese, on the other hand, had a more peaceful form of imperialism. They sought to maintain unity, stability, and security, relying more on trade and cultural relations. Under the Confucian governing system, the military occupied the lowest rank in the social order. Ethiopia also maintained this type of imperialist structure without the aggressiveness and wars that we commonly see with Western imperialism. In ancient Persia, Cyrus the Great commanded a great empire by governing through subordinate kings rather than military conquest. Respecting the traditions of subject peoples, he freed the Jews from captivity in Babylon and allowed them to return to Jerusalem and rebuild the Temple. Thus if we look at world history, we see that imperialism is not always directly associated with war.

The second category, economics, also appears to be a major cause of war. However, again, this is merely a surface problem. For example, a materially poor country like India—which certainly needs additional resources—is not necessarily drawn to war. This is the case for most poor nations in history, which also did not initiate wars for economic reasons. It is, in fact, the prosperous countries that have a tendency to resort to warfare. Studies have shown that international wars tend to be initiated by the rich nations in more economically optimistic months of more economically optimistic years.[6] These wars seldom end as quickly as anticipated, as in the case of the United States in Vietnam or the Soviet Union in Afghanistan. As a result, they often end up draining the more powerful country economically and spreading pessimism back home.

An examination of the other theories would also show that each is a superficial explanation for war. In *The Causes of War*, Australian economist Geoffrey Blainey concludes that all of the popular theories of war—including most of those mentioned above, as well as the balance-of-power theory (uneven power balance between countries promotes war) and theories that blame armaments manufacturers, dictators, monarchs, revolutionaries, or other individuals or pressure groups—"explain rivalry and tension between countries rather than war."[7]

THE BIOLOGICAL ORIGIN OF WAR

There is a more basic cause that underlies all these surface causes, one that has been almost entirely overlooked by historians, economists, psychologists, sociologists, generals, and pacifists. Human aggression and war have their origin largely in the biological, biochemical, and psychological condition of the people involved. In a symposium on the anthropology of armed conflict and aggression, Margaret Mead came close to identifying the main solution to the problem of war when she speculated that social measures necessary for the prevention of modern warfare might include "radical changes in diet."[8]

War is a disease, a social disorder, and cannot be understood apart from the physical, mental, and spiritual health of individuals and society as a whole. Like public health from which it is inseparable, peace is defined as a state of optimal social well-being and balance with the environment. Sickness—a disharmony arising between the individual and the environment—and war—a disharmony arising between societies and the environment—have been the legacy of humanity's failure to adapt to changing circumstances. Let us look at this process, starting with individuals (see Table 8.1).

TABLE 8.1 PROGRESSIVE DEVELOPMENT OF CONFLICT.			
	NORMAL CONDITION	**ABNORMAL CONDITION**	**CHRONIC CONDITION**	**DEGENERATIVE CONDITION**
Individual	Orderly	Colds	Cysts	Heart disease
	Healthy	Coughs	Swellings	Stroke
	Peaceful	Fever	Stones	Tumors
		Cloudy thinking	Hardening	Mental illness
		Slow reflexes	Depression	Infertility
		Emotional outbursts	Aggressive behavior	AIDS
Family	Close	Squabbles	Neglect	Violence
	Healthy	Arguments	Abuse	Divorce
	Loving	Disagreements	Separation	Breakup
Community	Healthy	Unrest	Decline of	Crime
	Prosperous	Delinquency	traditional values	Violence
	Tranquil	Absenteeism	Hedonism	Decadence
				Pornography
Environment	Clean	Littered	Abused	Eroded
	Beautiful	Neglected	Polluted	Desertified
	Flourishing	Misused	Vanishing	Extinct
Nation	Healthy	Political protest	Insurrection	Revolution
	Bountiful	Economic	Rebellion	Civil war
	Harmonious	stagnation	Depression	Economic collapse
World	Healthy	Raids	Famine	World war
	Peaceful	Feuds	Poverty	epidemics
	Unified	Sanctions	War	Global warming
		Embargoes	Crusade	and climate change

1. *Normal Condition.* In healthy individuals, dietary excess is discharged through normal bodily processes. The liver and kidneys, for example, filter toxins and excess acids from food and drink and discharge them through urination, respiration, and perspiration. The blood quality remains strong, natural immunity to

disease is maintained, thinking is clear and focused, and the individual is able to respond peacefully to changes in the environment.

2. *Abnormal Condition.* So long as the amount of excess is light to moderate, normal discharge mechanisms such as urination, bowel movement, breathing, and perspiration can handle toxins or excess waste that enter the circulatory system. But, if the quantity of excess is large and continuous, the body is not capable of discharging it smoothly, and various abnormal processes begin. Overeating, for example, often results in colds and fevers, coughs and chills, and other minor symptoms of imbalance. At this stage, thinking begins to cloud, reflexes slow down, and the emotions are less easy to control. These symptoms may occur at any time but often manifest themselves during a change in season, for example, at the beginning of spring or early autumn. At these times it is especially important to balance our food, change our clothing, and adjust our level of activity to accommodate the change in weather.

3. *Chronic Condition.* If the unbalanced way of eating and lifestyle continues unchanged, progressively more chronic symptoms develop, including high blood pressure, kidney or gallbladder stones, and swellings and cysts. The quality of the blood (including its relative alkalinity or acidity, balance of nutrients, and electromagnetic charge) begins to deteriorate, the lymph system weakens, and natural immunity to disease diminishes. At this stage, the individual is subject to the more serious infectious diseases transmitted by viruses or bacteria. Diseased or stressed organs and systems, including a poorly nourished brain and central nervous system, can also produce chronic mental and psychological disorders. Liver malfunction, for example, is associated with outbursts of anger. Kidney problems can give rise to fear and lack of will, while lung disorders are connected with depression and sadness. As a result of chronic dietary imbalance, ways of thinking and behavior become rigid and aggressive on the one hand (overly yang); unfocused and passive on the other hand (overly yin); or sometimes, both. Personal or social violence is often the result.

4. *Degenerative Condition.* After a period of chronic imbalance, the mind and body begin to experience degenerative changes, including hardening of the coronary or cerebral arteries, stiffening of the joints and bones, and the development of tumors and malignancies. These responses to dietary and environmental imbalances represent the body's final effort to isolate toxic excess and allow the body as a whole to function, even in a weakened state. Eventually, however, the heart attacks or strokes become more frequent, or the cancer metastasizes throughout the body, and the individual dies.

The process of social decline is similar to that of individual degeneration. In societies and civilizations, impaired public health and consciousness that arises from improper dietary and environmental practices results in a sequence of progressively more serious disorders.

1. *Normal Social Order.* Harmonious relations exist within society and among different societies. Health, peace, and prosperity prevail. Countries trade freely with one another and there is a high degree of cultural and social exchange. Disagreements are settled peacefully with a view to the welfare of the whole, not just one side or the other.

2. *Social Disorder.* Within a society, abnormal energy is discharged or expressed in family squabbles, juvenile delinquency, economic stagnation, and political unrest. Between societies, this can lead to the imposition of tariffs and trade wars, propaganda campaigns, economic sanctions and embargoes, military raids and reprisals, and other relatively moderate symptoms of social disharmony.

3. *Social Chaos.* If the underlying way of life, including basic ways of eating and orientation to the environment, remains unchanged, the fabric of society begins to tear. At the family level, parents, children, and other relatives abuse or batter each other, separate, or break off all communication. At the community level, traditional moral and religious values decline, crime rises, chaotic lifestyles flourish, and economic depressions become more frequent. Within society, this can lead to political insurrection, rebellion, or civil war. At the international level, nations seek territorial or ideological control, and a campaign of annihilation (such as a crusade or holy war) breaks out.

4. *Social Decline and Fall.* Eventually, the society or civilization collapses. This can happen from a depletion in the soil, a breakdown in the family, and the spread of epidemic diseases, or from military exhaustion and invasion by a superior force.

THE DIETARY CAUSES OF WAR

At the biological level, war may be viewed as (1) the periodic social discharge of toxins, stagnated energy, collective fear and anger, and other physical and psychological manifestations of longtime dietary, way of life, and environmental imbalances, or (2) an effort by society to recover balance through violent means. When a community, culture, or civilization has forgotten the secret of balancing itself internally through peaceful methods, such as through self-reflection on the part of its leaders or through sincere diplomatic efforts, external aggression is one avenue through which balance may be restored. But, unless the underlying way of life is changed, the harmony achieved by violent intervention is temporary and sooner or later leads to another, usually more deadly, outbreak of hostilities.

Closely connected with violence is fear. When an individual or community is unable to restore balance peacefully, fear arises. Fear takes two forms: (1) fear that our individual survival will not continue, and (2) fear that our species or offspring may become extinct. The second type of fear is the ultimate fear that everyone has. Compared with fear of hunger, poverty, oppression, and individual death, fear for the survival of one's children or human life as a whole can lead to desperation. If the big issue—humanity's destiny—is not touched, individual or group violence is usually regarded as crime. If the big issue is touched, however, everyone picks up a weapon, not to defend themselves, but to defend their posterity, the species as a whole. This is why women did not traditionally participate in battle. The next generation depended on their survival. Men rarely go to war to save their own lives. They go to war in the name of some religious, political, or cultural ideal. In many people, war brings out qualities of altruism, self-sacrifice, and courage. Ethically, it is very different from crime; however, the higher cause for which men stand ready to selflessly give their lives in war is usually very limited and not really essential to the species as a whole. This is especially true today. Everyone is opposed to modern war, in which no distinctions between men and women, parents and children, and military and civilians are made. But we accept it because of our deep inner fear for our children's and species' survival under another form of rule. Of course, nuclear weapons would destroy both sides in any conflict, so we cannot use them. We have no choice but to find a peaceful alternative.

In the past, eras of peace and harmony prevailed when societies and civilizations observed the natural order, including appropriate food selection and preparation. In most regions of the world, a balanced diet was traditionally centered on whole cereal grains as the staff of life, though the proportion and type of grain, as well as supplemental foods, differed with each climate and culture. Conversely, eras of fear, war, and disharmony prevailed when whole grains declined in central importance or when foodstuffs from radically different environments began to be eaten as daily fare.

Using yin and yang as a tool for review and evaluation, we may summarize the effects of different foods and combinations of foods on personal and social health in a temperate environment as follows:

1. The regular consumption of strong yang foods such as meat, eggs, poultry, chemically-refined salt, hard dairy food, and excess fish and seafood, as well as some extreme yin foods such as refined sugar and alcohol, creates more active energy that often finds an outlet in aggressive action or behavior.

2. The regular consumption of strong yin foods such as white flour, white rice, and other refined grains; too much fruit and fruit juice; tropical fruits and vegetables; sweets, spices, and soft drinks; and most drugs and medications creates more depressive energy that is perceived as weakness and attracts aggression.

3. The regular consumption of both strong yang and strong yin foods and beverages creates a cycle of imbalance that is alternately aggressive and defensive, violent and fearful.

The intensity and frequency of war varies primarily with the diets of the community, tribe, nation, or society involved. In primitive cultures and early civilization, where very little animal food was consumed and where most items in the
diet were local and seasonally grown, war resembled an adventure or a sport
more than a battle. European explorers and travelers marveled at the lack of both
defensive and offensive weapons among some native peoples in the New World.
In the early eighteenth century, a Spanish priest described the Arhuacos of Colombia. Members of this culture traditionally resolved their quarrels by going out to
the woods and beating their staves against a big tree or rock. The person whose
staff broke first was regarded as the winner, following which the two opponents
embraced and came home as friends.[9] In the Pacific Islands and Australia, we
find a similar pattern:

> Among the Melanesians there is a very mild form of war between related
> clans, seldom resulting in casualties, fought with clubs only, in the spirit
> of a game. With more habitual enemies there is a form of pitched battle
> which, while resulting in casualties, is surrounded by elaborate formalities
> and rules limiting its destructiveness and distinguishing it from the most
> serious type of war—ambushes or early-morning raids with the object of
> annihilating the village. Certain Australian tribes occasionally send out
> expeditions, ostensibly to procure medicinal plants and minerals such as
> red ocher hundreds of miles away. They usually have to fight their way
> through tribes on whose territory they trespass and return with thrilling
> tales of adventure rather than valuable commodities. These milder forms
> of war give an opportunity for working off aggressive impulses without
> danger to the social solidarity or economic welfare of either of the contend-
> ing parties.[10]

Primitive war, as this passage from *A Study of War* by Quincy Wright shows,
is very similar to modern sports. It is a socially sanctioned way to channel surplus
active energy. In this encyclopedic work, Professor Wright (who was a leading
authority in the field of international law and an adviser to the U.S. War Department and the Nuremberg trials) concluded that war—especially civilized war, in
which the taking of human life is a primary objective—is unnatural and that "the
trend of evolution has been toward symbiotic relations and perhaps toward vegetarian diet."[11] After researching the incidence of human aggression in nearly 600
primitive cultures, Professor Wright concluded that warfare is more prevalent
among societies in which animal food forms a major part of the diet than in societies in which a more vegetarian way of life is practiced (see Table 8.2 on page
115). This tendency toward war is called *warlikeness*.

Table 8.2 shows that pastoralists are the most aggressive group, with up to
three times the mean average warlikeness as a peaceful norm. Pastoralists observe

	POLITICAL WAR	DEFENSIVE WAR	SOCIAL WAR	ECONOMIC WAR	MEAN AVERAGE WARLIKENESS*
TABLE 8.2 CULTURE AND WARLIKENESS.					
Percentage of Primitive Peoples in Each Cultural Class Practicing Each Type of Warfare					
Lower Hunters	5	93	2	0	1.97
Higher Hunters	12	60	28	0	2.20
Dependent Hunters	7	66	27	0	2.20
All Hunters	8	75	17	0	2.09
Lower Agriculturists	15	61	23	1	2.10
Medium Agriculturists	1	61	32	6	2.43
Higher Agriculturists	1	35	42	22	2.85
All Agriculturists	4	52	33	11	2.51
Lower Pastoralists	0	35	65	0	2.65
Higher Pastoralists	0	11	68	21	3.10
All Pastoralists	0	24	67	9	2.85
All Peoples	5	59	29	7	2.38

* Where 1.00 is equivalent to peacefulness. • *Source:* Quincy Wright, *A Study of War,* 1965.

the most animal-based food pattern because of their arid, desert climate and environment and dependence on herds of cattle, sheep, goats, camels, and other animals. Agriculturalists are the next most conflict-prone, with about 2.5 times mean warlikeness. Agriculture introduced the concept of private property, leading to conflict over land use, water rights, and the rise of militias and armies. Hence, it led to a sharp rise in conflict. Hunters are the least combative, with only two times as much aggression. Hunters are primarily gatherers and eat large amounts of plant foods. They have no notion of individual ownership and often migrate from one area to another and are less inclined to defend specific territory. Overall, they are the most peaceful of the three groups.

Professor Wright further arranged the twenty-six historical civilizations from ancient to modern times according to degrees of warlikeness. This arrangement was based on twenty-five variables, including general social characteristics, frequency of battles, military techniques, and military characteristics. Once again, according to his listing, the vegetarian and semi-vegetarian civilizations generally fall into the peaceful category, while those in which substantial amounts of meat, poultry, fish, or other animal food was consumed tended to be warlike (see Table 8.3 on page 116).

TABLE 8.3 CIVILIZATION AND WARLIKENESS.					
WARLIKE		**MODERATELY WARLIKE**		**PEACEFUL**	
Babylonic	Andean	Hittite	Germanic	Orthodox	Chinese
Classic	Syriac	Arabic	Irish	Egyptian	Mayan
Tartar	Iranian	Scandinavian	Indic	Mesopotamian	Minoan
Japanese	Mexican	Western	Hindu	Sinic	
		Russian	Nestorian		
		Yucatec			

Source: Quincy Wright, A Study of War, 1965.

In modern times, the same general pattern holds true. We can divide the world population broadly between Western countries eating a diet high in animal food and Asian, African, and South American peoples eating predominantly vegetable-quality food. Since the end of the fifteenth century, we find that two-thirds of the wars fought took place in Europe. According to Professor Wright, 2,400 important battles were fought in Europe between 1480 and 1941, while only 359 were fought outside Europe. Thus what we find is Europe, representing a relatively small area and population of the earth, fighting throughout the rest of the world. Without understanding the biological and psychological nature of modern European people—particularly the Anglo-Saxon and Germanic peoples—we cannot understand the cause of war, especially in our modern age.

DIET, CLIMATE, AND WAR

From earliest times, human cultures and civilizations developed a way of eating that was centered around grains and vegetables, with a small supplemental amount of animal food. The two exceptions to this dietary pattern fall outside the temperate zones of the world. The first is in the colder and northern semi-polar regions, where the growing season is so short that over the millennia, a balanced diet evolved which was high in meat, fish, and seafood. The second exception is in the tropical and subtropical areas, where people adopted a more all-vegetarian diet higher in simply cooked foods, raw foods, fruits, and liquids. In colder and polar regions, about 25 to 30 percent of the traditional diet consisted of fish, seafood, walrus, caribou, and other sea and animal life. The cold and ice in northern areas naturally serves to preserve animal food from spoiling. However, in temperate climates, and to an even greater extent in tropical climates, animal food spoils rapidly and must be consumed rapidly or be smothered with salt, sugar, spices, or other ingredients with strong preservative qualities.

As long as ecological ways of eating were followed, societies and civilizations generally enjoyed good health and eras of peace. Over the millennia, however, as humanity journeyed through the dark half of the cycle of northern celestial energy, natural dietary boundaries between different regions of the world were repeatedly crossed, giving way to sickness, imbalanced judgment, and war. History records the accelerating violation of natural dietary order, as populations in temperate zones, tropical climates, and polar regions—as well as in islands, deserts, and other unique habitats—have increasingly consumed foods in improper proportions or foods that are more appropriate for an earlier epoch or another environment. In fact, we may say that the problems of disease and war are largely the result of adhering blindly to ways of thinking and eating that would be appropriate in another era (season, year, age, or epoch) or under other environmental conditions, but that are not in harmony with the present conditions and needs.

By eating foods suitable for another habitat, such as meat and sugar in a temperate climate, we begin to lose adaptability to our own environment. Outbreaks of infectious diseases have tended to follow waves of international food exchange between different climatic zones. The microorganisms associated with malaria, smallpox, bubonic plague, measles, and other scourges that have killed millions of people over the centuries almost all originated in tropical regions and diffused to temperate zones via overland caravan routes or international shipping lanes. The increasing amount of animal food consumed was also an important factor in the spread of epidemics. By today's standards, the amount of animal food consumed by traditional societies—about 10 to 15 percent by volume—was small. Without refrigeration, meat, poultry, milk, and other dairy food spoiled rapidly and, putrefying in the intestines, created a stagnant internal environment in which harmful bacteria and viruses could thrive. Until the introduction of refrigeration, both primitive and civilized people eating a small amount of animal food were subject to the frequent outbreak of infectious epidemics when they came in contact with foreign cultures.

Because strong yang attracts strong yin, it is not possible to consume regular amounts of meat and dairy food without seeking a rough balance with spices, sugar, or alcohol. In early historical times, a magnetic dietary attraction developed between the temperate northern half of the world and the tropical southern half of the world, expanding and accelerating contact with each other. Practically speaking, eating foods grown in the same general climatic zone, even those imported from hundreds and thousands of miles away, is not injurious to our health or consciousness so long as the environments are similar. Eating foods from a fundamentally different climate (even those imported from a few hundred miles away), however, may have serious consequences. Thus, historically, the East-West trade in which grains, beans, seeds, nuts, dried fruits, seaweeds, and salt were exchanged across long distances in temperate climates had a beneficial influence on human health and consciousness by providing variety in the diet and stimulating ecological diversity. Conversely, the North-South trade—in which animal food, hard liquor, and other foods more suitable for a cold climate crossed natural environmental boundaries with sugar, spices, tropical fruits and vegetables, and other foods more suitable for a hot climate—had adverse effects on personal health and social life.

As the historical spiral tightened, the frequency and magnitude of disease, war, and other personal and social disorders increased logarithmically. The dynamic interplay between temperate and tropical ways of eating—harmonious in their own climates but disharmonious in opposite climates—is one of the secret melodies underlying world history.

ENVIRONMENTAL CAUSES OF WAR

The day-to-day way of eating is the principal way in which individuals and societies establish harmony with their surrounding environment. Human destiny is also influenced by a variety of other environmental factors, including climate, relative direction, geography, season, and atmospheric conditions, as well as the social environment in which people live.

1. *Climate.* People living in warm (between 30 and 70 degrees Fahrenheit) and hot (above 70 degrees) regions such as savannas, steppes, the tundra, deserts, tropical rain forests, and hot seashores have the highest incidence of war, while people living in cold regions and cooler regions (average temperature below 30 degrees Fahrenheit), including cool mountainous areas, broadleaf and coniferous forests, and cold seashores, make less war.[12]

2. *Relative Direction.* In wars between North and South, the northern group usually defeats the southern group. For example, nomads from Mongolia and Manchuria have repeatedly threatened to overrun Chinese civilization for thousands of years. For protection, China erected the Great Wall running along the north for 1,500 miles, but periodically, the northern tribes would break through and seize large areas or even take control of the mainland of China. Meanwhile, in Europe, northern tribes such as the Goths and Vandals periodically migrated south and took control of large regions. As a whole, Europe has dominated Africa to the south. In North America, the North defeated the South during the Civil War, and the United States has traditionally dominated South America.

Meanwhile, in wars between East and West, the eastern group has usually prevailed. Both Napoleon and Hitler won steady victories to the west, but when they turned east and marched on Russia, they were defeated. By the same token, the Mongols' westward advance on Russia was successful, but their eastward invasion of Japan failed.

3. *Geography.* Island and coastal societies are more aggressive than continent-based and inland societies. In some cases, such as those of England or Japan, they are physically able to control or colonize large parts of adjacent continents. In other cases, such as those of Sri Lanka or Cuba, they are able to spread their ide-

ology (Theravada Buddhism and Castro's revolution, respectively) in the face of continental opposition.

4. *Season.* Most wars start in the spring or summer or have been fought most intensely during these times of year.[13] For example, the American Revolution, the Civil War, the Spanish-American War, and World War I began in April, the Mexican War began in May, the War of 1812 began in June, and the Vietnam War is usually thought to have started in August with the Tonkin Gulf incident.

5. *Atmosphere.* In traditional Oriental philosophy and science, there is a nine-year cycle of atmospheric change known as Nine Star Ki (see Table 8.4 below and Figure 8.1 on page 123). Many wars have started in a #5 year, in which the accumulated electromagnetic charge of energy in the atmosphere is greatest. These include the U.S. Civil War, World War I, World War II, and the Korean War.

TABLE 8.4 ATMOSPHERIC ENERGY CYCLE.								
#9	#8	#7	#6	#5	#4	#3	#2	#1
1910	1911	1912	1913	1914	1915	1916	1917	1918
1919	1920	1921	1922	1923	1924	1925	1926	1927
1928	1929	1930	1931	1932	1933	1934	1935	1936
1937	1938	1939	1940	1941	1942	1943	1944	1945
1946	1947	1948	1949	1950	1951	1952	1953	1954
1955	1956	1957	1958	1959	1960	1961	1962	1963
1964	1965	1966	1967	1968	1969	1970	1971	1972
1973	1974	1975	1976	1977	1978	1979	1980	1981
1982	1983	1984	1985	1986	1987	1988	1989	1990
1991	1992	1993	1994	1995	1996	1997	1998	1999
2000	2001	2002	2003	2004	2005	2006	2007	2008
2009	2010	2011	2012	2013	2014	2015	2016	2017
2018	2019	2020	2021	2022	2023	2024	2025	2026

Modern science has no unifying theory to explain these facts; however, yin and yang provide a useful compass. Unless we understand the interrelation of these dynamic opposites, we cannot really understand the origin and development of war and why different parts of the world give rise to different social and cultural expressions. For example, in the North (where people are more yang), thinking is more horizontal, material, pragmatic, and analytical. In the South (where people are more yin), it is more vertical, spiritual, idealistic, and intuitive. This has given rise to very different ways of life. Confucianism and Taoism, which originated in North Asia, are very practical compared to Hinduism and other southern religions that are more concerned with teachings about the afterlife. Just as the split in Buddhism into northern and southern schools reflected this natural orientation, in Europe, Roman Catholicism eventually divided in half. The theoretical, intellectual, rational north became Protestant, while the more aesthetic, ceremonial, ritualistic south remained Catholic. For the same reasons, in the twentieth century, communism split up between the more doctrinaire northern camp headed by Moscow and the more relaxed southern camp of Asian, African, and Latin American communist parties that looked to China.

Table 8.5 below summarizes some of the principal environmental factors according to yin and yang. From this chart, it is clear that war is usually more prevalent when strong yang environmental stimuli are present, and less likely when strong yin environmental stimuli are present.

TABLE 8.5 ENVIRONMENTAL FACTORS AND WAR.		
	YIN	**YANG**
Temperature	Cold, cool	Hot, warm
Climate	Humid, dark	Dry, sunny
Directions	North (in the northern hemisphere) West	South (in the southern hemisphere) East
Geography	Continent Interior Field	Island Seashore Mountain
Season	Fall, winter	Spring, summer
Atmosphere	Less active	More active

North vs. South and East vs. West

Because opposites attract, there is a natural tendency for people living in cold climates to move to warmer climates. Thus, the Russians have traditionally sought territorial expansion to the south in Crimea, Afghanistan, and warmer areas of Manchuria. In the same way, people living in high mountains have traditionally made balance with their difficult and dangerous environment by coming down to the valleys and plains, where life is easier. In ancient Egypt, for example, people came down from the high inland plateaus to the fertile Nile River Delta. In China, people came down from the Kunlun Mountains to the Yangtze River. In Europe, the Greeks living in rugged, hilly terrain came down to the low coastlines and fanned out to create colonies. Germanic tribes came down from the more rugged, wild areas toward the Mediterranean. Mountain people traditionally go down to the field and build; then society decays, and again mountain people come down and build. The process of civilization is just like water going downhill and evaporating all the time. This is the natural Order of the Universe.

In a contest between yin and yang people, the more yang side will dominate. Thus northern countries, eating a substantial amount of animal food, dominate southern countries, eating mostly vegetarian food. Eastern countries dominate western countries on account of the earth's direction of rotation. Island societies and coastal regions dominate continents and inland areas owing to a more yang diet, including fish, seaweed, and salty food.

There are exceptions to this rule. For example, the West was able to dominate the East in modern times because of the Industrial Revolution. This movement is against the natural order and cannot last very long. Already, after only three to four hundred years, a short time historically, Western influence and control are on the decline, and Eastern spirituality and culture are beginning to take root in the West.

But, the victory of yang over yin is always relatively short-lived. Externally, yang conquers yin, but yin eventually triumphs over yang from within. This is particularly apparent in North-South conquests where people from colder climates, eating meat and other stronger yang animal foods, invade warmer climates, where a more vegetarian way of eating is practiced. From the point of view of culture, the south is higher, so as soon as the north conquers, they quickly appreciate and adapt the higher southern culture. Culturally, spiritually, mentally, they become southern people. This happened to the Mongols in China, the Aryans in India, and the Germanic tribes in southern Europe. The same thing is now happening with East and West. Historically, the West was more yang, active, physical. With their armies and higher technology, they conquered the whole world. But mentally and spiritually, they were weak. The conquered people—the Indians, the Chinese, the Africans—were stronger mentally and spiritually. As a result, the West is surrendering to Eastern and Southern culture: Indian religions, Chinese cuisine, African music, and South American dance.

In the history books, statements such as, "This country or race won this war or this battle" often are recorded. This approach thinks only in terms of the physical victory. However, the war didn't end with the battle or the treaty. The yin war still continued. The yin war continues for a long period because the nature of yin is to prevail more quietly and have a long life. When Rome (to the north) conquered Israel (to the south), it was eventually conquered from within by Christianity, which came out of Israel. A gentle, peaceful religion (yin) triumphed over the greatest military empire (yang) in the world. In the beginning then, yang victory appears total, but it lasts for only a short time, while yin victory takes a long time to achieve and then is complete. Today when we talk of Rome, we don't think of Caesar. We think of the Vatican. The capital of the ancient Roman Empire is now the world capital of Christianity. This example teaches us that there is no victory in war, unless you win ideologically or spiritually. Every party that won physically and materially lost mentally and spiritually. This is the Order of the Universe.

Yin and yang also help us understand the relative speed of social change in different societies. In northern areas, where the natural environment is more actively changing, there is more stimulation for social change. Meanwhile in southern, warmer areas where the environment is less changeable, the pace of development is much slower. In Europe and China, for example, changes of dynasty or kingdoms usually took place every three or four hundred years, while in Egypt, Persia, and India, dynasties and kingdoms lasted much longer—seven or eight hundred years. Among dynasties, moreover, there are yin and yang distinctions. Yang dynasties, established by power, are very short, while yin ones, established by idea, continue longer. In the Hellenistic world, Alexander the Great's empire disappeared within a generation after his death. In Chinese history, the Mongols under Genghis Khan established a dynasty that lasted only three generations. Napoleon, Hitler, and other mighty military leaders all created empires that vanished quickly. In contrast, yin empires such as the Vedic, Incan, and Mayan endured for centuries. Still today, cultural values remain far stronger in southern regions than northern ones. Despite many reforms in India, the caste system there is still strong. In Arabia, despite the spread of modern technology and ideas, women still mostly wear veils and are expected to stay within the home. The South is very slow to change.

Humid vs. Dry

The relation between humid and dry cultures is a little more complicated. Usually, dry environments produce very simple societies. Like deserts, they are relatively inactive. In contrast, humid countries are more active. England is a very humid country—lots of mist and fog—and very active. Dry countries, as in the Sahara Desert or Persia or the Arabian regions, are frequently conquered and colonized by humid countries. However, the humid people cannot completely conquer the dry countries. The British and other Western people influenced the Arabic people—half-colonized them—but they couldn't colonize completely. The same thing happened with the Native Americans. While they were living in less dry areas such as the Northeast, the Plains, and the Pacific Northwest, they were conquered. But when indigenous people retreated to dry desert territory and high, dry mountains, they survived and couldn't be conquered. Food, of course, plays a complementary role with environment in these cases. In dry, arid regions, where agriculture is difficult, a more nomadic lifestyle is appropriate and more animal food is eaten. Thus, desert people are more yang (more physically strong). But because of the hot environment, the consumption of animal food easily produces aggressive behavior. This is why dry, hot areas such as the Middle East are the site of so many wars.

Active vs. Less Active Atmospheric Energy

Atmospheric conditions influence the development of society, including the likelihood of war. In the southern half of the world; in spring and summer, and during hot weather; and during years 3, 4, 8, and 9 of the atmospheric cycle (see Figure 8.1 and Table 8.4), air circulation is greater and the impulse to create, grow, develop, and expand is nourished primarily by centrifugal energy spiralling upwards from the rotation of the earth. The energy at these locations and times is experienced as going up and out, having an uplifting effect on individuals and society. This can make for great mental creativity and spiritual achievement. But if the way of life, including daily way of eating, is imbalanced, this upward energy can be very unsettling. Animal food in particular is more subject to discharge—to release excess, harmful, or extreme energy from the body in an abnormal way—at these times, making outbreaks of violence and war more likely. Hot and warm regions where this energy prevails are very hard to control. Thus in southern areas, such as Afghanistan or Central America, people are much freer and more independent by nature, and central authority is very hard to enforce.

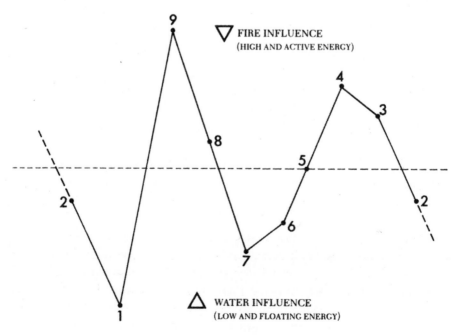

Figure 8.1. Nine-Year Atmospheric Cycle.

Conversely, in the northern half of the world; in the autumn and winter, and during colder weather; or during years 1, 2, 6, and 7 of the atmospheric cycle, air circulation is less active and the impulse to control, govern, and make order predominates, owing to the proportionate influence of centripetal energy spiralling downwards from the sun, the planets, the stars, and the infinite universe. This energy is experienced as going down and inward, exercising a more calming, stabilizing effect on the thinking and behavior of individuals and societies. At these times, war is less likely.

In #5 years (see Figure 8.1 on page 123 and Table 8.4 on page 119), the atmospheric energy moves to the center position in the cycle, where it is the strongest. Depending upon how the energy at this time is utilized, a strong tendency will emerge either to unify the whole environment or to destroy it. Furthermore, the atmosphere changes from yang to yin at this time, creating the highest degree of change and turbulence in the nine-year cycle. Like a "critical day" in biorhythms, crossing from one half of the atmospheric cycle to the other entails the greatest risk of accident, sickness, or other symptoms of imbalance. The risk of war breaking out is highest during these years, which include 2022. (See Appendix G.) The next-greatest danger of war is during #1 years, following the large swing of energy from yin (9) to yang (1). Also, #9 years are potentially explosive, because they represent the most expansive phase of the cycle. Number 9 years are governed by fire-like energy, which is very outgoing, impulsive, and passionate. Conflict at all levels is heightened at this time.

SOCIAL FACTORS

The question still remains as to why people think and behave differently when acting as individuals than when acting as members of a group. On a personal level, self-examination and daily observation show us that individuals on the whole tend to be peaceful and harmonious in their interactions. Occasionally, however, an agitated or upset condition occurs and extreme anger may impel the use of violence.

We can see this phenomenon on the battlefield. Almost without exception, when men are captured, they tend to have peaceful natures and are not necessarily interested in fighting. But when they act as part of a massive organization, like a nation or an army, they suddenly become killers.

In *War and Peace*, the epic novel about Russia during the Napoleonic War, Tolstoy describes how a totally different ethic, morality, and psychological and spiritual dimension takes over, transforming peaceful individuals into a violent mass. As a prisoner in his native Moscow, Pierre Bezukhov has made friends with a French corporal guarding him. One day, the French soldier enters the place where the Russians are confined and from outside Pierre hears the sharp rattle of drums. Recognizing his friend, he speaks up:

"Corporal, what is to become of the sick man? . . . " Pierre was beginning; but even as he spoke doubts arose in his mind whether this was the corporal he knew, or some stranger, so unlike himself did the corporal look at that moment. In the changed face of the corporal, in the sound of his voice, in the agitating, deafening din of the drums, Pierre recognized that mysterious, callous force which drove men against their will to murder their kind. . . . Pierre realized that this mysterious force had already complete possession of these men and that to say anything more now was useless.[14]

In such a situation, we can see the basic factors responsible for causing war. The first requirement is the leaders' verbal agitation of the people, whether they be monarchs or elected representatives. (In this case, both Napoleon and Tsar Alexander I exhorted their countrymen to war.) Secondly, war requires peoples' consent and approval of leaders' decisions, followed by their active participation. (The Russians and the French entered the War of 1812 enthusiastically, and both Napoleon and Alexander were idolized by their troops.) Third, weapons and other destructive instruments of war are needed. (Both sides were well equipped with infantry, cavalry, and cannon.) Fourth, a spirit of total agreement and an orientation under a single image, slogan, or ideology is required. (The French fought for Napoleon's dream of a unified Europe. The Russians fought to defend their homeland.)

In terms of yin and yang, leaders at this time are usually very yang, pulling the people toward war. They can't do this on a physical, material level only, so they need to create slogans appealing to patriotism, religious beliefs, or other ideological values to inspire their followers. In contrast, the followers are generally more yin types of people. They are led to war, spirited by the leaders in the form of propaganda. Of course, weapons and implements are needed on the physical level, but these are produced by industries and other economic units that are an integral part of the society.

To the factors influencing society that we have examined above, we can add the social factors outlined in Table 8.6.

TABLE 8.6 SOCIAL FACTORS AND WAR.		
	YIN	**YANG**
Group Dynamics	Followers	Leader
Social Unit	Individual	Group
Belief Structure	Views	Ideology

THE NAPOLEONIC WARS: A CASE HISTORY

Applying what we've learned about the underlying dietary and environmental causes of war, let us look more closely at an actual battlefield situation. According to the history books, either Napoleon's brilliant military genius or his obsession with power (depending on who is writing the account) is the main cause of the Napoleonic Wars. The basic reason for his defeat in Russia is said to be the cold weather. While these assertions are true, they are surface explanations rather than underlying causes. To understand this war, we must delve deeper into the biochemical and psychological nature of the people involved.

In examining their diets, we find that the Russians, a nation of strong, hardworking farmers and peasants, traditionally ate buckwheat as their staple grain, supplemented by rye, oats, and other hardy vegetable-quality foods. In contrast, the French soldiers and their allies were drawn more from urban environments and traditionally ate softer bread, more animal food, more sugar and spices, and more fruit and alcohol. In fact, modern food processing was inaugurated under Napoleon, who famously said that "an army marches on its stomach," and his troops were the first to receive tin cans of boiled beef, corned beef, mutton, and stew, as well as regular rations of refined white flour. In his *A History of the World*, Hugh Thomas stated:

> Napoleon's armies took white bread with them wherever they went in Europe as a banner of liberation from old dull bran or rye breads.[15]

In a contest between these two ways of eating, the Russians' diet was much more balanced and vital. It was also in harmony with their native environment, the cold northern plains and forests of Russia. This factor further accounted for the superior health and judgment of the Russians. In fact, on account of improper diet, the French troops were ravaged by typhus fever and lost a major portion of their army to disease. The approaching cold weather augmented Napoleon's deteriorating position, but was not the cause of his retreat. When they took Moscow, which was abandoned by the Russians without a fight in early September, the weather was unusually mild. Without an enemy, however, French discipline broke down, riotous living spread, and running short of supplies, Napoleon decided to reorganize his forces at a base camp several hundred miles away. On the way back, Russian guerrilla forces harassed the French columns, loaded down with their booty. When the cold finally intensified, the French lost all morale and the retreat turned into a rout. Only about 3,000 men of Napoleon's original 265,000-man army survived.

In *War and Peace*, Tolstoy observed, "Napoleon [is] like a child holding on to the straps inside a carriage and imagining that he is driving it." Searching for the underlying causes of historical events, Tolstoy depicts the carriage of human destiny as being driven by two complementary/opposite forces: freedom and necessity. "Everything changes and moves to and fro," Tolstoy writes, "and that movement is God." The novel's hero, Pierre Bezukhov, strives unremittingly toward "the infinite, the eternal, and the absolute." On their retreat from Moscow, the French troops take some of their Russian prisoners with them, including Pierre. Deprived of the rich food and other comforts to which he is accustomed, Pierre comes to a fresh, Zen-like awareness of reality. He realizes that peace and harmony are to be found in the ordinary, everyday things of life, including the traditional grain-and-vegetable diet of the Russian countryside.

> Here and now for the first time in his life Pierre fully appreciated the enjoyment of eating because he was hungry, of drinking because he was thirsty, of sleep because he was sleepy, of warmth because he was cold, of talking to a fellow creature because he felt like talking and wanted to hear a human voice. The satisfaction of one's needs—good food, cleanliness, freedom—now that he was deprived of these seemed to Pierre to constitute perfect happiness. . . .[16]

The spirit of the Russian people and army that Tolstoy extols in the novel rests on a firm biological foundation. As a whole, the Russians were physically, mentally, and spiritually stronger than the French.

Apart from the influence of diet and environment on the outcome of the war, we find that the Napoleonic Wars were begun for largely dietary/consumer reasons. For centuries, excessive meat-eating in Europe had created a strong counterbalancing desire for sweets, spices, and other tropical foods. The impetus to colonize the southern half of the world grew out of this biological desire. In 1806, Napoleon introduced the Continental System. Under this system, European countries were required to obtain sugar, coffee, and other imports exclusively from the French Empire and its overseas territories. To ensure compliance, Napoleon ordered a naval blockade of England, France's major imperial rival. Though the blockade was not successful, the French emperor threatened retaliation against any continental countries that resisted him. Napoleon's march on Russia six years later resulted when Tsar Alexander refused to abide by the Continental System and turned to England for coffee, sugar, and other imported foods.

Interestingly, 1806—the year the food boycott was started—was a #5 year in the atmospheric cycle. As we have seen, a #5 year is the most likely period for hostilities to break out in the nine-year atmospheric cycle. In addition to going against the Order of the Universe, by invading Russia to the north and east, Napoleon made the mistake of taking on England, an island society that was much more yang—physically strong and active—than the continent as a whole. Like Hitler a century later, Napoleon could conquer all the other countries of Europe except England and Russia.

Finally, Napoleon's own health and judgment must be considered. Endowed with a strong constitution, Napoleon had a native genius that could have been used for either the good or the detriment of humanity. For the first forty years of his life, his intuition remained strong and his iron will could not be deflected.

However, years of dietary neglect and a chaotic way of life took their toll. By himself, Napoleon customarily gulped down his food in six minutes, almost without chewing. In company, he stretched out meals to twelve minutes. In Russia, he took sick with cystitis and his judgment on the field began to falter. (Cystitis, a bladder disorder, is connected with loss of willpower and direction in traditional Oriental philosophy and medicine.) As one modern Western medical historian observed, "Napoleon died over five years after Waterloo and Waterloo was lost three years after the campaign of Moscow. But his own disastrous fall began and became inevitable when his own health and judgment started to fail."[17] Had Napoleon not abused his health, the map of Europe might be very different today.

SUMMARY

The causes of war are beyond the simple scope of imperialism or economics. Instead, if we strike at the root like Thoreau observed, it is generated, shaped, and influenced by biological factors, climate, environmental factors, by disease spread through ill-fitting foods, and other larger, deeper causes. These are a few of the ways we can look at history in a more comprehensive way. By studying the Order of the Universe, we realize that the whole world can never really be controlled by one individual, religion, nation, or way of life. Attempts to monopolize or dictate basic life processes—such as health, food, sex, clothing, and beliefs—cannot endure for very long because they go against the way of nature. To unify the world and end the threat of war, all different philosophies and social expressions must be embraced and respected. Like good health, from which it is inseparable, peace is the natural birthright of each and every human being and naturally follows from eating simply and living in harmony with the surrounding environment.

PEACE PROMOTER

Eric Zutrau and Tom Iglehart, Massachusetts

The public health movement in the United States began in Boston's Lemuel Shattuck Hospital in the early nineteenth century. The Shattuck had become a major state facility for the poor and homeless, the mentally ill, and the emotionally disturbed, as well as an inpatient clinic for state prisoners requiring medication. In 1980, Eric Zutrau and Tom Iglehart, two of my students in Boston, decided to initiate a macrobiotic food program in this historic hospital, whose usual food offerings (like most health care facilities in the country) were high in saturated fat, dietary cholesterol, animal protein, and sugar.

The administrators of the hospital, including director Paul Schulman, were open to new ideas of health. There was a lot of unfamiliarity with the new diet on the part of doctors, nurses, and other staff, however, and it was decided to introduce whole foods in the employees' cafeteria first, and then to the patients later. Eric and Tom were invited to become members of the hospital's dietary department and hired a full-time cooking crew of five for a two-month trial program. Operating from a little side kitchen, they set up a small macrobiotic lunch line side-by-side with the regular cafeteria line. "Many of the hospital employees were very conventional," Tom recalls. "They didn't even go to a Chinese restaurant. Fried rice was considered slightly communist." Eventually many of the physicians, nurses, orderlies, and housekeepers decided to taste the grains, vegetables, and other fresh foods in the macrobiotic line and liked what they tasted. Overall staff response was favorable and improved noticeably after the two serving lines were integrated, allowing items from both menus to be combined.

After the trial period, the program was extended, and by the second year, half of the food served each day in the cafeteria was prepared macrobiotically. Regular daily attendance in the cafeteria increased from about 60 at first to 200. At the noontime meal, from 70 to 90 percent of all meals served included, by customer request, at least one item from the alternative menu. "People who had never eaten in our line before would break down and say, 'Give me a little of the millet casserole.' Others told us, 'I've been eating your mixed vegetables for a year and a half and feel so much better,'" Tom notes. The kitchen crew included students from the Kushi Institute such as Paul Marks, a young man in his mid-twenties who had relieved childhood leukemia following the macrobiotic dietary approach. Several macrobiotic nurses, such as Virginia Brown, who reversed her own "terminal" case of malignant melanoma under my guidance, worked during this period in the psychiatric wards.

The success of the macrobiotic cafeteria line eventually opened the door for research with patients. Doctors at Tufts University School of Nutrition and Dr. Jonathan Lieff, Chief of Psychiatry and Geriatric Services at the Shattuck Hospital, became interested in macrobiotics' success in preventing heart disease and other sicknesses. They designed an experiment in the spring of 1982 to test the effect of the diet on long-term psychiatric and geriatric patients. Some of these people had been confined in the hospital for thirty years or more. In a double-blind study, in which neither the ordinary hospital staff nor the patients knew they were participating, macrobiotic foods disguised as "conventional" foods were introduced to a ward of nineteen patients over an eight-week period. Altogether, 187 food items were prepared on the macrobiotic menu, including mock chicken, coffee, and butter, which were hard to simulate. The research study was paid for by the Massachusetts Department of Public Health and serviced by the local macrobiotic community. In their report, the Tufts and Shattuck nutritionists noted medically significant reductions in psychosis and agitation among the psychiatric and geriatric patients over the two months they were on the diet. The patients took to the new food very well and only one person—a blind man—realized that the food had been changed from predominantly animal to vegetable quality. The project was also cost-effective, averaging sixty-one cents per meal, a 30 percent savings over usual food costs.

Although the Shattuck macrobiotic experiment ended after four years when funding ran out in 1984, it received enthusiastic support among administrators, staff, and patients at the hospital and served as a model for the development of alternative meals and effective nutritional therapies in other institutions. Eric, Tom, and their associates compiled a manual that hospitals and other service organizations could use to help make the transition to a more balanced diet, including menus, recipes, and advice on purchasing in bulk (including government surplus food). As a result of the Shattuck experiment and other macrobiotic community projects, Massachusetts Governor Michael Dukakis signed a state proclamation each autumn observing Holistic Health and Nutrition Awareness Month, encouraging residents of the commonwealth to increase their consumption of whole, unprocessed foods.

William P. Castelli, M.D., director of the Framingham Project (the nation's major cardiovascular research study), expressed hope that the Shattuck program could be extended to other institutions. In a letter, he wrote:

> I certainly applaud and support your effort to bring a well-balanced healthy alternative diet to the staff and patients of the Lemuel Shattuck Hospital.
>
> As you know our work in Framingham has revealed to us many of the details of the horrendous epidemic of coronary heart disease in this country, especially the fact that every fifth man and every seventeenth woman will have a heart attack before they reach age sixty.
>
> And yet, three-quarters of the people who live on the face of the earth will never have a heart attack; they live in Asia, Africa, and South America outside

of the big cities and they eat a diet like the one you are now offering your colleagues and the patients at the Lemuel Shattuck Hospital.

Dr. Robert Wissler, the professor and chairman of the Department of Pathology of the University of Chicago, fed the usual house diet of the Billings Hospital (the University of Chicago Medical School's major university hospital) to his baboons and they all lost their legs from atherosclerosis. How our patients are supposed to get well from this is beyond my imagination.

The major contributors to risk of coronary disease in Framingham are the blood fats and these are directly related to what you eat. A diet low in fat will greatly help in this regard and it is virtually unobtainable in most medical institutions in this country.

Many cancers are aided and abetted by high fat diets as well. Your efforts in this regard are much appreciated and hopefully some research will eventually come out of your program.

Vincent T. DeVita, Jr., M.D., director of the National Cancer Institute from 1980 to 1988, hailed the Shattuck dietary program as "consistent with the Interim Dietary Recommendations published by the National Academy of Science" and also expressed hope that other hospitals and public institutions would continue research in this direction.

Source

Kushi, Michio. *Diet and Crime.* Edited by Tom Iglehart and Eric Zutrau. New York: Japan Publications, 1987.

9.

Seeds of Civilization

The history of human culture and civilization is essential to understanding our origin and destiny as a species. Appreciating history's spiral rhythms and cycles allows us to transcend the linear model of growth and development that prevails today (e.g., the emphasis on gross national product, per capita consumption, and other metrics) and aids us in creating a healthy, peaceful, and sustainable future. In this chapter, we shall study how civilization has changed from the first farming societies to the emergence of globalization and trans-Atlantic trade (the mid-1500s), and how the gradual changes in human diet have affected the peacefulness of different cultures.

THE REBIRTH OF CIVILIZATION

The ancient scientific and spiritual world community declined with the emergence of Vega as the new Pole Star, ushering in an era of darkness and struggle. About 10,000 years ago, the glaciers began to recede in Europe, North America, and Northern Asia. In the era of transition before farming, as temperate forest replaced areas of frozen tundra, hunting continued; as the ice sheets melted, fishing became possible. The bow and arrow reached complete development, and the dog was domesticated to help in securing game. As the earth started to warm up again, settled human communities devoted to cereal grain cultivation began to reform (see Figure 9.1 on page 133). The domestication of plants made village and town life possible. Domestication of animals also began, and cattle, sheep, goats, and pigs were kept as a supplemental source of food in cold weather and for use during times of poor harvest.

In Anatolia and Mesopotamia, the warming trend transformed cool, dry steppe conditions to broadleaf forests, and a variety of flora—including concentrated stands of wild cereals and legumes—began to flourish. Cultivation of barley and wheat, along with lentils, peas, the broad bean, and vetches, lay the foundation for the rebirth of civilization between 8000 and 7000 B.C.E.[1] During the next 2,000 years, simple farming gave way to plow-based agriculture and large-scale irrigation, requiring centralized administration. By the late 4000 and 3000 B.C.E., urban city-states flourished, textile weaving and work with copper

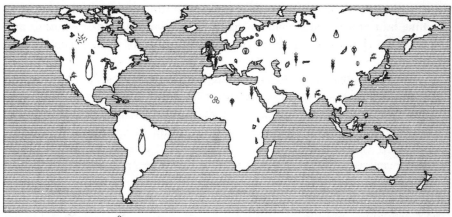

Figure 9.1. Whole Grains Around the World (Traditional Era to Present).

and other metals began, pottery developed along with the kiln for baking, and a counting method to record inventories of grain appears to have led to the invention of writing. The development of writing from a system of numerical notation to a way of expressing thoughts and ideas may be similar to the evolution of number processing into word processing in modern computing.

From the Middle East, farming spread north to Europe, and between 6000 B.C.E. and 4000 B.C.E. (when agriculture reached the British Isles), small farming communities that principally grew barley, wheat, and legumes spread rapidly across southern and central Europe. These agricultural communities were especially numerous in a corridor of loess stretching from modern-day Russia to France. Loess is a highly fertile dust laid down over the centuries by the wind around the perimeters of the former ice sheets. Hunting persisted in Alpine areas and in northerly climes, but generally gave way to the new agricultural way of life. Between the fifth and fourth millennia, megalithic culture—exemplified by Stonehenge—reached a zenith in the area to the west and north of the loess settlements. During the next millennia, fishing and seafaring trade—stimulated by milder environmental conditions and the domestication of grapes and olives along with barley and wheat—gave birth to the earliest European civilizations, the Minoan and the Mycenaean.

In the Far East, civilization reemerged in China in the fertile loess-lands of the north and northwest along terraces of the Yellow River that lent themselves to millet and rice production. The earliest-known millet culture dates to the early sixth or seventh millennium before our present era, while rice appeared about a thousand years later, especially in areas of central and south China. According to present data, millet, buckwheat, rice, soybeans, and other cultivated plants began to appear in Japan around 3000 B.C.E., though this date may be pushed further back as new archaeological evidence surfaces. In Southeast Asia, rice cultivation developed along with cultivation of taro, yams, the gourd, cucumbers, the water chestnut, and other garden vegetables. In India, wheat, barley, rice, peas, and lentils served as the staples of the Indus Valley civilization and its chief cities, Mohenjo-Daro and Harappa.

In Africa, periods of increased moisture (associated with glacial advances in Europe) ended about ten to fifteen thousand years ago, giving rise to wild strains of wheat and barley in the lower Nile. South of the Sahara Desert, which was habitable until the third millennium B.C.E., sorghum, millet, rice, pulses, yams, sesame seeds, watermelon, and other crops gradually came into cultivation over the next several thousand years. By C.E. 1000, most Africans were living in established farming societies, and centralized states conducted trade and diplomatic relations with Europe, the Middle East, and Southeast Asia.

In North America, milling stones about 12,000 years old suggest the significant dietary use of wild cereal grains and other plants following the retreat of the glaciers. Maize cultivation began in about 7000 B.C.E. in the region between Mexico and Guatemala. Over the next several thousand years, corn spread throughout Mesoamerica and formed the foundation for the Olmec, Zapotec, Maya, and Aztec civilizations. By about C.E. 800 to 900, most native peoples in North America—with the exception of desert, mountain, and sub-arctic regions, as well as the Pacific Northwest, where fishing and whaling prevailed—lived in settled, relatively peaceful agricultural communities, growing maize, beans, squash, and a wide variety of other vegetables and fruits.

In South America, where the climate was milder, early cultures supplemented wild plants with seaweed and seafood. Land animals were rarely consumed, as evidenced by the lack of hunting weapons found in the remains of prehistoric villages on the Peruvian coast. Two wild cereal grains, canihua and quinoa, were domesticated in the Andean highlands, possibly as early as the seventh millennium before our era. Maize reached Peru from Mesoamerica several thousand years later and, supplemented with beans, squash, tubers, and other domesticated vegetables, formed the foundation for a series of civilizations, culminating in the Inca Empire.

Memory of the previous ancient spiritual and scientific world community, or what we can call One World Civilization, was still strong in all of these early historical societies and continued to be passed down from generation to generation in myth, legend, and song as well as in architecture, technology, spiritual practices, and traditional arts and crafts.

THE INDO-EUROPEAN ADVANCE

On the Eurasian continent, the relatively peaceful development of early agricultural civilization was shattered by migratory waves of nomadic tribes from the northern and eastern steppes and semi-desert regions. These incursions began between the third and early second millennia B.C.E., several thousand years after civilization had begun in the Middle East and India and after farming communities had been established in Europe. The origins of the Indo-Europeans remain obscure. Historians usually locate them in the arid regions of the Russian Caucasus and Central Asia. Since the environment in these areas was not conducive to farming, the Indo-Europeans followed a pastoral way of life, migrating south and west in search of new grazing areas for their varied flocks of horses, asses, camels, and cattle. On the fringes of agricultural regions, this often led to violent conflict. The concept of private property also arose with pastoral surplus, and cattle served as the earliest form of monetary value. The word for war in ancient India, for example, is translated as "desire for cows."[2]

The domestication of the horse and the development of wheeled vehicles (eventually leading to the war chariot) gave the Indo-Europeans military superiority over farming regions and a means to enforce claims to their far-flung pastures. Although numerically smaller than the settled agricultural societies they overran, the impact of the Indo-Europeans on world history was immense. On the Indian subcontinent, they gave rise to Vedic civilization. In the Middle East, they gave birth to Iranian and Hittite civilization. In Europe, Indo-European migrations fanned out, creating Celtic, Germanic, Greek, Latin, Slavic, and Baltic culture. Though not Indo-European, Semitic culture in the Middle East, including that of the Arameans, Phoenicians, and Hebrews, also shared a semi-nomadic heritage, diet, and world view.

On the Indian subcontinent, the Indo-European diet—high in hardy cereal grains such as buckwheat; salt and other seasoning; animal foods such as beef, mutton, and dairy products; and other foods and cooking styles appropriate to a harsh, arid climate—rapidly returned to a regimen in harmony with a hot, moist environment. Wheat, rice, and more moderate grains formed the center of the diet, proportionately less salt and seasoning were used in cooking, more raw foods and liquids were consumed, and almost no animal foods were eaten. The new Sanskrit civilization gradually abandoned its nomadic origins and way of life, assimilating the gentler, more peaceful values of the former Indus Valley and Dravidian cultures that it displaced.

In the Middle East and Europe, however, the nomadic Indo-European diet established a lasting foothold, owing to less extreme geographical settings and to assimilation by both sides. The pastoralists by and large settled down in towns and cities, adopted some farming practices and substituted taxation for plunder. The farmers and urban city dwellers, meanwhile, increased their domestication of livestock, incorporated more baked flour products and animal food into their diets, and made use of the pastoralists' more advanced military techniques to expand their own influence and territorial control.

Although the waves of migrations and invasions ended in the first millennium B.C.E., world history is generally the story of the westward advance of Indo-European culture and values—including a diet high in processed grain and flour prod-

ucts, meat, and dairy food; a basic distrust of nature; a reliance on material technology; and a warlike ethic—across Europe, to the Americas, and to other parts
of the globe. In counterpoint to this dominant historical trend, traditional agricultural practices and values—including a diet centered around whole grains and
vegetables, faith in nature, trust in a nonmaterial reality, common ownership, and
a generally peaceful orientation—have survived and provided a spiritual counterbalance to the materialist orientation.

A distinctive feature of the Indian, European, and Middle Eastern way of eating
was the staple use of grain to make bread and other hard, baked flour products
from barley and wheat. Bread may have originated with nomadic cultures that
required an easily transportable staple food. Baking was also a very energizing
cooking method and one appreciated by ancient warriors. Meanwhile, in China,
Japan, and other areas of the Far East, millet, rice, and other grains were consumed
principally in whole form and cooked gently in pots with thick lids or stone
weights on top. In the East, whole grains were supplemented with softly-prepared
flour products in the form of boiled noodles and steamed dumplings. Physiologically, grains consumed in whole form contribute to an intuitive, integrative way
of thinking, while bread, cracked wheat, and other processed flour products contribute to a rational, analytic orientation. Similarly, Far Eastern styles of food
preparation, such as cooking under pressure, boiling, steaming, and stir-frying,
create more centered, peaceful energy than baking, frying, broiling, and other
heavier, more energetic cooking methods favored in the West. Along with differences in climate and environment, these different ways of preparing grain and of
cooking were primary causes for the different ways of life and thinking that developed in East and West in antiquity and that have continued to the present day.

THE AGE OF EMPIRES

The farming and nomadic ways of life have been the principal actors on the stage
of world history. From the stories of Cain and Abel and of Jacob and Esau to the
creation of Israel and Judah and the settling of the American West, the conflict
between cultivators and goat, sheep, or cattle herders has been a dominant theme
in mythology and literature. As responses to unique geographical and climatic
challenges, they originated out of natural, commonsense adaptations to the environment. Difficulties arose when celestial cycles, geological conditions, and the
climate and weather continued to change, but homo sapiens did not change.
Ways of acting and thinking remained fixed—often for centuries, and in some
cases for thousands of years up to the present.

Hunting as a way of life was a harmonious response to the coming of the ice
ages. Similarly, becoming pastoralists and adopting a diet moderately high in baked
flour products and meat and dairy food was a sensible solution to living in the
cold, arid steppes and semi-desert regions of Central Eurasia, where farming was
impractical. However, when the ice began to recede and the environment changed,

big-game hunting was no longer appropriate. When the search for new grazing lands brought nomadic tribes into warmer climates, livestock could no longer comfortably serve as a major portion of the diet. Just as the earliest human communities during the ice ages looked in vain to the vanished Golden Age for guidance on how to adjust to the new environment, so the earliest agricultural communities may have retained hunting and nomadic values harking back to the glacial era.

From the third millennium B.C.E., Eurasian farming and urban societies turned increasingly to tropical and subtropical foodstuffs to supplement their diet. This was in an effort to balance the consumption of meat, dairy food, and other animal products that continued long after the cooling trend had ended and that intensified with the Indo-European migrations and invasions. When nomadic cultures came in contact with agricultural civilization, bloodshed and war were often the result. Meanwhile, farming communities, overrun by nomads, turned increasingly to livestock production and included more animal food in their diet than was natural at the time in order to develop their own aggressiveness and repel the invaders.

As a supplement to grains and vegetables, animal-quality food helped to give early human civilizations the immediate burst of energy and strength that made it possible to expand territorially and develop material life and technology to new heights. In the long run, however, it lowered natural immunity to disease and reduced consciousness, vitality, and judgment, creating the foundation for disease, infections, pestilence, war, and social disorder. To balance meat, eggs, salty cheese, and other extremely yang or contracting fare, a strong desire for herbs, spices, tea, tropical fruits and vegetables, and other strong yin or expansive foods and beverages developed. By the second millennium before our era, Phoenician ships, as well as overland trade caravans to the East, began to transport foodstuffs between temperate and tropical zones. Protecting ships, trade routes, and eventually foreign colonies was a major impetus for the development of new weapons and the art of war.

During this age, the great empires of Mesopotamia, Egypt, the Aegean, and the Mediterranean—characterized by monumental architecture, the change from bronze to iron technology, and strong central authority—reached a zenith. Increased commerce and trade brought an influx of new foods from Asia Minor, Northern Africa, Gaul, and other distant lands. Eventually, the health and vitality of the city and rural populations started to decline as cultivated whole cereal grains—the foundations of these cultures—assumed a less central role in the daily diet and more flour products, animal food, and luxury imports were consumed. As traditional food patterns changed, frequent wars and civil strife developed, and the empires collapsed from internal or external pressures.

Weapons of war, such as agricultural implements, remained relatively primitive at first. Combat often resembled agricultural campaigns. Groups of farmers working together on collective irrigation projects donned battle dress and, along with domesticated animals and farm wagons, became the embryonic fighting force from which a professional military caste of infantry, cavalry, and chariots eventually developed. The development and use of iron in the second millennium B.C.E. made weapons more affordable, and spears, shields, and helmets spread rapidly to the lower classes.

Pestilence, or disease—the perennial companion to war—is often the forerunner of social decline. The infectious diseases that have plagued civilization were virtually unknown among preliterate traditional cultures, and are all believed to have originally been transmitted to humans from animal herds, especially domesticated livestock. For example, smallpox derives from cowpox; measles from canine distemper or rinderpest; and influenza from a viral infection common to pigs. Humans and cattle alone share fifty illnesses. Infectious diseases spread by rats, fleas, mosquitoes, and other rodents and insects are caused primarily by imbalanced ecological conditions, especially unnatural agricultural practices such as monocropping, deforestation, and other human intrusions into the environment that allow one species to proliferate at the expense of others. Overcrowding in cities and poor sanitary conditions further created a medium in which harmful bacilli and viruses could proliferate and be readily transmitted.

In Greece, plague broke out in Athens during its cultural zenith in 429 B.C.E., contributing to its demoralization and defeat by Sparta. According to Thucydides (an Athenian historian), the infection began in the tropics, spreading from Ethiopia to Egypt, Libya, and Persia before reaching Greece. The Peloponnesian War between Athens and Sparta was fought largely over control of dependencies and trade routes leading to the East and the subtropical rim of North Africa. Plato's *Republic*, describing a perfect society ruled by philosopher-kings, was a reaction to the decline of Mediterranean vitality. It was the chief embodiment of a series of ideal images inspired by the vanished Golden Age and developed by early Greek and later Roman writers and artists.

By the first century, the Silk Road—the overland caravan route between China and the Near East—had been established, and shipping routes between the Red Sea, the Bay of Bengal, and the South China Sea linked the Mediterranean with India and Southeast Asia. In the fifth century, Rome—the last of the early civilizations and weakened by a series of malarial plagues following the increased import of food from outlying provinces and distant lands—fell to local invasions. As a medical historian notes: "The story of the last centuries of Roman power is a long tale of plague. . . . The ultimate effects of this invasion [of malaria] were probably more catastrophic than the attacks of Goths and Vandals."[3] About C.E. 400, the ancient world came to an end with the collapse of the Roman Empire.

THE RISE OF CHRISTIANITY

Offering a simple grain-based diet, palm healing, and other spiritual practices that protected against pestilence and offered hope for a more peaceful society, the teachings of Jesus spread through the Hellenistic world. With the decay of Roman civilization, the network of granaries that supplied the Mediterranean region with wheat and barley disintegrated, the sanitation system broke down, and Christianity emerged as the main spiritual and temporal power. During the medieval era, grain consumption plummeted throughout Europe; preserved meat became the staple in many regions. Due to a lack of fodder, Europeans customarily slaughtered their pigs and cattle in the autumn, and the shedding of blood—human as well as animal—became a more routine part of life. Central administration broke down, the cities decayed, consciousness dimmed, and the early part of this epoch is remembered as the Dark Ages.

Still, the amount of animal food consumed was modest by present-day standards. The word *meat*, for example, originally meant "meal," staple food, grains and vegetables. At the end of the medieval age, almost a thousand years later, the word *meat* still referred to vegetable-quality food, as this passage from Genesis 1:29 in the King James Version of the Bible makes clear:

> Behold, I have given you every herb bearing seed, which is upon the face of all the earth, and every tree, in the which is the fruit of a tree yielding seed; to you it shall be for meat.

Only in modern times did the word *meat* come to mean exclusively animal food.

In medieval Europe, there were four times a year when little or no animal food was consumed for up to six weeks at a time (such as during Lent). During non-fasting periods, moreover, people (except for the nobility) consumed meat only a few times a month and in much smaller quantities than commonly consumed today. In general, nearly all food consumed during the early part of this period was locally grown and consumed in season or preserved naturally over the winter. The indigenous pattern of eating contributed to the rise of racial movements and kingdoms that characterized this era. The way of eating promoted by the Church during this age contributed to the moderation of violence. Laws of war were observed, protecting women, children, and clergy. Religious communities and houses of worship were respected as sanctuaries, and the doctrine of the just war was formulated, defining conditions under which a prince or ruler could morally resort to arms. The most ambitious attempt to curb violence was the Peace of God, instituted in France during the eleventh century. Under the Peace of God, fighting was banned between Wednesday evening and Monday morning—the days toward the end of the week, around Sabbath, during which limits on animal food were often observed. While the Peace of God was not always enforced, it served to moderate bloodshed and evolved into the King's Peace and the development of the modern state. The King's Peace referred to a central authority that could outlaw private warfare, feuds, and vendettas, and guarantee peace and safe conduct over a large territory.

THE DEVELOPMENT OF EASTERN CIVILIZATION

Like early Christianity, Buddhism held up vegetarian or semi-vegetarian ideals, which, if not always adopted by urban populaces, at least tempered their dietary excesses and exercised a calming and humanizing effect on daily life. Taken over from Jainism, another peaceful religion, the doctrine of *ahimsa*—nonviolence— became enshrined in the reigns of two Buddhist kings in India, Asoka (third century B.C.E.) and Harsha (sixth century C.E.). After leading their armies to great victories on the battlefield, both monarchs changed their way of eating, initiated dietary reforms in society, and renounced war.

Following a brief Golden Age under Harsha, India degenerated into a land of petty kingdoms and became engulfed in a wave of otherworldly religion. India's political decline and the rapid spread of the devotional cults in the medieval era, from about the ninth to the fourteenth century, followed the introduction of sugarcane into India from Southeast Asia.

Physiologically, sugar robs the body of needed nutrients, weakens the digestive tract, and unleashes erratic emotions by expanding the nervous system. At the individual level, regular consumption of sugar can give rise to unfocused thinking, hyperactivity, irregular heartbeat, nervous tension, and a wide variety of other physical, emotional, and mental disorders. Because of refined sugar's high potency, the human digestive system automatically strives to balance it with strong, contracting foods such as meat or temporarily soothing substances such as milk and other dairy products. At a social level, these symptoms are often manifested as wild, chaotic behavior, including ideological, political, and religious fanaticism.

In medieval India, where meat had long been taboo for health and religious reasons, Hindus appear to have turned to dairy food in the medieval period to counteract the injurious consequences of their rising sugar intake. Milk, ghee (clarified butter), and yogurt do calm down the nervous system, but at another high price: Dairy food leads to the buildup of fat and mucus within the body, contributing to overall physical stagnation and emotional dependency, especially in a warm or tropical climate. For the next thousand years, as a probable result of this change in way of eating, a weak and divided India remained under foreign domination and turned increasingly toward religious teachings that denied the importance of food, the body, physical health, and the material world.

In China, classical civilizations went through a similar advance and decline. During the first historical dynasty, that of the Shang (about 1900 to 1300 B.C.E.), Chinese culture reached a zenith. Though codified at a later date, the I Ching, the *Yellow Emperor's Classic of Internal Medicine*, and other classics are thought to date to this era. Millet and, to a lesser extent, rice constituted principal fare. During harvest festivals and other special occasions, these foods were prepared in ceremonial bronze vessels that have never been equaled in beauty and craftsmanship.

Though far below the cultural and artistic par of the Shang Dynasty, the succeeding Chou Dynasty (about 1300 to 221 B.C.E.) was notable for its social and economic consolidation. The amount of animal food in the diet, including fish and wild game, sharply increased during this era following the transition to an Iron Age technology, contributing to feats of great physical strength and endurance (such as the building of the Great Wall). Unified at great cost of human life and labor, the latter part of this age was remembered as the era of the Warring States. Toward the end of the Chou Dynasty, as decay and disorder multiplied, Confucius, Lao Tzu, Mencius, and other philosophers appeared, reawakening interest in the unifying principle of yin and yang and encouraging society to return to a simple grain-and-vegetable diet as a practical step toward peace and harmony.

The Han Dynasty (206 B.C.E. to C.E. 220), the first of the great international Chinese empires, saw the expansion of trade and commerce. Goods flowed freely to the Roman Empire, India, and Southeast Asia. In return for silk and spices, China received gold and silver and a variety of new foods, including tea, grapes, alfalfa, walnuts, sesame seeds, onions, caraway seeds, pomegranate, coriander, and cucumber. As territorial boundaries were pushed out, brown rice, the staple of southern China, was also enjoyed more in the north, where it was roasted and then steamed. The technique of making tofu and noodles was perfected. The introduction of these new vegetable-quality foods sparked an artistic and cultural reawakening that lasted for several centuries. From the north, however, China's traditional adversaries, the nomadic Hsiung-nu (also known as the Mongolians), threatened. The Mongolians' superior military technology included sturdier, faster, more maneuverable horses; sabers for use in close combat; stirrups; and the lance. The Great Wall could no longer restrain them. To combat the pastoral confederacy, the Chinese increased their consumption of meat, especially of pork and other domestic livestock. Though the frontiers were successfully defended, Han society began to decline from within following this change in the way of eating, and another period of conflict and disorder ensued.

The next major era, the T'ang Dynasty (C.E. 618 to 907), is remembered as a Golden Age. An innovative and efficient system of transportation and communication, including canals, waterways, and roads, unified a strong central empire, and China's boundaries were extended to areas of Manchuria, Tibet, Southeast Asia, and Korea. Buddhism, especially Zen, flourished during this period, and as the consumption of animal food ebbed, the Middle Kingdom enjoyed an unparalleled era of peace and stability. Arts and letters reached a new pinnacle; Christians, Jews, and Muslims were welcomed; and the bold, vivid lines and images of T'ang calligraphy, landscape painting, poetry, sculpture, and pottery set a new standard of excellence.

The scientific imagination also soared under T'ang rule. From antiquity until the start of the Industrial Revolution, nearly all of humanity's scientific and technical discoveries and inventions originated in China and slowly made their way west on the Silk Road across Central Asia to the Middle East and Europe. These included the wheelbarrow; the sailing-carriage; the wagon-mill; harnesses for draught animals; the crossbow; the kite; the technique of deep-drilling; the mastery of cast iron; the suspension bridge; canal lock-gates; the square-pallet chain pump; the edge-runner mill; metallurgical blowing-engines; the rotary fan and winnowing machine; the piston-bellows; the horizontal warp-loom and the draw-loom; numerous navigational inventions, including the fore-and-aft rig and the stern-post rudder; the magnetic compass; and porcelain. According to Joseph Needham in his monumental study, *Science and Civilization in China,* until the Renaissance and the advent of modern times, only four major mechanical techniques moved in the other direction (from West to East): the screw, the force pump for liquids, the crankshaft, and clockwork.[4]

Compared with India—whose lush tropical climate and vegetarian diet gave rise to a complex, expanded philosophy—the cool, rugged environment in China and the diet higher in grains and animal food led to development of a more practical culture. The seeds of China's brilliant output, which culminated in the development of paper, printing, and moveable type in the T'ang era, are the seeds of Far Eastern civilization itself: rice and millet. These two whole grains are the most biologically-developed plants in the vegetable kingdom. Unlike other cereal plants such as wheat, barley, corn, and oats, rice and millet are not divided in the middle with a seam. The celestial and terrestrial energy that they absorb and transmit is thus more whole and balanced, contributing to deeper intuition and more unity between the analytic left side of the brain and the more integrative, or synthetic, right side of the brain. Human beings and societies who regularly eat brown rice and/or millet develop very practical natures, devising many creative solutions to daily life.

From India and Southeast Asia, increased trade and communication brought sugarcane, spices, and other foods of tropical origin to China. By the seventh century, Yangzhou, a city of commerce and pleasure on the Yangtze River, became the center of indigenous Chinese sugar manufacture. From Mongolia and the West came dairy products, especially goat's milk and fermented mare's milk, and the polishing of rice and wheat, which also became widespread in Chinese urban communities during the later T'ang era. Boiling and steaming gave way to frying as the favorite method of cooking, and a gourmet philosophy developed that regarded practically anything, except a domestic animal that had died facing north, as edible.

The liberal expansiveness of the T'ang extended into the Sung Dynasty (C.E. 960–1279). The delicate yin nature of the Sung period manifested itself not only in the highly stylized and exquisite lines of its vases and other celebrated art objects, but also in the rising popularity of confections, pastries, and candied fruits. In one area of the Szechwan province, 40 percent of the peasants were employed in sugar production. Fruit was widely eaten at intervals during meals, as was cheese. As

Marco Polo recorded, this was a period in which food consumption revolved around restaurants and banquets. Yet amid this cosmopolitan milieu came voices of warning. Yang Fang, a Taoist commentator, complained that

> the sons and grandsons of officials had lost the way and will be unwilling to eat vegetables and will look on greens and broth as coarse fare, finding beans, wheat, and millet meager and tasteless, and insisting on the best polished rice, and the finest roasts to satisfy their greedy appetites, with the products of the water and the land and the confections of human artifice set out before them neatly in ornamentally carved dishes and trays.[5]

By the end of the thirteenth century, Chinese society had weakened from within and—following a series of plagues—became easy prey for external aggression. Invading Mongolian armies from the north seized large agricultural areas of millet and wheat, followed by administrative control of the country itself. As a footnote to the decline of this era, it is recorded that the "bad last prime minister" of the southern Sung was discovered to have hoarded several hundred jars of sugar and 800 jars of pepper. As in India, native independence ended and, except for a brief revival under the Ming Dynasty, China has been dominated by foreign rulers or ideologies ever since, including Marxist-Leninism.

THE RISE OF ISLAM

In the Middle East, Islam—which means "surrender" to God or the Order of the Universe—developed in the seventh century and expanded rapidly in Arabia, Persia, and North Africa following a series of epidemics that weakened the Mediterranean coastal regions. In Europe, Islam spread to Sicily, Cyprus, Malta, and Spain and threatened to overrun the entire continent until military defeats stopped its advance in northern Spain and in Constantinople.

As a reform movement among nomadic desert tribesmen, Islam was not as vegetarian or as pacifist in orientation as Christianity and Buddhism. However, its prophet, Muhammad, led a very simple life and served as a peacemaker among warring tribes. The Quran embodied a deep understanding of natural order and included many sections on the central importance of whole grains, even for nomadic communities. Yet the original teachings of Islam, like those of Christianity, quickly became institutionalized, and a religious hierarchy grew up, propagating the Prophet's message by Jihad, or Holy War.

The explosive growth of Islam—from a small tribal religion to a universal faith—within a century has remained a puzzle to historians. From our understanding of natural order and the spiral of history, we should look for a major change in food or environmental patterns preceding a shift in society. The answer to Islam's phenomenal growth may be found in the introduction of sugar refining to Arabia from India and Persia at about this time. "Sugar-making, which in Egypt may have preceded the Arab conquest, spread in the Mediterranean basin after that conquest," we read in one account. "Sugar followed the Quran."[6]

In the Middle East, where animal food formed a large part of the diet, sugar had different physiological effects on the nomadic Arab population than it had on the largely vegetarian population in India. In meat-eaters, sugar or other extremely yin substances (such as alcohol or drugs) can release the hardened yang energy accumulated from excessive consumption of meat, eggs, poultry, and dairy food (as well as the relentless dry heat of the desert sun), giving vent to periodic discharges of violence. Among desert nomads, who were eating large amounts of mutton, lamb, camel, poultry, and wild game, sugar had just such an explosive impact—unleashing wild and erratic emotions that were channeled into social and ideological ends. Advances in sugar processing also made available more highly refined sugar in the Middle East than in India. In Arabia, a crystallized solid form of white sugar was produced, while in India, raw sugarcane or a darker taffy-like sugar was prepared.

THE CRUSADES AND THE MONGOL ADVANCE

In England, France, Germany, the low countries, and elsewhere, excessive animal food—especially that which was preserved for a long time with salt—provided the impetus for the Crusades and centuries of warfare between Christians and Moslems. Europe's desire for sweet, bitter, and spicy items to balance its high consumption of salted meat and sour dairy food during the early medieval period resulted in the next great wave of international food exchange. The Silk Road and other old trade routes to the East, blocked by the Arabs, reopened in the eleventh century, and spices, sugar, and tropical fruits and vegetables flooded into the West through Genoa, Venice, and other Mediterranean ports. In conquered areas of Jerusalem, Acre, and Jericho, the Crusaders took over supervision of sugar production and later seized Arab sugar refineries in Sicily, Cypress, and Malta.

Meanwhile, in the East, traditional ways of eating fundamentally changed as the Mongols—a nomadic society eating a diet high in animal food—conquered China, Russia, and Central Asia in the thirteenth century and advanced as far west as Poland and Hungary before being stopped by the plague, internal rivalries, and the comforts of civilization. As with the Indo-European invaders of an earlier era, the Mongols brought new dietary patterns into southern and western agricultural regions, including the use of more dairy food and meat.

The dietary results of the Crusades and Mongol invasions were immense. Refined sugar, imported from tropical and subtropical climates, flooded into Europe; it was expensive and had such a devastating initial impact on temperate-climate nervous systems that it was locked away in apothecary shops for centuries and used only medicinally to counterbalance certain tight (yang) disorders. The introduction of sugar, spices, and other tropical food to medieval Europe, coupled with rising animal food production, weakened natural immunity and resistance to infection, leaving its population susceptible to plague and sudden death. In the period of the Black Death—the mid-fourteenth century—about one-third of Europe's people perished. The Black Death began in Caffia, a Crimean town on the Black Sea, at the intersection of the Mongol advance and the caravan route between East and West. In 1346, plague broke out among a Mongol army besieging the city. A company of Italian merchants in Caffia brought the plague to Genoa, from where it spread quickly through Italy, Central Europe, Scandinavia, and England. Though transmitted by flea-infested rats and poor sanitary conditions, the plague bacillus itself was the agent, rather than the underlying cause, of the scourge.

On the historical spiral, it is interesting that sugar and gunpowder—two chemically refined products—appeared at about the same time. The first primitive guns appeared in Europe in the early fourteenth century. The relation between gunpowder and a fuse is similar to that between meat and sugar. The harder substance (yang) needs only a soft spark (yin) to set it off. The explosive combination of extreme foodstuffs contributed to the Inquisition, anti-Semitism, and witch-hunting that swept Europe at this time. During the late Middle Ages, dualistic thinking reached a peak, as spiritual and temporal authorities enforced an uncompromising separation between God and the world; human beings and nature; body and spirit; and good and evil.

In the Orient, this way of thinking, culminating in religious intolerance, was unknown so long as grains and vegetables formed the staple of the diet. In China, the land of its origin, gunpowder continued to be used primarily for peaceful purposes. Westerners failed to understand why the Chinese did not take military advantage of this new technology. Matteo Ricci, the seventeenth-century Jesuit missionary, wrote that "in the month-long New Year celebrations [the Chinese] used up more saltpeter and gunpowder than we would need for a war lasting two or three years.'"[7]

In Europe, the invention of the cannon ushered in a new era of warfare. Castles and fortifications that had endured many years of siege could be demolished in a few hours or days. Arms races also intensified, as the competition to develop bigger and better gunpowder weapons replaced the duel between more efficient lances and shields and crossbows and breastplate armor.

DISCOVERY OF THE NEW WORLD

The global spiral of ever-widening dietary imbalance expanded in the fifteenth century, when Europe's craving for spices resulted in the discovery of the New World. For centuries, Europe had paid Asians in gold for their wares. With the failure of the Crusades, however, Arab middlemen along the overland trade routes commanded an increasing share of the profits. The trans-Saharan trade—in which Europe exchanged firearms, salt, and luxury goods with Africa for gold, leatherwork, and slaves—helped pay for some of the costs. But the prospects of opening a direct sea route to Asia appealed to the most imaginative rulers and adventurers.

Columbus's vision of Lost Paradise and dream of finding a shorter sea route to the fabled East was essentially realized on the continent he confused with the Indies and China. Armed forces—forts, garrisons, and warships—followed trade, and the early history of the Americas is a chronicle of the subjection of native peoples to provide sugar, alcohol, spices, and tropical fruits and vegetables to balance Europe's steadily rising consumption of meat, poultry, dairy food, and salt.

As a social institution, slavery played an important role in sugar production in the Near East and southern Europe. Sugarcane, a labor-intensive crop, requires up to twenty or more wettings from planting to cutting, as well as large amounts of mechanical or human labor to grind the cane, extract the juice, and process the syrup. After the Black Death, when agricultural labor was scarce, the use of slave labor expanded. To run their sugar plantations, the Muslims, Crusaders, Spanish, and Portuguese turned to the more gentle and peaceful cultures of the south for slaves. In the New World, sugar production reached new heights because of almost unlimited territory and ideal growing conditions, and the modern slave trade began. Columbus brought sugarcane to the Americas on his second voyage, and the first sugar mill was built in Santo Domingo in 1508. (See Figure 9.2 below for a map of sugar's expansion.)

In Mexico, sugarcane was the chief crop. The Spanish began bringing slaves from Africa to harvest the cane in 1520. In Brazil, the Portuguese began shipping sugar to Lisbon in 1526.

In addition to slavery, sugar and other new foods had other important demographic effects. Prior to contact with the Old World, the New World appears to have been free of contagious disease. However, following contact, including the introduction of sugar, alcohol, and other new foods, the common European and African childhood diseases took a heavy toll. Along with slavery, they reduced indigenous American populations by 95 percent within a century and a half. As one historian notes, "Clearly, if smallpox had not come when it did, the Spanish

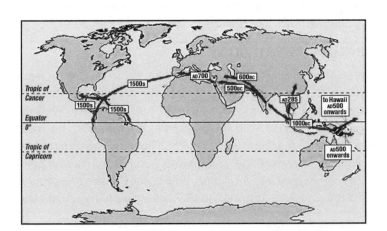

Figure 9.2.
The Spread of Sugar.

victory could not have been achieved in Mexico. The same was true of Pizarro's filibuster into Peru. For the smallpox epidemic in Mexico did not confine its ravages to Aztec territory. Instead, it spread to Guatemala, where it appeared in 1520, and continued southward, penetrating the Inca domain in 1525 or 1526."[8] A major factor in the spread of epidemic in the New World was the small, supplemental amounts of animal food consumed by native peoples. Though marginal to their overall diet, animal food, as we have seen, spoils rapidly and provides a breeding ground for infectious disease agents. The Indians' inability to hold alcohol—a traditional European balance for heavy animal food consumption—stemmed from their much smaller consumption of meat, eggs, fish, and other animal food.

In the sixteenth century, the modern era of territorial expansion and power began. Successive empires of the Portuguese, Spanish, Dutch, Germans, and English vied for control of the Sugar and Spice Islands (the Caribbean and the Maluku Islands, respectively), and spread the colonial pattern in the New World to other continents. Innumerable wars were fought to control the supply of cloves from the Maluku Islands, nutmeg from the Celebes, cinnamon from Ceylon, pepper from the Malabar Coast, and ginger from China. Each conquest resulted in new tropical products reaching temperate zones. In addition to spices, chocolate, coffee, tea, tomatoes and potatoes, citrus fruits, and other new foods and stimulants were transported back to Europe and North America. Once again, a new round of deadly diseases developed as principles of environmental harmony were ignored. Syphilis appeared for the first time and rapidly spread across the world.

At the ideological level, the wars of this period were fought between competing Protestant and Catholic doctrines, and intense missionary activity preceded the colonization of foreign countries. However, during the Renaissance, Christianity as a whole lost its grip on Western consciousness as new ideas of humanism, freedom of conscience and inquiry, and the scientific spirit took hold. Though usually a spur to religious consciousness, the increasing outbreak of disease, plague, and war further served to undermine the Church's influence by appearing to afflict the just as well as the unjust. The medieval era ended in the early 1600s with the international collapse of local and regional agricultural economies and ways of eating that had existed for thousands of years.

SUMMARY

As the eighteenth century French philosopher Jean Anthelme Brillat-Savarin observed in *The Physiology of Taste*, "The destiny of a nation depends on the manner it feeds itself." More and more national cuisines are disappearing as the world becomes more globalized. Indeed, the nation-state itself is vanishing as multinational corporations, including big pharma, agribusiness, biotech cartels, and other giant enterprises that monopolize seeds, farming, food processing, and medicine increasingly control what we eat, how we heal, and how we resort to violence to solve our problems. In the next chapter, we shall explore how this modernizing trend developed.

PEACE PROMOTER

Frank Kern, Virginia

In 1979, Frank Kern, assistant director at Tidewater Detention Center in Chesapeake, a state facility for juvenile offenders, decided to initiate some dietary reforms in prisons. After studying at the Kushi Institute and attending my lectures, he arranged an experiment in which sugar was taken out of the meals and snacks of twenty-four male teenage inmates. They had been jailed for offenses from disorderly conduct, larceny, and burglary to alcohol and narcotic violations. Coke machines were removed from the premises and fruit juice replaced soft drinks, while honey and other milder sweeteners replaced refined sugar.

The three-month trial was designed as a double-blind case-control study so that neither the detention center personnel nor the inmates knew that they were being tested.

At the end of the trial period, the regular staff records on inmates' behavior were checked against a control group of thirty-four youngsters who had been institutionalized previously. According to Stephen Schoenthaler, Ph.D., the youngsters on the modified diet exhibited a 45 percent lower incidence of formal disciplinary actions and antisocial behavior than the control group. Follow-up studies over the next year showed that after limiting sugar, there was "an 82 percent reduction in assaults, 77 percent reduction in thefts, 65 percent reduction in horseplay, and 55 percent reduction in refusal to obey orders."

"In the United States today," Frank Kern said, "it costs from $17,000 to $50,000 a year to take care of each inmate. . . . The medical model of criminal behavior and rehabilitation is not working. It still revolves around the concept of socioeconomics, family birth ranking, fixations, toilet training, and the entire spectrum of intrapsychic factors that exist for all of us.

"Entirely overlooked are the effects of the foods we eat. In addition to excessive amounts of meat and disastrous amounts of sugar, there are over four thousand chemicals in food that have never been tested on the central nervous system. People commit crimes when they feel bad. I've never met anyone yet who committed a crime when they felt well. Some of the worst diets exist in prisons. . . . Many inmates consume three to four hundred pounds of sugar annually. Simply changing menus has had dramatic effects. . . . We need to rethink our approach and introduce macrobiotics into prisons. Food is part of the rehabilitation. It truly works."

The response to the Tidewater experiment was immediate and positive. Following national publicity, Kern received some fifty letters a week—mostly from prison officials in other states—inquiring about his project. Further studies were conducted in corrections institutions, and equally dramatic findings resulted. Juvenile detention centers nationwide began to change their meal plans.

In 1985, Virginia state officials gave the go-ahead for a much larger macrobiotic food and educational program at the Powhatan State Penitentiary. Under the leadership of Roy Steevensz, former director of the East West Center in Hollywood, a small number of inmates started attending classes. Assistant Warden Tom Parlett was impressed: "We've tried many other types of rehabilitation and it hasn't worked. So why not try this? The ten or twelve inmates I've worked with are really excited. Their whole attitudes have changed." Parlett himself was convinced to change his diet. Macrobiotics, he said, "makes a lot of sense."

In July 1986, 400 people attended a macrobiotic banquet at the prison. Organizers hoped the Powhatan project would be a prototype for the Virginia Department of Corrections to investigate establishing new statewide nutritional and educational policies toward cost saving, short- and long-term health benefits, and the potential rehabilitative effects. State authorities also have found that the macrobiotic menus are consistent with every religious dietary canon observed by the inmate spectrum. Around the country, prisoners have filed litigation seeking special diets, costing state governments hundreds of thousands of dollars in court costs.

In the future, the Powhatan program will include alternative macrobiotic food service, education, and training for inmates, food-service staff, and key administrators. Miso soup, sea vegetables, and gomashio sea salt are already available in the prison canteen. Several tofu and miso companies expressed interest in establishing an agricultural-based prison industry, which will provide job training and skills that can later be used outside of prison to create healthy food. The U.S. Department of Agriculture, the American Farm Federation, and the Center for Innovations in Corrections endorsed this proposal.

In the years since, there have been many advances in diet and nutrition in the prison system. In California, for example, a private contractor won rights in 1997 to build a private prison and offered a vegan diet. At the time, California had a recidivism, or re-arrest, rate of 95 percent. The new facility (in Victory Valley) experienced a recidivism rate of less than 2 percent. According to prison officials, the vegan group's prison yard was no longer controlled by the most aggressive prisoners. Nor did inmates divide into typical groups separated by race or gang affiliation.

Sources

"The Diet-Behavior Connection." *Science News* 124, no. 8 (1983): 125.

Frazee-Walker, Diane. "Vegan Diet Impacts Recidivism." *Prison Law Blog*, May 20, 2013. http://www.prisonlawblog.com/blog/vegan-diet-impacts-recidivism

"Freedom Food." *The Richmond News Leader* (Richmond, VA), July 26, 1986.

Schoenthaler, Stephen J. "The Effect of Sugar on the Treatment and Control of Antisocial Behavior." *International Journal of Biosocial Research* 3, no. 1 (1982): 1–9.

"Special Issue on Diet Behind Bars." *East West Journal* (June 1982).

10.

The Modern Age

In the previous chapter, we covered human diet and thinking from the first civilizations to the emergence of globalization. But when did the modern ways of thinking and eating truly begin? We can say that this modern age began with the European Renaissance, which took place from the mid-fourteenth century to the mid-sixteenth century. The Renaissance spurned great thinkers such as Leonardo da Vinci and was the starting point for revolutions in painting, sculpture, astronomy, and classical learning. The universal unrest culminated in World Wars I and II, from which we have yet to fully recover. In this chapter, we will examine the roots of modern society and how we can shape our future in a positive light.

THE DEVELOPMENT OF THE RENAISSANCE

The Renaissance marks the beginning of the modern way of thinking and eating. *Renaissance* means "rebirth." The word was first used by Vasari in *The Lives of the Painters* to describe the brilliant rejuvenation of art and learning that flourished in Florence in the fourteenth and fifteenth centuries. Not since the Golden Age of Athens in the fifth century B.C.E. has the culture of a single city made such an imprint upon the Western imagination.

The spirit of the Renaissance was very close to that of China. In outlook, both cultures acknowledged the primacy of heaven and earth, yet were essentially humanistic. Both laid stress on everyday life and practical wisdom and relied for nourishment on the classics. This characterized these cultures' ethics, compared to medieval Europe's focus on abstract intellectual concepts and otherworldly religious doctrines. In science, both cultures emphasized direct observation and technical inventiveness. In art, both cultures excelled at landscapes and portraits detailing the flora and fauna of the natural world and strived to achieve precision of detail and immediacy of impact. In literature, earthly paradises such as More's *Utopia,* Bacon's *New Atlantis,* and Campanella's *City of the Sun* displaced the quest for the Holy Grail and Heavenly Jerusalem.

In the late Middle Ages, the transmission of technology from the East declined as the Mongols overran China, and the illustrious Sung Dynasty came to an end. But in Italy, the continuity of scientific progress was unbroken as several generations of brilliant thinkers, of whom Leonardo da Vinci was foremost, set in motion the gears and wheels of the modern world. In addition to drawings for manned flight, submarines, the tank, shrapnel, and other modern weaponry, Leonardo sketched twenty of the twenty-two principal components of modern machinery, including the lever, cam, pulley, and flywheel.

Leonardo's innovations in painting rivaled his contributions to mechanics and, like the latter, displayed peculiarly Oriental influences. As one modern art critic observed:

> [Although Leonardo] most certainly never saw a Sung or Ming painting, his somewhat Chinese feeling for distant mountains, for landscape as both a fact and a symbol, and for the wideness of the world led him in the *Mona Lisa* to reject converging lines and adopt a strikingly Chinese combination of aerial perspective with shifting viewpoints and parallel bands of scenery. His *sfumato* [shading] is comparable to the tonal technique of Chinese ink painting, his wall-stain notion is remindful of Zen blots, and his idea of the microcosm and the macrocosm, although thoroughly Western, is in exact agreement with part of the old Chinese outlook.[1]

By the fifteenth century, following the eastward march of the Crusades and the westward advance of the Mongols, the Italian city-states controlled the western termini of the trade routes to the East. Venetian and Genovese ships ruled the Mediterranean and carried the fabulous cargoes of silks, spices, cotton, and sugar to their final destinations in England, Flanders, and the German states. At the center of this commercial network lay Florence, the banking capital of Renaissance Europe. Florence's first family, the Medici, spun such an intricate web of connections (for example, financing both sides in the Hundred Years' War) that they seemed to complement the nearly invisible silkworms spinning their cocoons at the other end of the Silk Road.

Columbus's discovery of the Americas, Vasco da Gama's journey around Africa, and the explorations of Amerigo Vespucci at the turn of the sixteenth century marked the end of the old overland caravans and the Italian mercantile system. The economy of the Renaissance, built upon the wealth of Asia, collapsed, and the commercial center of power gravitated to Spain, Portugal, France, and England. Silk for men and women's apparel henceforth arrived from China in frigates sailing around Africa.

The Chinese fabrics and fragrances form the petals of the Renaissance flower, but for its roots we must look, as in an actual plant, to the soil. The seeds of that brilliance are the seeds of Far Eastern civilization itself: millet and rice. By Leonardo's time, the two grains that had nourished Chinese culture for millennia entered southern Europe and were cultivated along the entire rim of the Mediterranean coast (see Figure 10.1 on page 152). During Leonardo's time, Florence

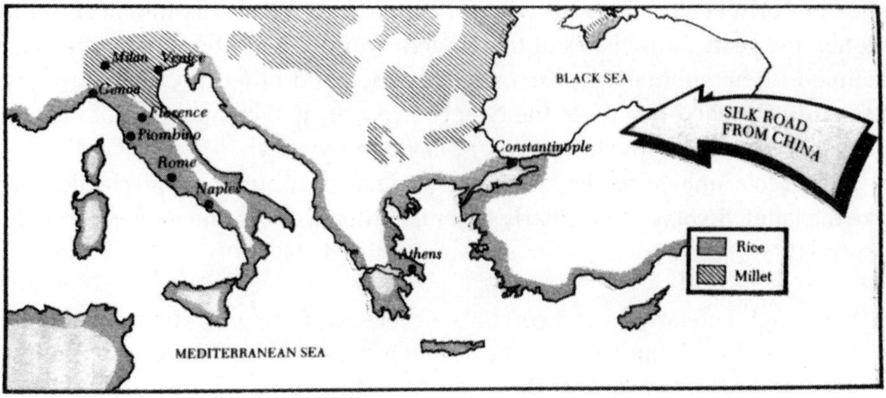

Figure 10.1. Rice and Millet Farming in Southern Europe, 1500.

occupied the geographical center of rice cultivation in the West, and millet grew in the area encompassing Milan and Venice. Leonardo's own diet consisted principally of grains and vegetables, and from notes in his diary recording scientific experiments with millet, we know that he kept a regular supply on hand. "The life of man is formed from things he eats," Leonardo wrote. "If you would keep healthy, follow this regimen: do not eat unless you feel inclined, and sup lightly: chew well and let what you take be well cooked and simple."[2]

Millet and whole brown rice appear to be the biological source of Leonardo's creativity. However, as he grew older, he also ate plenty of fruit, wine, and other expansive foods. These strong yin foods weakened his own health and judgment and set up a powerful attraction for their opposite. Although a pacifist, Leonardo lent his inventive talents to Cesare Borgia, the ambitious military leader in Romagna who was immortalized in Machiavelli's *The Prince.* In the summer of 1502, Leonardo and Machiavelli joined Borgia's encampment at Piombino and designed an engineering project to divert the course of the Arno River, making Florence directly accessible by sea and depriving Pisa, its rival, of water. Leonardo also pursued studies in the construction of a gigantic crossbow, rapid-fire artillery, and other weapons of mass destruction. However, after Borgia's treacherous military campaigns, resulting in the murder of his own officers, Leonardo left his service and returned to Florence and began work on *The Battle of Anghiari.* The sketches for this lost masterpiece of men and horses at war depict the infinite horror and anguish of battle in a mood reminiscent of Picasso's later *Guernica.* In this painting and the aptly named *Grotesque Heads,* Leonardo's figures display physiognomic signs of heavy meat, dairy, and sugar consumption—unlike the clear and balanced visages of his religious portraits and the *Mona Lisa,* the work that crowned his astonishing career.

Both the father of the modern world and the architect of its demise, Leonardo's military service reflected the split between intuition and reason that would widen in each successive century and reach a culmination in the atomic era. As a scientist, he betrayed an appalling callousness toward mass destruction. As an artist, he exhibited an infinite compassion and tenderness for life.

THE AGRICULTURAL REVOLUTION

As the amount of animal food, sugar, and spices in the European diet increased in the Middle Ages, traditional values and understanding declined, disease spread, and religion-sanctioned wars intensified. The integrity of the physical body and the rhythms of daily life were increasingly sacrificed to the tyranny of rigidified church structures and narrow interpretations of the spiritual life. With the Renaissance and the advent of the scientific and industrial revolutions, a new era of open inquiry and investigation began.

With the rise of meat consumption and the influx of new foods from Asia, Africa, and the Americas, European farmers began to experiment with artificial cultivation and breeding techniques, including the use of certain fertilizers, mixtures, and hybrids, to support the change in climate and soil conditions undergone by the new species.

In England, the center of the agricultural revolution, sheep's wool became a valued commodity for manufacturing. Enclosure laws transformed common farmland that was used to grow grains and vegetables into a checkerboard of rationally-planned private pastures for the breeding of sheep and growing of fodder. Hedging was also introduced on a large scale, permitting single crops to be grown without weeding, and cattle, traditionally used for plowing and turning millstones for grinding grain, were bred selectively for their meat and milk. The introduction of farm machinery, continuous cropping, and rock fertilizers increased agricultural yields and reduced rural populations. Refinements in milling made white flour widely available. From England, technological advances spread to other parts of Europe and the United States. By 1800, white bread, once limited only to the aristocracy, was eaten in manufacturing countries by nearly all the middle and lower classes, and sugar had ceased being a luxury and became a staple.

Though originally guided by conscience and a spirit of adventure, modern science soon narrowed its focus to the sensorially detectable world. As the diet declined, a new materialism prevailed, articulated by Hobbes' mechanistic political theories, Descartes' Cartesian rationalism, and Newton's linear physics. In respect to agricultural changes, a few dissenting voices were raised, such as those of the Diggers and Levellers in England, who upheld the freedom to till and plant the soil; common ownership of the land; and the primacy of grains and root vegetables. But by the eighteenth century, new farming techniques, patterns of food consumption, and modern dualist thinking began to diffuse around the world, separating humanity from nature, the body from the mind, the material from the spiritual, and the Occidental from the Oriental. The modern nation-state was one of the consequences of this analytical trend. The sovereignty of rulers to determine the law and religion of the population within their territorial boundaries was recognized in the Treaty of Westphalia, ending the Thirty Years' War in 1648.

THE POLITICAL REVOLUTION

The eighteenth century saw a further intensification of wars among the European powers and their foreign colonies. Although these rivalries were fought in the name of emerging nationalism and liberal political ideologies, control over international food exchange continued to be the primary underlying cause of the conflicts. In India, the East India Company challenged Portuguese and French mercantile interests, establishing large tea plantations involving millions of native laborers. In the Battle of Plassey, England triumphed over France, securing colonial control over India for the next two centuries.

In the New World, the Triangular Trade originally saw English finished goods going to Africa; African slaves going to America; and sugar, molasses, and other tropical commodities going to England. New England, however, began to cut into this lucrative trade and ship rum directly to Africa, bypassing England. "The maturation of this second triangle put the New England colonies on a direct collision course with Britain," a historian notes, "but the underlying problems were economic, taking on political import precisely because they brought divergent economic interests into confrontation."[3]

The American Revolution broke out against this economic background. Though born out of rebellion to English colonial duties on tea and sugar, there was also a creative political element. The architects of the fledgling United States believed that a sound food and agricultural system was the foundation of society and its future happiness. Benjamin Franklin adopted a meatless diet when he was sixteen, as he explains in his *Autobiography*, and his arrival in Philadelphia with two loaves of whole wheat bread has become part of our folklore.

Thomas Jefferson also gave up almost all animal food, using it primarily as a condiment. The principal author of the Declaration of Independence saw agricultural self-sufficiency and a nation of small farms as the indispensable foundation for the cultivation of life, liberty, and the pursuit of happiness. "The greatest service which can be rendered any country," Jefferson declared, "is to add a useful plant to its culture."[4] During a visit to France, Jefferson noticed that rice was used by many people as a staple, especially during religious holidays such as Lent when meat was not eaten. Most of the rice consumed in France came from Italy, so Jefferson went to Italy for the purpose of obtaining rice seed to send back to America, where the British had torched the rice fields and diminished the supply. He also went to see a newly developed rice-cleaning machine that Edward Rutledge had described to him in Congress in 1775. The Italian government, however, had strict laws prohibiting the export of rice seed. Determined to introduce this food item to North America, Jefferson risked a possible diplomatic scandal by hiring an Italian mule driver to illegally cross the border with several large sacks of seed from the best rice-growing district in Italy—the region between Turin and Milan, which had been growing rice since Leonardo da Vinci's time. The shipment was stopped at the border and turned back. Undaunted, Jefferson filled the large pockets of his coat with seed and carried it across the border himself. Upon arriving back in France, he sent the seed to Charleston, South Carolina, where it was divided among a select group of planters. Jefferson was so pleased with the outcome of this project that he later arranged for seeds of rice to be sent to the Carolinas from Egypt, China, and elsewhere.

The utopian spirit of the American revolutionary age, which found its zenith in Franklin and Jefferson's political ideals as well as their many practical inventions, harked back to the Renaissance. The biological source of this cultural flowering once again can be traced back to whole cereal grains.

Nevertheless, at the social level, meat and sugar continued to play a pivotal role in the development of the new republic. "I know not why we should blush to confess that molasses was an essential ingredient in American independence," John Adams wrote in 1775.[5] Six years later, the Revolutionary War ended when France, engaged in competition with England for control of sugar plantations on Dominica, Martinique, Granada, and St. Lucia, entered the war and provided the decisive margin of victory at Yorktown. In the view of one present-day historian of the period:

> The loss of the Sugar Islands to the French and their determination to get them back, explains the otherwise inexplicable willingness of the French government to enter the War of American Independence on the side of the Americans.[6]

THE INDUSTRIAL REVOLUTION

Sugar continued to play a central role in the development of modern civilization and contributed to the rise of capitalism (see Figure 10.2 on page 156). The sugar plantation is now viewed by historians as the bridge between the preindustrial shop and the industrial factory. In his book *Sweetness and Power*, Sidney Mintz wrote, "It may seem a topsy-turvy view of the West to find its factories elsewhere at so early a period. But the sugarcane plantation is gradually winning recognition as an unusual combination of agricultural and industrial forms. . . ."[7]

The sugar plantation was also a cauldron for revolution. In Hispaniola, France's dream of extending its empire in the New World floundered when 30,000 French troops who were sent to put down a rebellion on the sugar plantations succumbed to yellow fever. The black freedom fighters, led by Toussaint l'Ouverture, had a much simpler, more well-balanced diet than the French and were able to live in harmony with the environment. As a result of this defeat, Napoleon decided to cut his losses in the tropics and sell the Louisiana Territory to President Thomas Jefferson.

The taste for sugar

Sugar consumption per person in the UK and US has been steadily rising

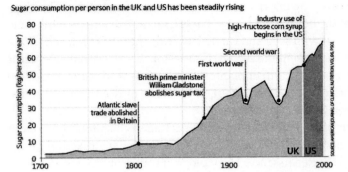

Figure 10.2.
Per Capita Sugar
Consumption in
the U.K.

The spread of industrialization in the nineteenth century further altered dietary patterns. In the early 1800s, a Hungarian flourmill introduced steel rollers that completely stripped the germ and bran from wheat, making available an even finer white flour. By the 1880s, this process had spread to the American Midwest. Commercially refined vegetable oils and margarine also came into use at this time. By mid-century, canning—first developed during the Napoleonic wars—reached the United States, and ready-to-prepare fish, seafood, tomatoes, corn, and other foods, as well as canned and condensed whole milk, made their appearance on grocery shelves.

Advances in transportation also wrought fundamental changes. The steamboat resulted in a rise in fresh milk and poultry consumption, as farmers could get their goods to the cities more quickly. The clipper ship made inexpensive tea widely available, and meat intake substantially rose with the coming of the railroad and refrigerated freight cars. In 1869, the Suez Canal opened, substantially shortening the journey of freighters from Europe to India and the Far East. By the time the Panama Canal opened in 1914—further stimulating commerce, especially the transport of tropical goods to northern countries—world trade had increased by ten times in about a century.

The agricultural, political, and industrial revolutions caused havoc in settled farming communities. Uprooted from their ancestral lands, millions of farm families flocked to the cities in quest of food and employment. In the process, they became mired in cycles of poverty and disease, hired themselves out for low wages in coalmines or factories, and formed the pools for standing armies and conscription. Throughout Europe, many of those who could not make the transformation from feudal to industrial society made a career out of military life. In Sweden and Prussia, disciplined fighting forces were developed using new techniques of drilling and patriotic oratory.

In England, Scotland, the German states, the Italian peninsula, Scandinavia, and many other European areas, farmers could no longer compete with American wheat and other foodstuffs that could be grown cheaply with new mechanical methods, shipped quickly abroad, and sold beneath market prices. Deprived of a livelihood, millions of European farm families left their homelands and emigrated to America, the land of opportunity and bountiful harvests. In some countries, such as Ireland, Belgium, and Germany, this process was accelerated by famine as the potato crop failed. Native to the tropical highlands of Peru, the potato was brought to Europe in the sixteenth century and in some regions, such as Ireland, almost completely displaced whole grains in the diet. The great potato blight began in Nova Scotia and Boston in 1842 and reached Ireland in 1845, destroying the potato crop and indirectly killing millions of people. Until the end of the century, European affairs, including the policies of Bismarck and Disraeli, revolved around tariffs on foreign food and the social effects of the great dislocations caused by industrialization and changing food patterns.

The plight of uprooted families in Europe generated an idealistic countermovement that found expression in the utopian social ideals and experimental communities of Robert Owen, Charles Fourier, Henri de Saint-Simon, and others. The writings of Karl Marx and Friedrich Engels also envisioned a new society in which work would no longer be dehumanizing and tried to provide a scientific basis for this notion's historical inevitability. Viewing life as perpetual conflict, Marx and Engels popularized the notion of incessant class struggle and war between the proletariat and the bourgeoisie. By the end of the nineteenth century, industrial workers had begun to demand reforms and organize unions and federations with millions of members. Violence and bloodshed broke out in mines, factories, and shops between representatives of labor and capital.

Meanwhile, millions of East Indians, Chinese, Javanese, and other Asian immigrants flocked to the Caribbean, South Africa, and other territories to handle sugarcane and other commodity crops following the cessation of Black slavery by the European nations. In the United States, millions of Chinese were imported to work on the railroads and in the fields. Friction among different racial and ethnic groups often resulted. Meanwhile, at gunpoint, the Western nations compelled China, Japan, and other traditional societies to open their doors to disadvantageous trade and market agreements. An anti-colonial reaction, beginning in the 1880s, set off a wave of bloodshed in Asia and Africa, culminating in the political freedom movements and social revolutions of the twentieth century.

Although the Industrial Revolution increased material prosperity, it also increased the pace of life, and infectious diseases (including typhus fever, smallpox, and measles) assumed epidemic proportions and became the leading causes of death in the European countries. Prior to this time, degenerative diseases were virtually unknown. In the late eighteenth century, individual cases of cancer, heart disease, and other chronic disorders began to emerge in the upper classes, which were most prone to dietary excess. Furthermore, as in past eras, disease and pestilence followed waves of international food exchange. During the nineteenth century, waterborne diseases such as typhoid, dysentery, and cholera, as well as fly-borne diseases such as malaria and yellow fever, became epidemic in the manufacturing countries and their foreign colonies. Continued quantification and specialization in science led to the rise of metabolic theory and advances in surgery and drug use. Chemist Justus von Liebig, the "founder of modern nutrition," classified nourishment into categories and subcategories. The superiority of animal protein gained general acceptance, and simple carbohydrates that give quick energy, such as white flour, refined sugar, and potatoes, became even more desirable.

WORLD WAR I

"It is the exhaustion of the cereal seeds that causes the weakening of the seed of humanity," Emile Zola warned at the end of the nineteenth century, as modern civilization reaped the first fruits of mechanized agriculture.[8] Industrial society, however, remained blind to the admonitions of the French author, as well as those of other early health reformers such as Christoph W. Hufeland, the German physician who revived and popularized the term "macrobiotics"; Rev. Sylvester Graham, a crusader against refined flour; and Ellen Harmon White and John Harvey Kellogg, the Adventist leaders who opened a vegetarian healing center in Battle Creek, Michigan.

By the beginning of the new century, Europe and North America's desire for excessive yang food increased, and livestock producers (such as the ranchers in the western U.S., Argentina, and Australia) could not fill society's demand for beef. A further round of yin stimulants, pacifiers, and narcotics brought back by Western military expeditions in Cuba, the Philippines, the Congo, and elsewhere began to have devastating social consequences in the industrialized nations. Even alcohol, a longstanding yin balance to meat and animal food, grew out of control; a movement to prohibit it spread in the industrial countries because of its effects on family life. Pasteurized milk became available, and the invention of the cream separator, the milking machine, and advances in commercial refrigeration launched the modern dairy industry. Between 1875 and 1915, sugar consumption doubled to eighty pounds per capita, and Coca-Cola and other soft drinks became widely available, with their popularity increasing with each new decade.

In 1914, the assassination of an Austrian archduke lit the fuse that set off fighting among the European states locked in a bitter competition to colonize Africa and Asia and control the Suez sea routes to the East. In 1917, the United States joined the war when German U-boats threatened to starve England into submission by sinking food vessels off the south and west coasts. On the other side of the Atlantic Ocean, U.S. Food Administrator Herbert Hoover purchased the entire U.S. sugar and hog crops to save Britain.

For nearly a century following the Napoleonic wars, statesmen and diplomats made concerted efforts to prevent another continental war in Europe. These included the Congress of Vienna in 1815 and the Hague Conferences in 1899 and

1907. Citizens, authors, and artists also played a leading role. Key figures included Leo Tolstoy (whose writings on nonviolence influenced Gandhi); Alfred Nobel, the inventor of dynamite who established a prize fund to prevent war; and Austrian novelist Bertha von Suttner, author of *Lay Down Your Arms* and the first woman to receive the Nobel Peace Prize. Across the Atlantic, Henry David Thoreau's essay, "On Civil Disobedience"; the World Parliament of Religions in Chicago in 1893; and the Ford Peace Expedition at the beginning of World War I were valiant efforts at reconciliation and world unity. But none of these attempts succeeded.

From a biological perspective, World War I represented an explosive discharge of stagnant metabolic energy that had been accumulating in Europe for many decades as a result of dietary and environmental excess. The increasing mechanization of modern life at this period reflected the increasing mechanization of the modern food and agricultural system. The advent of skyscrapers; the use of glass as a primary building material; and the development of the automobile, luxury liner, and airplane coincided with the increasing use of metal and glass in canning, bottling, and other packaging. When war came, these vehicles were transformed into tanks, battleships, and fighter planes. Developments in long-range striking power (rifles, machine guns, artillery) also paralleled rises in meat and sugar consumption, and the introduction of poison gas followed the chemical adulteration of commercial food. Advances in the manufacture of ammonium nitrate led to the rise of both chemical fertilizer for farming and a key ingredient for explosives.

In 1909, German chemist Fritz Haber developed a way to synthesize nitrate from air through a high-temperature, energy-intensive process. Carl Bosch, another German chemist, subsequently perfected the method, and it came to be known as the *Haber-Bosch process*. The discovery led to advances in armaments manufacture and in chemical agriculture, both of which use nitrates. As investigative journalist Tom Philpott observed, "Before it made it onto farm fields in a big way, Haber's breakthrough fueled the U.S. and European munitions industry, particularly in World War II. In that way, the industrialization of farming shares roots with the industrialization of killing represented by modern war."

By the end of the Second World War, America constructed ten large nitrate factories to make bombs. After the war, the chemical industry shifted from armaments to fertilizer and chemical inputs soared. High-yielding new hybrid strains of corn fueled this rise. Today, 30 percent of U.S. farmland is devoted to corn, most of which now is genetically engineered. In the Third World, the Haber-Bosch process led to the Green Revolution and a population explosion. Hybrid corn, rice, wheat, and other crops resulted in record harvests, and the world population doubled from 2.4 billion in 1950 to 4.4 billion in 1980. By 2000, it rose to 6.1 billion, and in 2015 it reached 7.3 billion. It is thought that the expanding crop harvests played a large factor in the world population increase.

On the one hand, chemical fertilizer has reduced hunger and starvation and raised living standards, as well as enabled the number of people on the planet to multiply several times. However, it has also contributed to major environmental destruction. Chemical fertilizers have resulted in steep declines in soil vitality and the emission of nitrous oxide, a greenhouse gas that is 300 times more destructive than carbon dioxide. Along with arsenic-based pesticides, fertilizer has poisoned the water table in Bangladesh and other South Asian regions and led to massive pollution of the Mississippi River, including dead zones in the Gulf of Mexico and elsewhere.

The myth of Western progress and European superiority was shattered by the First World War. By the time global fighting ended, nearly 40 million people had died, about half from direct fighting and about half from an epidemic of influenza that swept the world. Few lessons were learned from this war as the trend toward greater mechanization in all aspects of life continued. But the fundamental role of diet as the hidden mechanism of history was not lost on a few prophetic voices. Sir William Osler, the father of modern medical education, observed, "More people are killed by overeating and drinking than by the sword."[9] Cancer researcher William Howard Hay, M.D., concurred, "White flour and white sugar have cost more lives than all the wars of all time."[10]

WORLD WAR II

After World War I, the efforts to balance extreme foods reached a new plateau. The creation of mammoth incubators led to the mass production of poultry. In the 1920s, home refrigeration came into vogue, and prepackaged frozen foods reduced the consumption of fresh garden produce. Refined, canned, and dehydrated foods also took an increasing share of the market. In the 1930s, the vitamin industry developed, selling back to the consumer the nutrients removed in processing grain. Artificial colors, chemical preservatives, and other additives found their way into daily food as new synthetic flavors, cosmetic appearance, and extended shelf life replaced wholesomeness and nutrition as primary concerns. Monoculture—itself a departure from traditional farming techniques—failed to meet the rising demand for unseasonal fare, and modern society began to turn to chemical agriculture to increase production, stretch quantity, and meet demand. These changes, along with increased consumption of beef and other animal foods high in saturated fat and dietary cholesterol, laid the foundation for the modern epidemics of heart disease, cancer, and other degenerative diseases that developed in the middle of the twentieth century. The rise in commercial cigarette smoking, increased industrial pollution, and a more sedentary way of life resulting from the spread of the automobile and other modern conveniences contributed to the increased incidence of these diseases.

In the 1930s and early 1940s, chaotic dietary habits spread around the world. As their intuition and common sense declined, populations in the industrialized countries became subject to delusional ideologies and the manipulation of rigid or unstable political and military leaders. The end result was another world war. In the case of Germany, a dietary heritage of sausage, wurst, and other processed meat helped to transform society into a slaughterhouse, while heavy consumption of beer, sugar, chocolate, and other extreme yin substances created a magnetic attraction to the Aryan ideal—the archetypal symbol of extreme yang.

In the case of Japan, the principal biological factors leading to aggression, war, and doctrines of racial superiority included the adoption of modern German nutritional and medical standards at the beginning of the Meiji era (emphasizing the importance of animal protein), in order to compete with the West; rising sugar and tropical fruit consumption following the colonization of Taiwan; the spread of white rice, MSG (monosodium glutamate), refined salt, and other highly processed foods; and excessive consumption of fish and seafood. Fish-eating, for example, produces a way of thinking that is cool, collected, and sharp, but lacks width and depth; a fish is narrow and moves in a straight line. Japan's attack on Pearl Harbor was very shortsighted. At the end of the nineteenth century, the polishing of rice had led to outbreaks of beriberi (thiamine deficiency) aboard ships, and the Japanese Navy had adopted a semi-modern diet, including high amounts of enriched white bread, canned food, sugar, and fish. The excesses of Japanese forces in Manchuria, China, Southeast Asia, and elsewhere can be attributed physiologically to these dietary extremes and environmentally to the generally volcanic temperament of the Japanese people.

In the case of the United States and its allies, mental inflexibility and cloudy thinking resulting from too much meat, sugar, white bread, soft drinks, and other articles in the modern diet led to official indifference toward the plight of the Jews; racial prejudice; the removal of citizens of Japanese ancestry to detention centers; and the strategic bombing of civilian population centers in Dresden, Hiroshima, and elsewhere.

EINSTEIN AND THE DEVELOPMENT OF ATOMIC ENERGY

In the popular imagination, the atomic age is associated with Albert Einstein more than any other figure. In 1905, as a young scientist, he devised the famous equation $E=mc^2$, theorizing that matter could be transformed into energy. Although this formula did not directly anticipate nuclear energy, Einstein's work, along with that of Rutherford, Joliet-Curie, Fermi, and other physicists in the early part of the century, set in motion the events that culminated in the splitting of the atom.

Einstein also wrote the historic letter to President Franklin D. Roosevelt in 1939, warning of the need to develop an atomic bomb before the Nazis did. This appeal led to the Manhattan Project. Germany, however, had surrendered by the time the first American atomic bombs were ready, and instead they were used on Japan in August 1945. Einstein deeply regretted his involvement in the creation of the bomb, feeling the destruction of Hiroshima and Nagasaki was morally unjustifiable. He devoted the rest of his life—ten years—to world peace and world government activities.

To help understand Einstein's pivotal role as midwife to the nuclear age, it is important to review his environmental, dietary, and medical history. Born into a German family of Jewish origin in 1879, young Albert grew up with a boundless love for nature, music, and the simple ways of the Swabian countryside. The farmers in the surrounding area were very peaceful and moderate, like their Swiss neighbors. Once, at age four, Albert broke into tears while watching soldiers drill in uniform. Although his parents had turned away from orthodox religion, at about ten years of age Albert began to study the scriptures and for about two years adhered to a more balanced Kosher diet, refusing to eat pork and some other animal foods. Later, his parents moved to Munich and then to Italy for several years, where Albert embarked on a program of self-study in museums, churches, fields, and forests and developed a lifelong taste for Italian foods, including noodles and pasta. In 1896, at age sixteen, he enrolled in a famous technological institute in Zurich and became a Swiss citizen. Here, in one of Europe's greatest scientific academies, Einstein showed none of the reticence or dull-mindedness he had displayed in Catholic elementary school and the lyceum in Germany. In Switzerland, he worked at the Patent Office in Berne, married in 1903, and wrote occasional scientific papers. In 1919, astronomers at the Royal Society in London announced that photographs of a total eclipse of the sun had verified Einstein's general theory of relativity. Overnight he became world famous.

During the period in Europe when some of his most brilliant scientific thinking was accomplished, Einstein was divorced and cooked for himself. He ate simply, making mostly soup and hard-boiled eggs. Eggs are the most condensed (yang) food in the usual diet and produce powerful theoretical faculties when prepared in this way. Later, his cousin, second wife, and housekeeper cooked for him, and like most modern women of this period, they prepared substantial amounts of meat, sugar, and other highly processed foods. As an international celebrity, he was also the guest of honor at many banquets featuring rich, gourmet fare.

For the rest of his life, Einstein suffered periodic personal and family illnesses brought about chiefly by chaotic eating. In 1917, he came down with a serious stomach ulcer that continued for several years. In 1928, he suffered a heart attack, probably brought about by his fondness for eggs as well as other animal foods high in saturated fat and cholesterol, and his doctor put him on a fat-and salt-restricted diet. In the early 1930s, his younger son, Eduard, was diagnosed as schizophrenic and spent most of his life in a Swiss sanitarium. In 1936, shortly after their arrival in the United States, his second wife, Elsa, died from heart and kidney disease. By the time Einstein wrote his historic letter to Roosevelt, he no longer attended most public functions, citing poor health. In 1946, he was diagnosed with acute anemia, and two years later doctors found an aneurysm in his abdominal aorta. In 1955, after years of pain, fatigue, and sorrow, he died of complications from pneumonia, anemia, and a weak heart.

In his later years at Princeton, I had the opportunity to visit Einstein and discuss world government activities and the peace problem with him. In person, as in his photographs, Einstein's overall features showed a strong inherited constitution. His basic intuition and insight came from generations of ancestors who ate plenty of whole grains and vegetables and who had survived many difficulties because of their religious heritage. Nourished also by the fields and forests, lakes, and mountains of his native and adopted homelands, he had a deep love for nature and the universe. He detested machines and balanced his mental activity by playing the violin and by sailing. Einstein's love of the natural world led him to devote his life to explaining its order. He spent the last decades of his life searching for a unified field theory to explain the nature of light, energy, gravity, and matter. His inclination to vegetable-quality food contributed to this quest, as well as to his insight, compassion, and dedication to peace.

Like most modern thinkers and artists, Einstein did his best work in his early years, drawing on and exhausting the strengths he had inherited from his ancestors and leaving low reserves to fuel him in his maturity and old age. As a typical yang intellectual who craved solitude and space to pursue his studies, he had a weakness for strong yin, such as sugar, coffee, fruits, and sweets, which contributed to his celebrated absentmindedness and the inability to realize his dream. Had his strong constitutional reserves not been weakened by a chaotic and excessive diet, he might have foreseen the destructive uses to which his name and formulations were put. Near the end of his life, he turned toward a more plant-based diet:

> Although I have been prevented by outward circumstances from observing a strictly vegetarian diet, I have long been an adherent to the cause in principle. Besides agreeing with the aims of vegetarianism for aesthetic and moral reasons, it is my view that a vegetarian manner of living by its purely physical effect on the human temperament would most beneficially influence the lot of mankind.[11]

Had he eaten more whole grains, he might have discovered the logarithmic spiral as the universal pattern unifying the four known physical forces of the universe. For example, his theory that light bends and that space is curved is a modern formulation of traditional cosmological understanding, which intuitively grasped that the speed of light is not constant but approaches infinite velocity and that space, like other phenomena, moves in a spiral.

Like Leonardo da Vinci, Einstein blended the scientific with the artistic and musical, and the natural with the ethical and moral. In private and public forums, he constantly sought to balance opposites and show the interconnectedness of all phenomena. "Science without religion is lame," he declared. "Religion without science is blind." Like Leonardo, Einstein was a lifelong peace promoter who, in a period of poor health and judgment, lent his genius to the forces of mass destruction. Fortunately, like his Renaissance predecessor, Einstein quickly realized his mistake. After the bombing of Hiroshima, he told Leo Szilard, the physicist who prevailed upon him to write the letter to Roosevelt, "You see now that the ancient Chinese were right. It is not possible to foresee the results of what you do. The only wise thing to do is to take no action—to take absolutely no action."[12]

THE FAST-FOOD REVOLUTION

Of course, the atomic age is the culmination of a powerful tendency within history, not brought about by a single individual. A change of food precedes a change of society. In the past, dietary patterns were affected primarily by changes in natural environmental conditions, as well as by trade and advances in transportation. However, since the late nineteenth century, changes in food quality arose largely as a result of technological intervention in the processes of farming, food processing, and cooking. The artificial splitting of the atom coincided with the creation of synthetic food.

Following World War II, the final artificialization of modern agriculture, food production, and medicine took place. Chemical farming became nearly universal in industrialized countries as inexpensive petroleum-based fertilizers, herbicides, and pesticides became available. For example, DDT, a powerful insecticide that proved successful in reducing malaria during the war, was introduced as a common pesticide. Sulfa drugs, penicillin, Atabrine, and other powerful drugs that had proved successful in treating wartime infection entered into general pharmaceutical use. Synthetic antibiotics, hormones, and preservatives further weakened the quality of meat and poultry, and more animal products had to be consumed to maintain the same level of energy and sensory satisfaction. The consumption of soft drinks and citrus juices, which are very yin, skyrocketed and helped to balance this overly yang intake.

Beginning in the 1950s, mass television advertising campaigns began to sell the appearance of food, including its packaging and social status, rather than the quality of the food itself. Beef, milk, cheese, ice cream, and other products of the cow completely replaced whole grains, bread, noodles, and pasta as the staple in most of the industrialized world. Through artificial insemination and growth hormones, the cattle population soared until there was one cow for every two people in the United States. By the 1960s, a majority of the world's grain was fed to livestock rather than used for direct human consumption. With the introduction of fast food and TV dinners, as well as the growth of neighborhood drive-ins, pizza parlors, and hamburger chains, the home-cooked family meal became the exception rather than the rule. Meanwhile, the vast majority of modern women gave up breastfeeding for infant formula. The medical profession and the dietetic associations lent their seal of approval to the new way of eating, promoting imbalanced nutritional theories such as the Basic Four Food Groups and generally endorsing the superiority of enriched, processed foods over whole, natural foods, including mother's milk.

For the first time in human history, daily cooking in most parts of the civilized world left the home and became largely the responsibility of people outside the family. Automats, vending machines, and other mechanical, assembly-line techniques insulated much of the food that was served from any human contact. Electricity and the microwave replaced wood and gas as main methods of cooking, subjecting food to further artificial electromagnetic vibrations, loss of natural energy, and even changes in molecular structure. Grace, or giving thanks for the bounty of the earth—a custom that had sustained generations of ancestors and bound them with the creation—largely disappeared from the family dinner table, along with real food. If modern people thought about their way of eating at all, they recognized a vague allegiance to a godhead of protein, fat, and carbohydrates; a devil called calories; and a minor pantheon of vitamins and minerals. Television replaced the hearth as the center of the household. The nightly news—featuring the nuclear arms buildup, hostilities between the U.S. and U.S.S.R., and regional wars around the world—supplanted ordinary dinnertime conversation. An atmosphere of global fear and crisis surrounded the meal, further contributing to feelings of isolation and despair.

THE COLLAPSE OF MODERN SOCIETY

As the end of the twentieth century drew near, signs of the approaching collapse of modern civilization multiplied rapidly. Generations of cheap fossil fuel and the overuse of chemical pesticides and fertilizers that depleted the topsoil finally backfired in the 1970s with the Arab oil squeeze. This was when OPEC (Organization of the Petroleum Exporting Countries) first raised oil prices, which triggered a major wake-up call that there wasn't unlimited cheap oil. Modern society has discovered that the topsoil has eroded; seed vitality has diminished; acid rains threaten the remaining forests and wildlife; toxic wastes imperil the rivers and waterways; and global warming and climate change threaten to transform much of the world into a desert or other wasteland.

In the tropical regions of Africa, Asia, and Latin America, the world's rainforests—containing one-third of all the plant and animal species on earth—face final destruction from beef-raising, mining, and logging. The destruction of the rainforests also threatens major global climatic and weather changes by cutting off the oxygen supplied by mahogany trees and other tropical plants. The fertility of the land, stretching back to the time of Moses, has been nearly exhausted in a single lifetime. New disease-resistant pests developed to challenge the hegemony of chemical sprays. By 1980, two-thirds of all folk varieties of wheat and garden vegetables once grown in North America and Europe had disappeared.

A generation later, an estimated 25 to 50 percent of all species of plants and animals around the globe are imperiled.

In the developing countries, modern agriculture proved disruptive on an even larger scale. Cattle grazing, use of marginal lands, and the export of cash crops overturned traditional patterns of farming and cultural life. Thousands of species of grains and vegetables that had flourished since Egyptian Dynastic, Vedic, or Incan times disappeared with the spread of monocropping. For example, more than 5,500 varieties of rice were once cultivated in India. Since the mid-1960s, when four new, high-yielding hybrid seeds were introduced as part of the Green Revolution, most of these hardy, disease-resistant types of local seed died out. In Bangladesh, arsenic from insecticides poisoned the water table, contaminated the rice, and continue to cause thousands of deaths each year. Tens of millions of families, uprooted from their ancestral lands by beef producers, coffee plantations, and other agribusiness enterprises, flocked to metropolitan centers such as Cairo, Mexico City, and Sao Paulo in quest of employment and opportunity. The vast urban slums created by this exodus from the land offered only poverty, hunger, and emergency relief—consisting of infant formula, refined foods, and immunizations and artificial population-control techniques—that ultimately further contributed to disease and destitution.

During this period, the latest turn in the international food exchange spiral had Western soldiers (the most physical or yang element of society) returning from Vietnam, Afghanistan, Lebanon, El Salvador, Iraq, and other tropical and semitropical regions with marijuana, cocaine, heroin, and opium. Once again, the influx of extreme yin from the tropics had seriously undermined family life and social order in the industrial northern nations of the world. Legislative efforts to prohibit illicit drugs proved as futile as did the efforts of previous generations to control sugar or alcohol.

As a result of tampering with the elements and refusing to abide by the limits of the four seasons, cancer, heart disease, and other chronic disorders proliferated through the modern world, reaching epidemic proportions between 1950 and 1980. In the early twenty-first century, they (along with the modern diet) spread to the developing world and today eclipse infectious diseases as the major threat to public health.

THE AGE OF BIOTECHNOLOGY

The modern age, which began with the agricultural revolution in the seventeenth century, is ending in the early twenty-first century with the worldwide triumph of refined, processed, and artificial food. While this way of eating provided unparalleled variety, convenience, and sensory fulfillment, its effects on personal and social health and consciousness have proved devastating. Now, at the end of the modern age, families are beset with conflict and division, with one out of every two marriages ending in divorce. Schools have become places of confinement rather than instruction and discovery. Modern medicine is unable to reverse the epidemic of chronic and immunodeficiency diseases. Millions of relatively healthy women of childbearing age have consented to have their uteruses, ovaries, or breasts surgically removed as a preventive measure against cancer. Religious frenzy, self-mutilation, and sacrificial death marked the end of earlier epochs. The wave of hysterectomies, mastectomies, and other usually unnecessary operations, as well as the spread of immunodeficiency diseases and the shunning of AIDS and Ebola patients, harks back to the plagues and panic that accompanied the decline of past civilizations.

At the societal levels, crime, assassinations, kidnappings, suicide bombings, and terrorist activity have become routine. Economies have stagnated and political ideologies have lost their adherents. Worldly cults and otherworldly sects have flourished as despair, fear, and apathy spread. Wild, erratic behavior, delusional thinking, and other chaotic manifestations of underlying physical and psychological imbalance have become commonplace at all levels of life. Nation states have proved unable to overcome their fear and mistrust of each other and halt the spread of nuclear weapons and other weapons of mass destruction. The developing countries have embarked on the construction of nuclear reactors that could be converted to producing fissionable plutonium. The earth itself lies dying, its topsoil eroded, its forests and plains plundered, its waters and atmosphere polluted, its animal and plant life on the verge of extinction. The fragile system of nourishment that has taken 4 billion years of evolution to perfect has broken down.

The irradiation of food has now also spread as growers and merchandisers seek to further retard the ripening of grains, vegetables, and fruits and extend their shelf life. Under this practice, the food's cells, including the genes, are changed or destroyed, through a process which bombards the food with electrons from a nuclear accelerator or—the more common approach—exposes it to high-energy gamma rays given off by radioactive cobalt and cesium. In the early 1980s, the U.S. FDA approved the irradiation of most common foods so long as they were labeled "picowaved," and the Department of Energy endorsed this innovation in food technology as an excellent way to use spent nuclear fuel. Nuclear energy has arrived on the dinner plate.

In the face of the collapse of natural human beings, scientists and genetic engineers have begun to tamper with the basic quality of human life itself. With the development of the artificial human heart in the early 1980s and GMO foods in the 1990s, the latest, and possibly final, act in the human drama—the Age of Biotechnology—began to unfold.

ROOTS OF THE MODERN CRISIS

The Second World War marked the end of human civilization's horizontal movement. In the atomic bombing of Hiroshima and Nagasaki, West met East and the limits of modern technology became obvious. The new weaponry made obsolete territorial exclusivity, national sovereignty, and the materialist trend of the last several thousand years. From now on, humanity could expand vertically into outer space and inwardly into mind and consciousness. The desire to control the world by money, by power, and by ideas would continue into the next century, fueled by the momentum of the past. The yang spiral of the dark half of the cycle of Northern celestial energy is clearly ending as the twenty-

TABLE 10.1 WORLD AGES AND HUMAN DEVELOPMENT			
	ANCIENT SCIENTIFIC AND SPIRITUAL WORLD COMMUNITY	ANCIENT AGE	MEDIEVAL AGE
Biological Foundation			
Agriculture	Natural	Organic	Organic
Staple Food	Wild cereals Foraged plants	Whole grains and vegetables	Whole grains Salted meat Spices
Cooking	Sun-baked Wind-dried	Wood	Charcoal
Technology	Natural and cosmic force	Wind Water Solar energy	Animal and muscular power
Personal and Family Life			
Basic Unit	Family	Tribe; Empire	Kingdom
Family Type	Global	Clan	Extended
Health and Sickness	Healthy and energetic	Pestilence	Plague
Medicine	Vibrational	Diet Acupuncture Massage	Herbs
Social Organization			
Social Relations	Harmonious Peaceful	Stable	Volatile
Conflict	Adventure	Raids Reprisals Conquest	Crusade
Ideology	Way of nature	Mythological	Religious
Dream	Paradise	Golden age	Millennium

first century unfolds, even though life will continue to speed up and contract for another generation.

The atomic bomb made one world inevitable. Mass explosion is one possible way for this one world to come about. The second is forming a unified world. Global nuclear war would likely result in the end of all human life and even the planet itself. Building a world community would start a new spiral, going in a slower, wider, more harmonious direction.

MODERN AGE	RECENT AGE	BIOTECHNOLOGICAL AGE	AGE OF HUMANITY
Industrial	Chemical	Biogenetic	Organic and Natural
Refined grains Meat and Sugar Tropical foods	Meat and sugar Refined and processed foods	Chemicalized and artificial food Genetically engineered food	Whole grains and vegetables
Coal Gas Petroleum	Electrical	Microwave Irradiated food	Wood Charcoal Gas
Mechanical Steam	Oil Electric Nuclear	Artificial electromagnetic radiation	Natural and cosmic force
Nation	Individual	Cell and DNA	Family
Extended	Nuclear	Artificial	Extended and global
Infectious disease	Degenerative disease	Immunodeficiency disease	Healthy and energetic
Surgery Drugs	Surgery Drugs Radiation	Transplants Artificial organs	Diet Vibrational Spiritual
Fragmented	Violent	Chaotic	Harmonious Peaceful
Balance of power alliances	Revolution World war	Biochemical Genetic	Adventure
Humanistic	Scientific	Cybernetic	Spiritual Way of nature
Utopia	Classless society	Automation	One peaceful world

Dawning realization that humanity shares a common origin and destiny has led to more universal conceptions of paradise. In the twentieth century, the utopian impulse shifted from small land-based communities to global villages and arcologies. Visionary architects and planners, including Le Corbusier, the Soviet Constructivists, Frank Lloyd Wright, Buckminster Fuller, Marshall McLuhan, Paolo Soleri, Antoni Gaudi, and Frank Gehry started to conceive and dream in planetary terms.

Following World War II, a global meeting of East and West—intuitive, spiritual thought and analytic, material thought—began, as the Pole Star shifted back toward its ancient location. The reconciliation of these two ways of life will not represent the triumph of one over the other, but a broader and deeper synthesis of the strengths in each. If the misuse of science and technology, as well as religion and ideology, could be avoided, the foundation for One Peaceful World could definitely be established.

Table 10.1 on pages 168 and 169 provides a visual example of how human development has changed with each historical world age.

SUMMARY

At the biological level, the future of our species depends upon preserving the traditional strains of whole grains and vegetables handed down from generation to generation since the first harvest and setting aside the artificial foods created from new hybrid strains and from products engineered in a laboratory. The choice of seeds that humanity sows in the days and years to come, as in the past, will guide and shape human destiny and determine whether the earth becomes an inferno or a paradise.

PEACE PROMOTER

Hildegard Lilienthal and Adelbert and Wieke Nelissen, Germany and the Netherlands

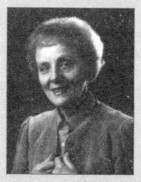

Hildegard Lilienthal

In 1979, Hildegard Lilienthal, a German housewife and nurse, entered a hospital in Hanau, a suburb of Frankfurt. For years she had been suffering from rheumatism, arthritis, and a heart condition. She could no longer walk, work, or care for her family. Doctors prescribed surgery and drugs, including infusions of gold. As a nurse who had worked for many years in the same hospital, she knew that her prognosis was grave. Concerned about her husband and two teenage sons, she declined medical treatment and determined to find an alternative.

Across the street from the hospital, she visited a small health food shop. The woman who worked there told her that her own milder symptoms of arthritis had disappeared on a macrobiotic diet. Hildegard decided to try this approach and cooked whole, natural foods, especially brown rice, for several months. She also applied a hot ginger compress on her kidneys, intestines, arms and hands, and legs and feet. The ginger compress, a traditional macrobiotic home remedy, stimulates circulation and reduces pains and aches. Quickly Hildegard's condition improved. She could walk again, and she was no longer confined to her home.

Looking back on her own childhood in what is now Poland, Hildegard recalled that her family ate very simply—mostly dark bread, grain porridge made from wheat or barley ground fresh daily, garden vegetables, sauerkraut, grain coffee, and apple cider. Animal food was eaten very seldom (usually just a little bacon was mixed in for flavoring). In the mountains, the people traditionally ate millet, lentils, dried pea soup, and sauerkraut. Hildegard remembered meeting one old woman who was 104 years old and who attributed her longevity to avoiding sugar, dairy foods, and other rich fare.

After World War II, German food patterns dramatically changed. "I worked in an American hospital and was amazed at the vast quantities of milk, white bread, chicken, potatoes, and milk," Hildegard recalls. "For breakfast, the U.S. officers would eat up to ten eggs apiece. But they were very wasteful. They would eat just the middle of the bread or part of the chicken and throw away the rest. We were so poor. It was the first time we saw so much food.

"After the war, American money poured in, and Germany got fat. We started eating meat every day, especially sauerbraten made with beef, as well as sausage and meatloaf. We also regularly started eating cheese, white bread, butter and jam, marmalade, sugar, and lots of cakes, especially the creamy ones. I went back to work and had no time to clean or cook for my family. I'd come home and cook for ten minutes, mostly ready-made foods, or set out oranges and bananas. Each year illnesses and misunderstandings increased, and our family grew further and further apart."

At first, the rest of Hildegard's family was not interested in her new way of eating. Then one day, her younger son, Uli, picked up a book his mother had been reading by George Ohsawa. Attracted to the Far East since childhood, Uli was fascinated with Ohsawa's adventurous spirit and dynamic philosophy of health and longevity. The next day he decided to stop eating meat and sugar. A few months later, Jorg, his older brother, also started eating macrobiotically.

The simpler way of eating did not appeal to their father, Johannes (Hans), and Hildegard continued to cook sausage, eggs, cheese, and other foods he was accustomed to. Over the next couple of years, she gradually began to incorporate whole grains, vegetables, and other better-quality foods into his usual meals. In 1981, Hans' chronic leg problem flared up, and he was admitted to the hospital. Doctors told him that the artery in his leg was clogged from the use of too much tobacco and would require amputation from below the thigh.

Hildegard, Uli, and Jorg brought brown rice and other food to the hospital for Hans and gave him ginger compresses. Mother and sons were convinced that a long-time diet of sausage and other extremely contractive (yang) foods was the main cause of their father's problem, and that smoking (also yang) only aggravated the condition. By greatly reducing saturated fats and dietary cholesterol in Hans' diet, they reasoned that the underlying cause of his circulatory problem could be eliminated. The ginger compress would help restore circulation and reduce the pain. Thanks to their ministrations, the thrombosis in the leg eased and surgery was not necessary.

Grateful that his leg was saved, Hans started to eat macrobiotically at home with the rest of the family. Soon he was back on his feet again, but at work, he continued to observe the usual German diet. As the manager of a large mine that supplied stone to the construction industry, he held an important position and was expected to socialize with his co-workers. However, one day, Hans announced that he would bring his lunch to work. Despite isolation and ridicule by other workers, he stuck to his decision.

Meanwhile, Hildegard had become the center of a growing network of macrobiotic activities in Frankfurt. Except for stiffness in one finger, her rheumatism and arthritis had completely disappeared. Her iron count, calcium levels, and other mineral and blood levels had all returned to normal. In addition to giving cooking classes and informal dietary consultations, she organized seminars for visiting macrobiotic teachers from other parts of Europe and America.

Both Uli and Jorg attended the Kushi Institute in Amsterdam, and Uli worked at Manna Foods, a large macrobiotic food company. In the basement of the family's three-storied stone house in suburban Frankfurt, Uli set up a small tofu and tempeh factory with the help of his brother. Using the highest-quality organic and natural ingredients, they began to produce about 300 cakes of tofu and 100 packages of tempeh in a typical workday.

Later that year, Hans retired from the stone quarry and decided to manage his wife and sons' activities. The new company was named Atlantis and expanded to distribute brown rice, miso, shoyu, and other macrobiotic staples. "In addition to delivering to food stores and restaurants, we deliver tempeh and tofu to one of the big banks in Frankfurt," said Hans, who handled all of Atlantis's finances and deliveries.

Sharing the same food and dream, the Lilienthal family became much closer together than ever before. "Growing up, I was very weak and withdrawn," Uli observed. "Before, I might communicate with my father only once every three months even though we were living in the same house. Now we talk and work together every day. Family relations all around are much better."

One of the macrobiotic teachers who regularly came to Frankfurt to lecture and give seminars was Adelbert Nelissen. Adelbert first became active in macrobiotics in the late 1960s, when he was organizing demonstrations in his native Holland against the war in Vietnam. Since then, he and his wife, Wieke, along with their five children, devoted all their activities to spreading macrobiotics in Central Europe. They founded Manna Foods, which became one of the largest natural foods manufacturers and distributors in Europe, employing about fifty people in their warehouse and bakery in Amsterdam. They also published translations of macrobiotic books and established the Ost-West Zentrum in Amsterdam, which housed a restaurant, administrative offices, consultation rooms, and martial arts facilities. Beginning in 1980, Adelbert directed the Kushi Institute there as well, offering macrobiotic programs and cooking classes in both Dutch and German.

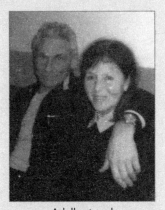

Adelbert and
Wieke Nelissen.

At a Peace Symposium in Frankfurt organized by the Lilienthals, Adelbert explained his own transformation from a leader of protest marches to a macrobiotic teacher. "I have become much more peaceful since I stopped eating meat and sugar. When we eat the same way, we are cooperating with each other, not against each other. By eating grains and vegetables, we add to and complete each other. I found that in conversation, I respond to the other person by saying 'and' rather than 'but.' With meat and sugar, coffee and other modern foods, there is a strong desire to compete and win. I realized that in fighting for peace I was fighting for power and control. I was very angry and exclusive.

"All movements have this in common: they don't change personally. They all feel, 'I am right, you are wrong.' However, our thinking, feelings, and beliefs are constantly changing. Our mind changes something like the temperature. We are hot or cold depending on our own condition, our level of activity or exercise. It's very relative.

"On the other hand, we often get stuck. When our bloodstream becomes full of fat and mucus, our thinking as well as intestines becomes constipated. We can't concentrate, can't hear, can't remember, can't express, and can't envision. We become preoccupied and don't react naturally. We feel attacked. Our stagnation creates frustration, and we project our fears onto others. Mind and body can't understand each other. Man and woman can't understand each other. East and West can't understand each other. This is the root cause of war.

"A tragic example of this occurred here in Germany. Hitler was a vegetarian, but he ate mostly sugar, fruits, and drugs. He didn't understand the ancient swastika symbol with its intersecting arms. He didn't understand balance. He was a sugar addict and received regular injections of amphetamines. He went mad and became attracted to very meaty people. Like wild animals, the Nazis became possessive and territorial, cruel and destructive.

"In post-war Germany, everyone has relatives in the eastern and western halves of the country. The feeling of family unity is still very strong. My hope is that macrobiotics will eventually take root in East Germany and lead to mutual understanding. Germany is the intellectual and spiritual center of Central Europe, and the dialectical tradition of Goethe, Hegel, and Marx is still very strong here. Macrobiotic teachings of yin and yang, based on a deeper understanding of dialectics as well as family unity, could appeal to the East Germans."

In the early 1980s, macrobiotic teachers in Western Europe began to make contact with interested individuals and small groups in Poland, East Germany, and Czechoslovakia, and lectures and cooking classes started in Romania and Yugoslavia. In Eastern Europe, it is difficult to get information about any foreign ideology or movement, and the state-run economy is oriented to meat and dairy products, so grains, beans, and vegetables are often in short supply. Macrobiotic literature was translated into Russian and distributed in parts of Moscow and Leningrad.

The Lilienthals, the Nelissens, and thousands of other macrobiotic families in Europe spread a way of life that, following the collapse of Communism, helped reunify a divided continent, and ushered in a bright new era of peace and harmony between the Eastern and Western blocs. Over the next twenty-five years, Adelbert and Wieke Nelissen continued to develop macrobiotic education throughout Europe, the Middle East, and other regions. Along with colleagues in America and Europe, they developed the Ideal Food Pattern—a clear, concise graphic presentation of the standard macrobiotic diet—and lay the foundation for *Macropedia*, an online encyclopedia. Unfortunately, Adelbert passed away suddenly in 2014 at age sixty-five year after an exhausting cycling trip, and *Macropedia* remains to be completed. But he left behind a strong legacy and bright vision of the future.

Sources

Alex Jack, visit to Germany, October 1985.

Amberwaves (Winter 2015).

Uli Lilienthal, personal letter, March 1986.

11.

Increased Violence
in the Twenty-First Century

O ver the last generation, conflict, violence, and war have continued to spread through many once peaceful societies. As the Spiral of History (see Chapter 7) reaches a climax, the pace of life is accelerating, all boundaries are dissolving, and everything is converging. All familiar institutions are breaking down: the family, the church, the school, the hospital, the brick-and-mortar store, the union, even the nation-state. Age-old concepts of race, sex, gender, the consciousness of plants and animals, and the relation of mind, body, and spirit are in flux. Advances in communication, transportation, and other areas of life have wrought tremendous changes for the better, including the Internet, cell phones, jet travel, and other extraordinary useful and efficient devices and technologies. At the same time, they have led to widespread anxiety, confusion, and chaos, as well as increased physical, mental, and emotional imbalance. The sections in this chapter discuss the reasons for and trends toward increased violence and war in the early twenty-first century.

THE SPREAD OF NUCLEAR WEAPONS AND POWER

With the end of the Cold War, the threat of global thermonuclear war greatly lessened. It did not disappear, however, as the Crimea crisis showed. In 2014, Russian President Vladimir Putin seized the Ukrainian province and forcibly incorporated it into the Russian Federation. In turn, economic sanctions and other countermeasures by NATO (the North Atlantic Treaty Organization), the U.S., and the European Union threatened to internationalize a regional conflict. The downing of a civilian airliner further heightened tensions, and the world faced a possible nuclear confrontation for the first time since the Cuban Missile Crisis a half-century earlier. The following year, the deployment of Russian troops and planes to Syria intensified big power involvement in the Middle East and the risk of an armed clash.

Similarly, the explosive rise of extremist Islamic terrorism after 9/11 increased the likelihood of a nuclear "suitcase" or "dirty" bomb. Such an event could destroy a city and set off a chain of retaliatory measures by the United States,

Israel, or other targeted states whose arsenals include even greater weapons of mass destruction.

Nuclear energy itself continued to spread worldwide, with no effective way to safeguard against accidents, sabotage, or the leakage of radioactive waste. As the Fukushima disaster in Japan in 2011 showed, a single nuclear accident imperiled a modern industrial economy and released harmful fallout that encircled the world.

The manufacture of nuclear warheads and bombs and their conversion into fuel for electricity have generated enormous amounts of nuclear waste. As of 2016, it was estimated that there were over 15,000 nuclear weapons in the world. Other sources of harmful, potentially lethal radiation include uranium tailings, depleted uranium (recycled in weaponry), medical waste (high in cobalt-60 and other deadly isotopes), and food irradiation (widely used on spices and other foodstuffs).[1]

According to proponents of nuclear energy, one person's lifetime nuclear waste would fit in a Coke can. This claim is technically true but misleading. Once the atomic genie has been released into the environment, it is impossible to put it back into the bottle. As the Department of Energy (DOE) states, there are "millions of gallons of radioactive waste" as well as "thousands of tons of spent nuclear fuel and material" and also "huge quantities of contaminated soil and water."[2]

The DOE launched an ambitious campaign to clean up all contaminated sites by 2025. In Fernald, Ohio, for example, there were 31 million pounds of uranium product; 2.5 billion pounds of waste; 2.75 million cubic yards of contaminated soil and debris; and a 223-acre portion of the underlying Great Miami Aquifer with uranium levels measuring above drinking standards in the year 1989, when the site shut down. In total, the United States has over 100 similar sites, some encompassing thousands of acres.[3]

Safe storage and disposal of nuclear waste remains one of the most intractable problems of modern society. "Considering we have only had 10,000 years of written history, we must realize how long future generations will suffer from the onerous legacy left by present societies," stated Wolfgang Gründinger of the Foundation for the Rights of Future Generations. "Only a few decades of using nuclear energy leave hazardous nuclear waste for an unimaginable number of future generations."[4]

NEW VIRAL EPIDEMICS

HIV, the Ebola virus, and other deadly viruses emerged in Central Africa in the 1970s and 1980s following major changes in agriculture and regional food patterns. Chemical farming, including the use of pesticides and fertilizers, substantially increased, and traditional natural and organic farming decreased. New hybrid seeds with higher yields began to replace traditional open-pollinated varieties. Commodity crops and monocultures (the growing of only one crop in a space) replaced wild polycultures (the raising of multiple crops in the same space). Clearing of forests for agriculture or urban development and advances in mining also involved the introduction of new chemicals and unsustainable techniques. These changes increased yields and raised living standards, but at a long-term cost to human health and the environment. They upset the delicate checks and balances in the soil biota and in local ecosystems, as well as in the microflora in the intestines, giving rise to virulent new strains of microbes (including Marburg virus, Ebola virus, HIV, Zika, and others).[5]

This syndrome is not unique to Africa. Ebola also appeared on farms in the Philippines in 1989. In South America, herbicides introduced into the pampas in the 1950s altered the ecology, leading to the emergence of the corn mouse—the carrier of a deadly new virus that produced Argentine hemorrhagic fever (AHF), a disease similar to Ebola. In Central Africa, widespread poverty, sickness, and cultural decline in the colonial and post-colonial eras led to the decline of traditional agriculture and of diets based on brown rice and millet as staple foods. Cassava, a root crop imported from South America to Africa in the sixteenth century and traditionally consumed as an emergency crop during periods of famine and scarcity, became a principal food. Brown or lightly polished rice also gave way to white rice and highly refined grain products. Increased intake of animal protein, dairy food, and sugar, as well as other commodity crop foods such as bananas, coconut, palm oil, and coffee, further led to the decline of native diets and decreased health and vitality.

Following independence from Belgium, France, and Britain in the 1950s and 1960s, social problems and epidemic disease continued throughout Africa, including widespread hunger, political instability, malaria, tuberculosis, sickle-cell anemia, and other infectious or wasting conditions. Well-meaning international relief efforts (including the donation of foods high in sugar, white flour, powdered milk, etc.) saved lives, but resulted in nutritional deficiencies and a further decline in health and well-being. Mass vaccination campaigns had a similar impact, protecting people in the short run but weakening their resistance to disease over time. The constitutional strength and conditional vitality of Central Africans steadily declined. After coming into contact with animals infected with Ebola virus, SIV (Simian Immune-deficiency Virus, the precursor to HIV), and other pathogens—or eating contaminated bush meat—people in this region acquired natural immune deficiency, and Marburg (1967), Ebola (1976), AIDS (1981), and other lethal diseases took hold and began to spread.

Central Africa is also a major site of uranium; during the Cold War, the United States and Soviet Union competed aggressively for resources from Zaire (the former Belgian Congo) to replenish their nuclear arsenals. Mining, transport of radioactive materials, and accidental release of toxic materials further weakened the population. A similar catastrophe was experienced by the Navajo in the desert Southwest. As a result of these trends, diminished health, vitality, and consciousness gave rise to further political, economic, and social instability across Central Africa in the 1980s, 1990s, and early 2000s. Following a legacy of slavery and colonialism, agribusiness, mining, and deforestation contributed to widespread upheaval, including civil war, disputes over blood diamonds and other conflict minerals, and genocide. By the early twenty-first century, Africa, the cradle of humanity, was transformed into a graveyard. The entire region became ground zero, or the epicenter, for a historical spiral that imperils human survival on the planet.

RISE IN SCHOOL SHOOTINGS

Another trend in recent years has been the alarming increase in school shootings and other mass violence against students, teachers, and the general public. While there have been isolated cases of community violence in past decades, the Columbine High School massacre in 1999 marked a turning point. It was the first mass killing in double digits (leaving fifteen dead and twenty-one injured). Since then, there have been over 150 other school shootings, as well as mass murders in movie theaters, shopping malls, and other locales. Highly publicized massacres in Russia, Germany, Norway, and other countries are part of this trend. Many factors have contributed to this dramatic rise in school and community violence, including increased availability of guns, dysfunctional homes, violent movies and video games, drugs and medications, and bullying.

Medications, especially SSRIs (Selective Serotonin Reuptake Inhibitors), have been associated with violence and aggression. From 1988 to 1994, and 1999 to 2000, the use of these powerful drugs to treat depression and anxiety tripled. Thirty-eight million young people alone worldwide were prescribed Prozac, one of the most popular drugs in this category, since it was first introduced in 1988. In the U.S., 10 million children are on psychiatric drugs for depression or to treat educational and behavioral problems. These medications alter brain chemistry, elevating mood for some patients, but lowering it for others. According to the Diagnostic and Statistical Manual of Mental Disorders (DSM) IV, the most authoritative source of diagnostic information for mental health professionals, "All antidepressants can cause mania" which is a "potentially psychotic condition of intense mental and emotional excitement."[6] Feelings of invincibility, extreme power, farfetched and elaborate plans, as well as the urge to commit violence, often accompany this condition. In 2004, a federal panel of drug experts warned that antidepressants "could cause children and teenagers to become suicidal."[7] Ed Harris, one of the Columbine shooters, was being treated with Luvox, an SSRI medication. Another teen, Jeff Weise, upped his dosage of Prozac in the week before killing nine people and himself. Joseph Wesbecker, another Prozac user, shot and killed eight co-workers. The deadliest American mass shooting, at Virginia Tech, was committed by Cho Seung-Hui, who reportedly took medication for depression before slaying thirty-two people. Dr. David Healy, a British psychiatrist and author of *Let Them Eat Prozac*, estimates that 90 percent of school shootings are linked to SSRIs.

Serotonin, a hormone associated with relaxation and well-being, is modulated by SSRI and other mood-altering drugs. Lack of serotonin causes insomnia, over thinking, anxiety, and worry. Though linked with the brain in popular psychology, serotonin is produced in the large intestine and 90 percent of the body's supply is located in the digestive tract, where it regulates intestinal movement. The remainder is located in the central nervous system, where it regulates mood, appetite, and sleep, as well as memory and learning.

Serotonin is naturally produced by grains, beans, nuts, seeds, and other plant foods. Conversely, stimulants, refined carbohydrates, and excessive animal protein adversely affect its levels. White rice, white flour, sugar, coffee, turkey, eggs, and similar substances give a temporary rush of serotonin, but then block its effects. It is far preferable to treat depression, anxiety and other symptoms of low serotonin with dietary adjustments and modification than with psychiatric drugs.

THE GMO THREAT

Genetically modified organisms (GMOs) are another potential trigger for sudden, explosive violence. Genetically modified foods were introduced in 1996, and over the next decade, GMO soy, maize, cottonseed, and canola oil displaced up to 90 percent of their conventional counterparts. Combining the nuclei of different species is extremely difficult, as nature resists the artificial combining of genomes. Genetic engineers unsuccessfully tried physical, chemical, and biological means. Finally, at the University of California at Davis, scientists developed a "gene gun" to combine the DNA of two species. Specially designed guns were fitted with microbullets containing the DNA-coated gold particles of the novel species. The gene gun was then fired at high velocity into a petri dish containing the DNA of the target or host species. Only in this way were scientists able to combine nucleic material.

From an energetic view of "you are what you eat," we absorb not only the nutrients, DNA, and other physical components that we ingest—we also take in the food's *Ki*, or life energy, including the waves, vibrations, and other influences of its environment. Hence, eating factory farmed beef, pork, and chicken exposes us not only to saturated fat, animal-quality protein, and rapid growth, but we also take in the fear, sorrow, hopelessness, and other emotions the animals experienced while confined or caged in the factory right up to slaughter.

Similarly, when we consume GMO food or ingredients, we absorb the violent energy from the gene gun that gave birth to that particular line of altered foods. The explosive discharge, blast, searing heat, and pain that went into the seeds or target DNA in the petri dish is replicated and passed on to future generations of GMO plants. Compare that energy with the peaceful, gentle energy of natural seeds growing in the earth.

An estimated 75 percent of all processed supermarket foods contain transgenic soy, corn, or cotton ingredients. Most nonorganic beef, pork, chicken, fish, and other conventionally-grown or farmed animal products also contain GMO corn, soy, or cotton used in livestock feed. Milk and other dairy products are widely made with bovine somatotropin (BST), a genetically-engineered growth hormone. No studies have been done on the possible relationship of GMOs to the rise of school, workplace, and family violence, but the timing of the introduction of GMO foods in the mid 1990s and the rise in school shootings in America coincide. It is highly probable that the young men in the tragic cases mentioned above regularly ingested GMOs in breakfast cereal, bread, meat, chicken, milk, and other ordinary staples, and they may have contributed to or tipped the balance of serotonin in the brain and gut.

Recently, some biotech foods have been developed with novel viral DNA that is inserted or spliced into the soybean, corn, or other target species. The novel species are designed to give herbicide resistance or another such benefit to the plant or animal being modified. In these cases, altered foods are still potentially violent and explosive. For example, in 2015, the World Health Organization designated glyphosate—the active ingredient in Monsanto's Roundup Ready herbicide—a probable carcinogen (a substance that can cause cancer). Many scientific and medical studies have concluded that GMOs contribute to toxicity and liver troubles, allergies and other respiratory problems, digestive ills, and reproductive abnormalities.[8] The negative emotions associated with these conditions are frustration and anger (originating in the liver); sadness and depression (lungs and intestines); anxiety and mistrust (spleen, pancreas, and stomach); mania (heart and circulatory); and fear, paranoia, and lack of will (kidney and reproductive). All of these can contribute to a violent mind or behavior.

In addition to soy, corn, cotton, and rapeseed, several additional foods have recently been genetically engineered. These include beet sugar (that now comprises a majority of the sugar used in the United States), alfalfa (fed to livestock), and papaya (in Hawaii). Potatoes and apples have also been approved by the U.S. Department of Agriculture, and salmon—the first GMO animal—has been approved but, as of 2016, has not been released, pending a labeling controversy in Congress. Thirty-five other animals, including cows and pigs, are in development. The introduction and spread of GMO seeds, crops, and foods in the U.S. and around the world represents one of the gravest threats to human health and well-being and to the natural evolution of our species.

In 2015, two-thirds of Europe announced plans to ban GMOs after the EU agreed to let its twenty-eight individual countries and regions opt out of producing genetically-engineered foods. The nineteen countries included Austria, Bulgaria, Croatia, Cyprus, Denmark, France, Germany, Italy, Hungary, Greece, Latvia, Lithuania, Luxembourg, Malta, Netherlands, Poland, and Slovenia, as well as Scotland, Northern Ireland, and Wales and Wallonia in Belgium. Russia also prohibited cultivation of GMOs, and Pope Francis questioned them in his encyclical *Laudato Si,* warning that transgenic food was contributing to the spread of oligopolies, global warming, and other environmental destruction.

ELECTROMAGNETIC FIELDS

The electronics and digital revolutions reach into every aspect of our lives. The vast majority of people on the planet today have a cell phone, as well as access to a refrigerator, stove, computer, MP3 player, radio, car, and other consumer goods and products that are electronically linked to satellites, high-voltage towers, and Wi-Fi networks. The artificial electromagnetic radiation from all of this activity saturates the globe. In most big cities, turn your tablet or smartphone on and you will discover you are in range of a dozen or more mobile networks. Virtually everywhere we go, we are subject to spy satellites that listen in to our phone calls, tags on products that emit radiation whenever we shop, and GPS signals that track our every movement. The artificial energy we are exposed to is staggering.

The latest generation of motor vehicles is one of the leading sources of EMFs (electromagnetic fields). In addition to built-in wireless devices such as GPS, Wi-Fi, and keyless entry, the engine and wiring create large magnetic fields in most current vehicles. Most homes have a background level of 1 to 3 milligauss of radiation. New cars measure about 10 milligauss. Electric and hybrid cars typically have six times higher magnetic fields than non-electric or non-hybrid vehicles.[9]

Electricity distribution lines and electrical wiring in walls create EMFs in homes, offices, stores, and other structures. About a third of the electricity circulating is lost while it loops between the transformer on the street and the building. Commonly, this leakage electrifies the water and the ground underneath, which is a good conductor and serves to attenuate electrical and magnetic fields.

Food cooked with microwave radiation, another ubiquitous feature of modern life, is particularly unhealthy. "Atoms, molecules, and cells hit by this hard electromagnetic radiation are forced to reverse polarity 1 to 100 billion times per second," pediatrician John Kerner and colleagues at Stanford University explained in an article in *Pediatrics.* "There are no atoms, molecules, or cells of any organic system able to withstand such a violent, destructive power for any extended period of time, not even in the low energy range of milliwatts."[10] In 1992, researchers at the Swiss Institute of Technology tested macrobiotic subjects who consumed microwaved food and reported a sharp decline in blood quality and immune function. Changes included a decrease in hemoglobin, an increase in hematocrit and leukocytes, higher cholesterol, and a decrease in lymphocytes. The microwaved food also increased the activity of certain bacteria in the food, and altered cells resembled the pathogenic stages that occur in the early development of some cancers. After objection by the food industry, the study was withdrawn from the scientific journal in which it appeared.[11]

Radio transmitters in walls, shelves, floors, and highways read microchips hidden in consumer products and credit cards. These embedded devices are known as Radio Frequency Identification (RFID) tags. Tires now have chips that measure highway speed, and airports scan the chips in the soles of travelers' shoes. RFID chips are also woven into many clothes and are scanned by marketers to profile their customers. Checkout counters scan merchandise, and cell phones now include apps that track steps, walking and running distance, and other health data.

Hospitals and medical centers are another major contributor to EMFs. Medical tests such as the CT scan, X-ray, magnetic resonance imaging (MRI), mammogram, and ultrasound, as well as treatments such as pacemakers, diathermy, and chiropractic lasers, all scan organs, functions, tissues, and cells.

From airport security checks to routine checkups at the doctor, from streaming movies to Smart Boards in school and university, we are bombarded with artificial radiation that takes a tiny, but cumulative toll on our health and psyche. The long-term effects of EMFs are unknown. There simply hasn't elapsed enough time to know what impact a smartphone or tablet will have over the course of an average lifetime, much less its genetic effects on the next generation.

Apple, Google, Microsoft, Amazon, and other giants in the digital field make tens of billions of dollars in revenues each year. But aside from gross toxicity tests, the IT industry has sponsored little if any comprehensive research on the impact of these new technologies on human health and the environment. Like GMOs, which also have no effective oversight, EMFs represent a vast, uncontrolled experiment on our species that may have dire, long-range results. Small, independent studies suggest that the global vanishing of the bees may be caused, in part, by EMFs, and that wild animals exposed to power lines and microwave towers also suffer widespread death and disability. But as a society, we don't want to know. The Siren song of instant messaging, unlimited playlists, cloud computing, and must-have apps may be luring us to our doom.

Conditions linked to EMFs include Alzheimer's disease, anxiety, attention deficit disorder, asthma, autism, birth defects, blood spasms, brain fog, cataracts, chronic fatigue, headache, macular degeneration, miscarriage, neuropathies, rashes, sleep problems, thyroid problems, and tinnitus. EMFs can affect all tissues of the body, leading to direct DNA damage, oxidative impairment, and disruption of neurotransmitters, cell division, signaling, metabolism, enzyme function, and protein synthesis.

Ionizing radiation can cause cancer, especially leukemia, lymphoma, and thyroid cancer. An EPA report originally designated EMFs as a class B1 carcinogen, the same as cigarettes, in 1990.[12] From an energetic perspective, EMFs are not always the primary cause of these ailments, but they are often major contributing factors.

GLOBAL WARMING AND CLIMATE CHANGE

Global warming has emerged as one of the greatest threats over the last generation. The earth has warmed about 1.4 degrees Fahrenheit since 1880, causing the average global sea levels to rise 8 inches. The rate of warming is also rising. The last two decades of the twentieth century were the hottest in 400 years. Eleven of the twelve years between 2004 and 2015 were among the dozen warmest years since 1850.[13] Arctic ice is disappearing rapidly, imperiling polar bears, seals, and other animals. Coral reefs face massive die-offs because of warmer waters. The seasons no longer follow an orderly sequence, and erratic weather is commonplace. Extreme weather events are on the rise, including wildfires, heat waves, tornadoes, and strong tropical storms. In California, the worst drought in 500 years reduced snowmelt in the Sierra Nevadas to 2 percent of normal, threatening agriculture in the Sacramento Valley (center of organic rice production in North America).

Twenty to 40 percent of all plant and animal species face extinction in coming decades because of temperature shifts affecting patterns of migration, food resources, photosynthesis, and other interrelated factors. Snowmelt in the Himalayas threatens the rice crop in India, China, and Southeast Asia that sustains billions of people, potentially leading to widespread hunger and famine. Aridity in Africa, Australia, and elsewhere endangers staple foods in those regions, and fresh drinking water will be scarce everywhere.

Anthropomorphic activity, beginning with the Industrial Revolution, is the principal cause of rising temperatures over the last 150 years. Fossil fuels are the chief cause of rising greenhouse gases, including carbon dioxide (CO_2) from petroleum, coal, and natural gas. Transportation, manufacturing, and other smokestack industries are main contributing factors. But as *Livestock's Long Shadow*—the landmark report of the United Nations' Food and Agricultural Organization (FAO)—concluded, the modern food and agricultural system is the biggest contributor to greenhouse gases. Eighteen percent of all fossil fuel use goes into producing beef, chickens, dairy food, processed sugar, and other high-energy foods. "This is a higher share than transport [which accounts for 13 percent]," the report concluded. In other words, production of processed foods accounts for about 40 percent more fossil fuel use than the energy used for all the cars, trucks, buses, trains, ships, and planes combined. The meat industry is "one of the . . . most significant contributors to the most serious environmental problems, at every scale from local to global [including] problems of land degradation, climate change and air pollution, water shortage and water pollution, and loss of biodiversity."[14]

Another sizable percentage of the energy used in society is indirectly linked to food in the form of refrigeration and air conditioning (as meat heats up the body more than plant foods), trips to the supermarket or restaurant in the family car, and other related costs. Taking these other factors into account, the Worldwatch Institute and other environmental groups estimate beef, dairy, and other animal food production causes as much as 51 percent of carbon, methane, and other atmospheric buildup. Conversely, a macrobiotic or vegan-oriented diet would eliminate about 60 to 90 percent of this fossil fuel use. It would also produce substantially more grains, beans, and other staples that could be used for direct human consumption and thus reduce poverty, hunger, and starvation.

At the 2015 international climate conference in Paris, the modern food pattern was the elephant in the room. As the nations of the world convened to prevent global warming, the single greatest cause of climate change was conspicuously ignored. The modern energy-dense way of eating is also a major cause of terrorism. Yet not a word about a plant-based diet or organic agriculture—the clear, simple, sustainable solution to the crisis—appeared in the final Paris Agreement. Commitments to reducing emissions from the livestock sector appeared in only twenty-one of the 120 national plans submitted in advance of the gathering. None called for a reduction in meat eating. On the eve of the conference, the U.S. announced that the 571-page Scientific Report of its own Dietary Guidelines Advisory Committee, linking the standard American diet with environmental destruction and climate change, would not be on the table.

The French hosts of the conference, meanwhile, arranged special cuisine to facilitate diplomacy that ironically raised CO_2 levels. As *The New York Times* reported, "At the French climate conference, negotiators from the United States, China, Russia, and India are dining together over duck confit, boeuf (beef) bourguignon, and French wines."

Despite this myopia, the Paris Agreement was historic. For the first time, the planet came together and adopted goals to limit the use of fossil fuels and mitigate the worst consequences of climate change.

Yet as 2015 ended, with Russia's military intervention in Syria, the flight of millions of refugees into Europe, and the deadly massacres in Paris and San Bernardino, a golden opportunity to address the paramount issues of our era now converging was missed. In the shadow of the French conference, fear, anger, and suspicion rippled around the world, and the war on terror moved to the forefront of the 2016 U.S. presidential election.

In 2014, the Pentagon reported that climate change posed an immediate threat to national security, with enhanced risks from terrorism, infectious disease, global poverty, and food shortages. It also predicted increased demand for emergency military disaster responses as extreme weather creates more global humanitarian crises. "Destruction and devastation from hurricanes can sow the seeds for instability," Defense Secretary Chuck Hegel observed. "Droughts and crop failures can leave millions of people without any lifeline, and trigger waves of mass migration."

Nowhere has this more evident than in the Middle East, where drought, the collapse of the wheat harvest, and competition for scarce water resources have contributed to the rise of extremist groups like ISIS. From 2006 to 2011, 60 percent of Syria experienced one of the worst droughts and severe crop failures in history.

In Hassakeh, a province in the northeast, three-quarters of wheat and other crops failed, and herders lost 85 percent of their livestock. During this period, according to the United Nations, nearly 1 million Syrians lost their livelihoods and flocked to Damascus and other cities to find food and work. Already burdened by a large Iraqi refugee population, the Assad regime was unable to cope with the massive influx of displaced persons. Its authoritarian nature and response only aggravated an unmanageable situation.

Similar patterns in other Arab countries contributed to the Arab Spring in Tunisia, Egypt, and Libya. Twelve of the world's fifteen highest water-scarce countries are in the Middle East: Syria, Algeria, Libya, Tunisia, Jordan, Qatar, Saudi Arabia, Yemen, UAR, Kuwait, Israel, and Palestine. In Libya, the number of "drought days" per year is projected to rise from more than 100 to 200—an enormous and potentially devastating increase whose impact is already contributing to the economic, political, and social chaos and hundreds of thousands of climate refugees fleeing to Europe.

"Young people [in the Middle East] have gone to big cities looking for work," notes Bill Nye, an expert on global warming and author of *Unstoppable: Harnessing Science to Change the World.* "There's not enough work for everybody, so the disaffected youths, as we say—the young people who don't believe in the system, believe the system has failed, don't believe in the economy—are more easily engaged and more easily recruited by terrorist organizations and then they end up part way around the world in Paris shooting people."

Record-breaking heat waves, floods, and droughts in other key wheat-growing countries, including Ukraine, Russia, China, Canada, and Australia, "contributed to global wheat shortages and skyrocketing bread prices," according to Oxford University geographer Troy Sternberg. Global wheat prices doubled from $157 per metric ton in June 2010 to $326 per metric ton in February 2011. Wheat is the major staple in the Middle East, used for pita bread, couscous, bulgur, and other basics. The steep rise in wheat prices caused average food expenditures to rise from about 10 to 35 percent of household income, further contributing to malnutrition, poverty, illness, family conflict, and social unrest. Of the world's major wheat importing countries, nine are in the Middle East. Following the sharp spike in wheat prices, seven of these nations had political upheavals resulting in civilian deaths.

In Saudi Arabia, internal unrest has largely been averted by funding radical Islamist movements outside the country. Twenty years ago, the Saudis prided themselves in being food self-sufficient when they used their fabulous oil wealth to tap an aquifer deep beneath the desert to produce irrigated wheat. However, most of the water is now gone, and the country no longer grows much grain. Instead, the kingdom is investing in farmland in Sudan and Ethiopia that is endangering water from the Nile River Delta, making it more vulnerable to sea level rise and saltwater invasion. With the world price of petroleum at record lows and North American oil production at record highs, the desert kingdom may be in for a rude awakening as its coffers run dry.

The birth rate in the Middle East is also a worrisome factor. As of 2015, one-third of the population is under fifteen years old. By 2030, it will more than double. The region also has the fastest growing rate of diabetes and other chronic diseases in the world. With the influx of hamburgers, soft drinks, and other convenience foods, children as young as seven are now contracting adult-onset diabetes for the first time anywhere in the world.

As the major players in the region face off—including the U.S., Russia, Turkey, Iran, Saudi Arabia, Israel, ISIS, Hamas, and Hezbollah—diet, fossil fuels, climate change, and terrorism are emerging as the four modern horsemen of the apocalypse.

Though not quite as extreme as in the Middle East, a similar dynamic prevails in Mexico and other parts of Central and South America. The Intergovernmental Panel on Climate Change (IPCC) Fourth Assessment Report found that a rapidly changing climate will lead to the replacement of tropical forest by savannas along with replacement of semi-arid vegetation by arid vegetation in most of central and northern Mexico. In tropical forests, species extinctions are likely, including 2 to 18 percent of mammals, 2 to 8 percent of the birds, and 1 to 11 percent of the butterflies. The iconic Monarch butterflies that winter in Mexico are especially endangered. Coastal vegetated wetlands are also at risk from rising sea levels.

However, the major catalyst for social unrest in Mexico has been NAFTA, the North American Free Trade Alliance. The 1994 pact deregulated all agricultural trade except for corn and dairy products. As a result, the U.S. government subsidized large corporate farms by $25 billion per year. Maize prices in Mexico plummeted, affecting millions of family farmers who were unable to compete with imported corn.

Over 60 percent of the cultivated land is planted with maize, and 18 million Mexicans rely on corn for their livelihood. One of three tortillas is now made with U.S. corn, including increasingly GMO corn that threatens native heirloom species as well as further weakens public health. The end result is that hundreds of thousands of rural families have flocked to Mexico City for food, work, and shelter. In most cases, they have found only poverty, disease, prostitution, and employment with murderous drug gangs. Another half-million food and/or climate refugees cross the border into the U.S. illegally every year.

Similar scenarios are playing out in the Carpathian Region, encompassing Croatia, Hungary, Slovakia, Czech Republic, Poland, Ukraine, Romania, and Serbia. Heat waves have become more frequent, longer, and more severe over the last generation. A rise in humidity resulting in flooding is projected for the Carpathian area, while southern and southeastern Ukraine may experience lengthy droughts and desertification of vast territories.

In the short run, wheat yields in Ukraine (the "breadbasket" of Europe) will rise because of mild warming. But in the long run, climate change will have a disastrous impact. GDP is forecast to drop, insect infestation will rise, and fertility of the soil will be damaged by erosion and desertification as the climate becomes more arid. Droughts in the country have already led to decreased production of buckwheat, potatoes, beetroots, cucumbers, cabbage, and other staples. Water shortages are frequent.

Amid the political and economic turmoil in the region, Monsanto, Dow, and other biotech companies have invested hundreds of millions of dollars in Ukraine, with a clear goal of making it a new hub of GMOs in Europe. The EU and NATO generally support this trend. In retaliation, Russia has prohibited genetically engineered foods and promoted organic agriculture as a solution to personal and planetary health.

Throughout the world, it is much the same story. In Asia, massive flooding and droughts (from a decrease in snowmelt in the Himalayas) are having a devastating impact in Bangladesh, India, China, and other countries. In Africa, drought and desertification across much of the Sahel threaten traditional agricultural and pastoral livelihoods, contributing to urban congestion, poverty, illness, civil war, and the massive flow of migrants. In the United States, Hurricanes Katrina and Sandy, widely attributed to extreme weather events and climate change, resulted in catastrophic economic damage and loss of life.

Global warming and climate change are also taking a large toll on the modern diet. The vitamin and mineral content in most common garden vegetables and fruits has declined by 25 to 50 percent in the last generation.[15] Similarly, the percentage of macronutrients has also altered. According to a groundbreaking study of the effect of rising CO_2 levels on the global food supply, protein and nitrogen concentrations are down up to 25 percent in wheat, rice, and other major staples, mineral and trace element content has fallen 8 percent on average in 130 common crops, and carbohydrate content has soared from 10 to 45 percent. The dramatic increase in starch and sugar content may be the main cause of "hidden hunger" (a lack of nutrients in the food people eat) and the global obesity epidemic.[16] The end result is people today have to eat more food than ever before to stay fit and healthy. Researchers conclude climate change is one of the primary causes of the overweight and obesity epidemic. Today, two out of three adults and one out of three children in America and other modern societies are overweight or obese. There are many factors contributing to this trend, including a more sedentary way of life, exposure to EMFs that affect the thyroid and hence alter metabolism, and supersize portions of food. But global warming may be a leading factor. Since this impact is widely unrecognized, even by nutritionists, virtually all food labels and nutritional data are obsolete. Food manufacturers, sellers, restaurants, schools, and other institutions that prepare nutrient profiles and plan menus and recipes accordingly typically rely on U.S. government food composition data that do not account for these nutrient declines.

As for violence and war, as we have seen earlier, studies show that conflict, violence, and war are more prevalent in hotter temperatures and climates and during extreme weather conditions. In a study examining the link between local climate variations and civil conflict, *Nature* journal found that the rate of armed conflict doubled—from 3 to 6 percent—during El-Nino related climate swings.[17] In *Tropic of Chaos: Climate Change and the New Geography of Violence,* Christian Parenti contends that climate change is amplifying historic crises all over the world. In this "belt of economically and politically battered post-colonial states girding the planet's mid-latitudes," writes Parenti, "the current and impending dislocations of climate change intersect with the already-existing crises of poverty and violence."[18]

Another study, "Heat in the Heartland: Climate Change and Economic Risk in the Midwest," found that "Rising heat is also one factor in higher violent crime rates, with as much as a 6.4 percent increase in crime likely (and a 1-in-20 chance of more than a 8.1 percent increase) in the Minneapolis-St. Paul metro area by the end of the century." The study made similar predictions for Indianapolis, Dayton, St. Louis, Columbus, Cincinnati, Chicago, and other urban areas.

With the start of the Cold War, the *Bulletin of the Atomic Scientists* journal created a "Doomsday Clock" estimating how close the world was to nuclear annihilation. The original clock was set to seven minutes before midnight in 1947. In the decades since, experts have periodically reset the clock—e.g., forward during the Cuban Missile Crisis and back following the collapse of the Soviet Union. With the rise of global warming, the clock was set to three minutes before midnight in 2015, the closest to doomsday since 1984.[19]

CONFLICT MINERALS

Another widely unrecognized cause of violence and conflict is competition over scarce or rare metals. In Central Africa, civil war and strife have claimed the lives of millions of people over the last generation. At the heart of the genocide is a struggle for control over mining and the lucrative trade in gems and scarce resources. The United Nations and governments, including the United States, have instituted laws prohibiting the trade in "blood diamonds" and most recently "conflict minerals." These include tin, tantalum, tungsten, and gold from parts of the Democratic Republic of Congo and neighboring countries. These strategic metals are used by companies worldwide to make medical devices, cell phones, airplanes, machine tools, and other consumer and industrial goods. Almost all of these indispensable materials are slated to run out in the next couple decades, driving prices—and the propensity to violence and war—sky high.

Ordinary metals are also a cause for alarm. In the Persian Gulf, a Japanese ship carrying zinc and lead was seized by Somali pirates in 2008. In Britain, theft of scrap metals from railroads increased by 500 percent in 2010. In Philadelphia, 2,500 manhole covers and sewer grates were stolen in 2007 as scrap metal prices soared.[20]

THE LONG WAR

In *The Shield of Achilles: War, Peace, and the Course of History,* Philip Bobbitt traces the history of combat and conflict resolution and contemplates the future. He characterizes the major conflicts of the twentieth century as a Long War that extended from World War I in 1914 through World War II, the Korean War, and the War in Vietnam, to the end of the Cold War in 1990.[21] He envisions the Long War as a single global conflict waged over the form the nation-state would take: communist, fascist, or parliamentarian. Today, he suggests, even the nation-state is obsolete, rapidly being replaced by the market-state, a geopolitical order that promises to maximize the opportunity of individual citizens rather than the material well-being of nations. It is a quantum shift to a new world order based not on territoriality but on opportunity and access. Its sudden arrival on the international scene is like the change from brick-and-mortar stores and heavy manufacturing industries to digital ecommerce and information technologies. The emerging market-state is privatizing many state activities and making representative government more responsive to the market.

In a subsequent book, *Terror and Consent: The Wars for the Twenty-First Century,* Bobbitt describes the rise of outlaw states (such as the Islamic caliphate) as the mirror image of the market-state, capitalizing on the borderless nature of globalization and the faceless commerce of online communication. Through the Internet, outlier states and networks can communicate anonymously, use social media to obtain new recruits, plan terrorist attacks, and wage cyberwar.

Unfortunately, Bobbitt's solution—including an effective counteroffensive using increased electronic surveillance, enhanced interrogation, and other extrajudicial procedures—is not as insightful as his analysis, and only perpetuates a dualist "us/them" mentality.

SUMMARY

In the twenty-first century, we have witnessed firsthand the spread of nuclear weapons and violence, new diseases, and school shootings. Genetically modified foods and electromagnetic fields are becoming more pervasive in everyday life. As these and other troublesome trends suggest, as we reach the very center of the historical spiral, forms of violence and war in the early twenty-first century are rapidly mutating. They potentially affect every individual, family, community, and region of the planet as a whole and will present humanity with very different challenges than any time in its long past.

PEACE PROMOTER

Michio Kushi and Martha Cottrell, M.D., New York

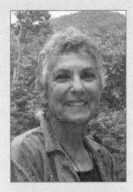

Martha Cottrell

Arrogance, greed, exclusivity, hate, anger, prejudice, and discrimination—the common defects of the human race—are directly connected with war. What makes such minds? Since coming to the United States, I have learned to center my thoughts and feelings by living a more natural way of life and eating whole, unprocessed foods. In the span of thirty-five to forty years, I rarely experienced anger. However, an observation caused me to become very angry inside for the first time in many years. I couldn't control my feelings regarding some health professionals and community leaders who treated young men with AIDS—Acquired Immune Deficiency Syndrome—as untouchables. Although these people were supposed to help others, they were afraid that they would become contaminated from contact with people with AIDS. At the time, it was thought that AIDS was highly contagious and incurable. Many hospital personnel wore heavy protective masks and gloves when dealing with AIDS people. Employers dismissed them, landlords evicted them, and even their own friends and family often treated them as lepers. Of course, here and there, a few people—including some doctors and nurses, some relatives and friends—treated AIDS people compassionately, though many of them were powerless to reverse the course of their illness.

I became very sad about the AIDS situation and decided to help. Beginning in the summer of 1983, I went to New York City every month or every other month to meet with AIDS friends and lecture about macrobiotics and natural order. I explained to them that AIDS is essentially a degenerative blood and lymph disorder, resulting from long-time disorderly and chaotic eating and living. It is not primarily a viral or bacterial disorder, though certain strains of microorganisms may activate the spread of the disease once the blood and lymph systems have become weakened through years of dietary abuse. From my observations, it was apparent that AIDS friends tended to eat cheese, sugar, chocolate, and greasy, oily foods of all kinds. In almost all cases, they had not been breastfed and thus lacked the natural immune factors found in mother's milk. In many instances, they had also taken drugs or medications for many years, and many had hepatitis. I explained that if they changed their way of eating and recovered an orderly way of living, there was nothing to worry about. Brown rice and other whole grains, miso soup, fresh vegetables, beans, fish, and other whole, unrefined foods—well balanced and carefully prepared—would strengthen their blood quality, and their condition would naturally stabilize and even possibly clear up. I impressed upon them that like other sick people, they were not victims. They were responsible for creating their sickness and now they were responsible for relieving it—peacefully.

In Greenwich Village, we set up cooking classes and about 200 to 300 men attended. Although we usually met in a very dark place because no one wanted to lend us their space, we introduced a balanced way of eating. We sang songs together and talked about strengthening the mind and spirit through difficulties and adversity. In the beginning, the AIDS people were amazed that I would shake hands with them, hug them, touch their bloody eruptions, and never wash my hands. Some of the AIDS friends came back with me to Boston, and soon they were in the kitchen helping prepare dinner with my wife, Aveline, for our household. Gradually, in New York and Boston, the men began to change their blood quality and their immune systems began to stabilize or improve. After several months, Dr. Martha Cottrell, the medical director of the Fashion Institute of Technology in New York, along with physicians in Boston, started monitoring their condition. The results—including the ratio of normal to abnormal T-cells and other blood values—indicated that slowly but steadily, some AIDS friends were stabilizing their condition. In May 1986, medical researchers at Boston University reported that the average survival time of AIDS friends eating macrobiotically had surpassed any known control group (thirty-one months vs. twenty-nine months). Many friends in the homosexual and heterosexual communities began to work together to educate the public on the relation of diet and AIDS, and a lasting solution to this disease may be on the horizon.

Several years later, I collaborated with Dr. Cottrell in writing *AIDS, Macrobiotics, and Natural Immunity* (New York: Japan Publications, 1990), and she became one of the leading macrobiotic teachers and counselors. In her late eighties, she writes and teaches in Ashville, North Carolina, where she lives as part of the macrobiotic community.

Source

Kushi, Michio. "Symposium on AIDS and Diet." Lecture at Boston University, Boston, MA, May 23, 1986.

12.

Diet and the Decline
of Violence

The threat of global catastrophe rose sharply in the twentieth century. The development and spread of nuclear weapons and energy; the rise of terrorism; the introduction of industrial chemicals and toxins; the spread of artificial electromagnetic fields, pesticides and GMOs, and psychiatric medicines; and the rise of global warming and climate change imperiled life on earth. How we meet these challenges will decide the future of our species. Paradoxically, at the same time that the threat of global annihilation has increased, daily life for most individuals and families living in many countries is safer and more peaceful today than ever before. As a plant-based diet spreads around the world, we can expect the planet to gradually turn away from violence and war.

DECLINE IN WAR BRUTALITY

In *The Better Angels of Our Nature: Why Violence Has Declined,* Steven Pinker, a cognitive scientist at Harvard University, contends that the Human Rights Revolution of the last several centuries has led to a dramatic decline in violence against blacks, children, women, gays, and other historically marginalized or abused groups.

Tribal warfare was nine times as deadly as war and genocide in the 20th century. The murder rate of Medieval Europe was more than thirty times what it is today. Slavery, sadistic punishments, and frivolous executions were unexceptionable features of life for millennia, then suddenly were targeted for abolition. Wars between developed countries have vanished, and even in the developing world, wars kill a fraction of the people they did a few decades ago. Rape, battering, hate crimes, deadly riots, child abuse, cruelty to animals—all substantially down.

How could this have happened, if human nature has not changed? What led people to stop sacrificing children, stabbing each other at the dinner table, or burning cats and disemboweling criminals as forms of popular entertainment? The key to explaining the decline of violence is to understand the inner demons that incline us toward violence (such as revenge, sadism, and tribalism) and the better angels that steer us away. Thanks to the spread of government, literacy, trade, and cosmopolitanism, we increasingly control our impulses, empathize with others, bargain rather than plunder, debunk toxic ideologies, and deploy our powers of reason to reduce the temptations of violence.[1]

In support of his thesis, Pinker reviews many historical, medical, psychological, and sociological sources and new research. While television is frequently decried today for its mindless, violent content, he cites a study in the *Archives of Childhood Diseases* that traditional nursery rhymes—the main childhood entertainment in times past—contained fifty-two scenes of violence per hour compared to 4.8 on TV today. *Grimms' Fairy Tales*, as well as Snow White, the Punch and Judy puppet show, and Mother Goose, he reminds us, are saturated with gore and bloodshed.

Deaths in warfare and homicide have substantially gone down in the modern era compared with times past. The twentieth century was an era of genocide, mass famine and starvation, and other catastrophes. But the actual percentage of people affected by these horrendous events was larger in the Middle Ages and early modern era. The Crusaders murdered 1 million Jews on the way to Jerusalem and then millions of Muslims in the ancient Holy Land. The Spanish Inquisition killed an estimated 500,000 Jews and Conversos, many by burning alive. The Aztecs sacrificed an estimated 1.2 million persons to the sun god between 1440 and 1524. The Thirty Years' War (1618–1648) between Protestant and Catholic Europe led to 5.75 million deaths. The percentage of casualties in the English Civil War (1642–1651) was greater than in World War I, when Britain lost the flower of its young men to trench warfare and futile campaigns like Gallipoli. The Taiping Rebellion in China, a civil war against the ruling Manchus in the mid-nineteenth century, resulted in 20 million deaths, one of the deadliest military conflicts in history.

From the seventeenth century on, the rise of Enlightenment values in Europe, the American Revolution, and other early democratic movements dramatically improved the quality of life and lessened violence. Capital punishment was abolished for petty offenses, torture and mutilation were largely prohibited, slavery was gradually ended, and animal welfare, including vegetarian and antivivisection movements, gained in popularity.

Since the end of World War II, Pinker asserts, the world has enjoyed the longest peace since the Roman Empire. Conscription (war drafting) is down 50 percent around the world. Battle deaths are down 90 percent. Unlike most empires that ended in violence, the Soviet Union peacefully self-destructed. The rise of terrorism, though shockingly brutal and murderous, has killed or injured only a relatively small number of people as a whole—on average, 2,500 per year worldwide since 1998, which is about 10 percent of the annual highway fatalities just in the U.S.

At a community level, rape in the U.S. fell 80 percent between 1973 and 2008. Corporal punishment halved between 1975 and 1992. Assaults against children, including kidnappings, fell between one-half and two-thirds between 1990 and 2007. Crime rates, too, have fallen sharply. In New York, once the murder capital of the country, homicide rates dropped 80 percent from the 1990s to the 2010s. Compared to traditional societies, the homicide rate in modern society is substantially less (see Figure 12.1 below).

What is to account for these dramatic changes over the last generation? Pinker cites the civilizing influence of commerce, science and technology, and rising IQs. The only mention of food or diet in his 800-page book is a brief section endorsing the conventional, now outmoded view that meat played a crucial role in human evolution and was largely responsible for our anatomical structure, strength, sociability, and intellect. Except for pointing out the corrosive effects of alcohol in sparking violence, predominantly in men, Pinker ignores the biological or spiritual roots of health and well-being, including the effects of specific foods on consciousness and the emotions. Curiously, he devotes a large part of his survey to looking at brain chemistry and specialized regions of the central nervous system that have been linked to competitiveness, aggression, and violence. But other than theorizing

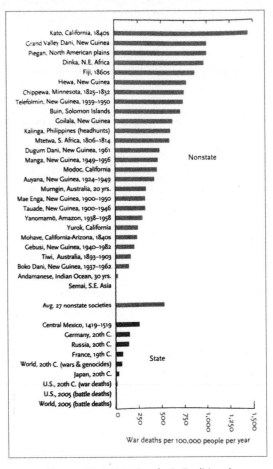

Figure 12.1. War Deaths in Traditional and Modern Society.

that some violent traits are genetic and passed on from parents to children, he doesn't look systematically at what influences neurological differences or how food affects what Abraham Lincoln called "the better angels of our nature." Still, the book makes a strong case that violence has diminished exponentially in recent centuries—and especially over the last generation—for most individuals, even as the threat of collective or global catastrophe has heightened.

SAPIEN JOURNEY

Sapiens: A Brief History of Humankind by Yuval Noah Harari offers another account of our species' steady conquest of violence and war. An Israeli historian, Harari challenges the view that human ancestors lived peacefully in harmony with nature. All around the world, he shows, ancient people slaughtered and drove to extinction animals and plants. In North America, native people hunted to extinction thirty-four of forty-seven genera and in South America fifty of sixty genera of large mammals, including saber-tooth tigers, giant ground sloths, native horses and camels, giant rodents, and mammoths. The Maoris in New Zealand, Arctic tribes, and other tribal societies also engaged in relentless destruction of native flora and fauna. The violence against animals carried over to violence within human society. In contemporary New Guinea, violence accounts for about 30 percent of male deaths. In Ecuador, up to 50 percent of adult Waoranis meet a violent death from fellow tribesmen. In contrast, the world average for urban society is 1.5 percent, according to Harari's 2015 commentary.[2]

Harari contends that the Agricultural Revolution—the trend toward wheat cultivation that began around 11,000 years ago—"kept more people alive under worse conditions." Although violence declined by about half, the average farmer "worked harder than the average forager and got a worse diet in return." Farming led to food surpluses and to the rise of elites dominated by kingship and priesthood. The stratification of society into clans, castes, and classes gave rise to property, money, and then guards, police, and armies to defend land and possessions. Monocropping proved vulnerable to crop losses, leading to periodic famine and disease.

As an aside, the oldest clay tablet that names an individual curiously bears the name of Kushim. The writing appears on an account of an inventory of barley in Uruk, an ancient Sumerian city on the Euphrates and the capital of Gilgamesh, the Babylonian epic hero. In family tradition, the ancestors of the Kushi family, my forebears, came from Sumer. In the Bible, Kush was the eldest son of Ham and grandson of Noah, and the Kushites lived in the land of Kush, believed to be on either or both sides of the Red Sea.

There are other resonances with *Sapiens* and our approach. In a breathtaking narrative, Harari traces the accelerating pace of history in terms similar to the Spiral of History: "As time went by, the conquest of knowledge and the conquest of territory become ever more tightly intertwined." "History is moving relentlessly toward unity," he observes. "The sectioning of Christianity and the collapse of the Mongol Empire are just speed bumps along the way." Although the world is still divided by religious, ethnic, and racial classifications, "today almost all humans share the same geopolitical system (the entire planet is divided into internationally recognized states); the same economic system (capitalist market forces shape even the remotest corners of the globe); the same legal system (human rights and international law are valid everywhere, at least theoretically); and the same scientific system (experts in Iran, Israel, Australia and Argentina have exactly the same views about the structure of atoms or the treatment of tuberculosis.)"

Money is the historical motor of trade, commerce, peace, and tranquility, Harari argues. However, he concedes, as Marx and Engels showed, money has a dark side. It is impersonal and heartless. "The first religious effect of the Agricultural Revolution was to turn plants and animals from equal members of a spiritual round table into property." More recently, free-market capitalism led to the slave trade and the oppression and suffering of tens of millions of people to provide sugar for "sweet tea and candy" in England and its colonies. Since the Industrial Revolution, "plants and animals were mechanized. Farm animals stopped being viewed as living creatures that could feel pain and distress, and instead came to be treated as machines."

"Today humankind has broken the law of the jungle," Harari continues. "There is at last real peace, and not just absence of war." Although there is a sharp decline in violence against other humans, global warfare has ended, and large-scale famines have been eliminated, "modern industrial agriculture might well be the greatest crime in history."

Similar to many of the chapters in this book, *Sapiens* demonstrates how ideology largely governs modern society. Laws, money, gods, and nations, the author asserts, have no objective reality. Though imaginary, they are "intersubjective." So long as people believe in them, they work and constitute the vibrational foundation of civilization.

The last part of *Sapiens* envisions the future. Again, similar to our model, Harari foresees the trend toward bionization and psychonization, or the introduction of artificial body parts and technological mind altering. "We stand at the brink of becoming true cyborgs, or having inorganic features that are inseparable from our bodies, features that modify our abilities, desires, personalities, and identities." In general, he sees this trend as positive and waxes eloquent about genetic engineering and the "law of natural selection being replaced by the law of intelligent design." He also believes "the road to the perfect medicine stands before us." Still, he is undecided where the momentum of history is leading. "We are consequently wrecking havoc on our fellow animals and on the surrounding ecosystem seeking little more than our own comfort and amusement, yet never finding satisfaction."

In the end, *Sapiens* opts for a secular, quasi-Buddhist solution to humanity's ills by mastering our cravings for creature and consumer comforts. Deeply sympathetic to the plight of animals, Harari yearns for a prehistoric animism in which "there is no barrier between humans and other beings. They can all communicate directly through speech, song, dance, and ceremony." Though nonreligious himself, he extols a "polytheism that is inherently open-minded and rarely persecutes 'heretics' and 'infidels.'"

Of the many contemporary books on human nature, *Sapiens* comes closest to intuiting the pulse of history and the alternating yin/yang eras of development by territoriality and force and universalization by idea or knowledge. Food plays an essential role in its narrative, and from the beginning this chronicle recognizes that "not withstanding the popular image of 'man the hunter,' gathering was Sapiens' main activity, and it [plant food] provided most of their calories, as well as raw materials such as flint, wood, and bamboo... In most places and at most times, foraging provided ideal nutrition. That is hardly surprising—this had been the human diet for hundreds of thousands of years, and the human body was well adapted to it."

FOOD CHANGES

From a macrobiotic perspective, the decrease in violence and war in modern society is directly related to changes in our way of eating. In the first edition of this book, we looked at the pulse of history and the positive and negative trends through 1980. Since then, the biggest biological, social, and spiritual change on the planet has been the transition from an animal- to a plant-centered diet. At a societal level, this change began with *Dietary Goals of the United States*, the landmark 1976 report of the U.S. Senate Select Committee on Nutrition and Human Needs that linked six of the top ten causes of death with the modern diet and a "wave of overnutrition" that was as dangerous to human health and longevity as malnutrition.[3] The McGovern Report, as it came to be known, sent shock waves through the scientific-medical community and the nation as a whole, leading to the Food Guide Pyramid in 1992. The Pyramid, with grains at the foundation of the recommended diet, replaced the Basic Four food groups guide, which included meat and dairy food as the superior sources of protein in the American diet.

As the guidelines accompanying the Pyramid suggested: "Use plant foods as the foundation of your meals. There are many ways to create a healthy eating pattern, but they all start with the three food groups at the base of the Pyramid: grains, fruits, and vegetables. Eating a variety of grains (especially whole grain foods), fruits, and vegetables is the basis of healthy eating. Enjoy meals that have rice, pasta, tortillas, or whole grain bread at the center of the plate, accompanied by plenty of fruits and vegetables . . ."[4]

Every five years, the Pyramid has been revised and inspired similar high-fiber, low-fat grain-vegetable-fruit-based guidelines by governments and medical organizations around the world. By 2000, whole grains replaced grains as the preferred form of cereal products; tofu, tempeh, and other high-protein soy foods were recommended; and a vegan diet that completely avoids all animal foods, including dairy food, was deemed healthful (even without vitamin supplementation). In 2015, the advisory committee recommended that foods be labeled according to their impact on planetary health as well as personal health. By this yardstick, grains and other plant foods lead to up to 90 percent more benefits to the air, soil, water, and wildlife than animal foods. The advisory report concluded:

> The major findings regarding sustainable diets were that a diet higher in plant-based foods, such as vegetables, fruits, whole grains, legumes, nuts, and seeds, and lower in calories and animal-based foods is more health promoting and is associated with less environmental impact than is the current U.S. diet. This pattern of eating can be achieved through a variety of dietary patterns, including the Healthy U.S.-style Pattern, the Healthy Mediterranean-style Pattern, and the Healthy Vegetarian Pattern. All of these dietary patterns are aligned with lower environmental impacts and provide options that can be adopted by the U.S. population. Current evidence shows that the average U.S. diet has a larger environmental impact in terms of increased greenhouse gas emissions, land use, water use, and energy use, compared to the above dietary patterns. This is because the current U.S. population intake of animal-based foods is higher and plant-based foods are lower, than proposed in these three dietary patterns.[5]

According to the U.S. government, the following changes in per capita intake of major foods have taken place over the last generation:

TABLE 12.1 CHANGE IN PER CAPITA FOOD CONSUMPTION, 1980–2009.*			
	1980	**2009**	**CHANGE**
Red meat	124	106	Down 16%
Chicken	32	56	Up 75%
Milk	28 gallons	22 gallons	Down 27%
Cheese	18	33	Up 83%
Fats and oils	57	79	Up 39%
Flour and cereals	145	195	Up 34%
Caloric sweeteners	120	131	Up 11%
Fruits and vegetables	588	708	Up 20%

* Pounds consumed annually per capita
Source: U.S. Census Statistical Abstract of the U.S., 2012

Organic food has exploded over the last generation in the U.S., Europe, and other modern societies. In 2014, 45 percent of the American people bought organic foods on an occasional or regular basis. Brown rice consumption increased 41 percent between 2006 and 2011. Almost all the natural foods that the macrobiotic community introduced in the 1960s to 1980s have now gone mainstream. Supermarkets today sell brown rice, millet, and other whole grains; miso, tofu, and tempeh; daikon, shiitake, and other Far Eastern vegetables; and shoyu, sea salt, sesame oil, and other seasonings and condiments. Even seaweed is beginning to make inroads, and many grocery stores today have fresh sushi counters or packaged sushi to take out, as well as nori for those who want to make it at home.

From an energetic view, the decline in American meat consumption is the most significant trend. Yang governs yin, and a reduction in meat, eggs, and other heavy animal foods leads to corresponding declines in extreme yin intake. Reduced intake of saturated fat, dietary cholesterol, refined sugar, and other highly processed foods has further led to declines in chronic and degenerative diseases. According to U.S. Mortality Data, the rates of major causes of death have dropped dramatically since 1960 (see Table 12.2 below).

TABLE 12.2 DECLINE IN DEATHS FROM CHRONIC DISEASE, 1960–2009.*				
DISEASE	**1960**	**2009**	**CHANGE**	**LIVES SAVED ANNUALLY**
Heart disease	559	180	Down 68%	1,137,000
Cancer	194	174	Down 10%	60,000
Strokes	178	38.9	Down 78%	417,300
Diabetes	22.5	20.9	Down 7%	4,800
Liver disease	13.3	9.2	Down 31%	12,300
Pneumonia	53.7	16.2	Down 70%	112,500
Accidents	62.3	37	Down 41%	75,900
Suicide	12.5	11.7	Down 6%	2,400

* Deaths per 100,000 people (age-adjusted to the 2000 US population)
Source: Centers for Disease Control and Prevention, "Fifty Years of Progress in Chronic Disease Epidemiology and Control," 2011

While there are many factors contributing to this decline, including better medical detection and treatment; a sharp decline in smoking; and improved socioeconomic conditions, especially for blacks and other minorities, a shift from an animal to a plant-based diet lies at the heart of this trend and in turn shapes and influences these co-factors as well.

Unfortunately, this positive direction is offset by an opposite trend in the developing world. As Third World countries become more affluent, they eat richer food, and their rates of chronic disease are climbing, surpassing those in developed countries. In China, for example, meat consumption between 1989 and 2009 soared 58 percent.[6] Today, cancer is the leading cause of death in China, followed by heart disease and stroke. Along with dietary changes, the country's alarming air pollution from coal-fired industries, chemicals used in manufacturing, and other toxins is a major factor in increased illness and mortality.

END OF THE COLD WAR

The pivotal dietary changes that took place in the early 1980s, 1990s, and up to the present may have contributed to the ending of the Cold War. In March 1985, President Ronald Reagan was diagnosed with colon cancer. The National Cancer Institute had just reported that radiation therapy and chemotherapy were ineffective and in some cases produced toxic side effects as follow-ups to surgery in the treatment of cancer: "Except possibly in selected patients with cancer of the stomach, there has been no demonstrated improvement in the survival of patients with the ten most common cancers when radiation therapy, chemotherapy, or both have been added to surgical resection."[7] The ten most common cancers are lung, colorectal, breast, prostate, uterus, bladder, pancreas, stomach, skin, and kidney. Shortly after the report was published, its author, Dr. Steven A. Rosenberg (the NCI's chief of surgery), operated on President Reagan's colon cancer and, instead of chemotherapy or radiation treatment, put him on a predominately plant-based diet.

Meanwhile, macrobiotic food was prepared at United Nations functions by Laura Masini, who had recovered from breast cancer with the help of macrobiotics and who served as hostess for her brother, Vernon Walters, the U.S. ambassador to the U.N., who was a bachelor. In Washington, Blande Keith, wife of a former Republican congressman from Massachusetts, was also influential in introducing macrobiotics to the Reagan family and staff of other government officials. Over the years, many governors, senators, congressmen, and heads of state came to me or other macrobiotic teachers or counselors for advice, especially when cancer struck themselves or their families.

Nancy Reagan, the president's wife, was also interested in nutrition and holistic healing. She secretly arranged for President Reagan to go on a trip to Germany for treatments with laetrile, a nutritional therapy based on the active ingredient in apricots. Laetrile has proved effective in treating some cancers, but had been banned in the United States.[8]

Not only did the more plant-based dietary approach help Reagan recover from cancer, but it made him more peaceful. Until this time, he had been a hardliner toward the Soviet Union, characterizing it as an "Evil Empire" and threatening to escalate the nuclear arms race with an expensive anti-ballistic missile shield from coast to coast. Meanwhile, the U.S.S.R. was going through major changes under new President Mikhail Gorbachev. In November 1985, several months after Reagan's surgery, the two heads of state met for the first time in Geneva. In October 1986, they met in Reykjavik, the capital of Iceland, where they concluded the agreement that would effectively end the Cold War between the two superpowers. Commentators were astonished at Reagan's willingness to make such a sweeping accord. From a macrobiotic view, it is clear that the change in eating released stagnation and blockages from the past and allowed Reagan to adopt a more conciliatory approach and keep a calm, peaceful mind. His often-quoted aphorism, "Trust but verify," was a commonsense response that won approval by both sides.

Some years later, during the Clinton presidency, Bill Clinton enjoyed cheeseburgers, French fries, and other fast food. But his high-cholesterol, high-fat diet eventually took a toll, and he underwent multiple surgeries for heart disease. The first was a quadruple bypass to restore blood flow to his heart, and the second involved implanting two stents to open one of the veins from the bypass surgery.

In the White House, the Clintons were introduced to shiatsu and a healthy way of eating by Patrick McCarty, a macrobiotic teacher and counselor in Orlando. After leaving office, Clinton gave up all animal food and became vegan on the advice of his physicians. He replaced hamburgers with soy burgers and gave up dairy food, as well. In the years since, he lost weight, regained vitality, and led an active life as head of the Clinton Global Initiative.

While campaigning for his wife, Hillary, Bill acknowledged that his plant-based diet "changed my life. I might not be around if I hadn't become a vegan. It's great." Following further medical advice, he widened his way of eating to include organic salmon once a week, but observed, "I'd just as soon be without it. The vegan diet is what I like the best. . . . I have more energy, I never clog. For me the no dairy thing, because I had an allergy, has really helped a lot. And I feel good."

The forty-fourth president of the United States, Barack Obama, eats organically (although not vegetarian). His wife Michelle started an organic garden on the White House grounds. His Administration had been vigilant against terrorism but reluctant to engage in the open-ended wars of his predecessors or use the violent, combative rhetoric of victory. On the Republican side, Dr. Ben Carson, a longtime vegetarian, ran for president in the 2016 election and attracted widespread support because of his calm, peaceful demeanor.

SUMMARY

In the coming years, as a plant-based way of eating continues to spread, we can expect it will have a further moderating and stabilizing effect on world leaders as well as the general public. In this way, the planet is moving toward a healthier, more peaceful, and sustainable future.

PART III

Transforming Ourselves and Society

In her days, every man shall eat in safety,
Under his own vine,
what he plants;
and sing the merry songs of peace
to all his neighbors.

—SHAKESPEARE

13.

Preventing Violence and Mechanical Thinking

There are many traditional accounts of the relation among food, conscious-ness, and behavior. In the late nineteenth century, six Zuni Indians from the American Southwest accompanied anthropologist Frank Cushing on a visit to Boston, where they were wined and dined at the Palmer House, one of the city's best hotels. According to Cushing, the Indians "suffered, literally, miseries untold" from the new food. After one meal, one of the elders exclaimed, "What is it in American food, my son, that fills the insides with much fighting?" For the rest of the journey, the Indians dined on dried corn that they had brought for just such an emergency.[1]

In the modern world, mental and psychological problems—including violent and aggressive behavior—are approached as though they were independent from physical problems. As we see in traditional philosophy and medicine, the approach to mental problems is not separate from the approach to physical prob-lems. Physical sicknesses are immediate causes of mental disturbances, and men-tal troubles immediately affect the physical condition. Mental and physical problems are two different manifestations arising from the same root: a dishar-monious way of life, including the habitual practice of improper diet, and a lack of balance in mental and physical activities.

From an energy point of view, everything we take in from our environment may be classified as food. In the human body, the digestive system and the nervous sys-tem perform complementary antagonistic functions. The digestive system is rela-tively simple, open, and hollow in structure, while the nervous system is highly complex, diverse, and compact. The more expanded (yin) digestive system breaks down and absorbs physical food—the most condensed or material (yang) form of energy. Meanwhile, the more contracted (yang) nervous system, especially the brain, processes information or "mental food" from the surrounding environment in the form of vibrations—the most expanded or nonmaterial (yin) form of energy.

If our digestive system is sluggish or overworked, there is a corresponding decline or impairment in our ability to perceive and assimilate information from the environment. This is especially true when we eat too much food, when we eat poor quality food, or when we eat food that is not appropriate for the climate we live in, the season of the year, our level of activity, or other personal conditions and needs. At these times, our alertness drops, our perception dulls, our memory fades, and our responses to the environment are erratic or confused. Conversely, if our digestion is proceeding smoothly, we respond to our surroundings intuitively, spontaneously, and appropriately. If we skip a meal or fast occasionally, the clarity of mind, inner calm, and determination that we need to accomplish what we set out to do are direct benefits of resting overburdened digestive functions.

THE ORGANS AND EMOTIONS

Food is energy, vibration, and movement. The body is composed of and restructured by food. Food simultaneously creates physical and psychological manifestations. If we change our physical condition, psychological changes result almost immediately. If we change our psychological conditions, physical changes can come about, although this takes much longer.

In Oriental medicine, it has been traditionally known that each major organ in the body is connected with mental, emotional, and spiritual manifestations and that each organ is nourished by special kinds of foods (see Table 13.1 on page 207). For example, liver dysfunctions, arising from excess sugar or fat consumption, can produce a volcanic release of energy that we call violence. High blood pressure; irregular heartbeat; hardening of the coronary, cerebral, or peripheral arteries; and other types of cardiovascular disease can result in exaggerated, impulsive behavior or rigid, compulsive thinking and activity, depending upon the form the disorder takes. An overworked spleen can lead to deterioration in blood quality along with corresponding feelings of a lack of resourcefulness. When the blood is well oxygenated, the brain performs at its maximum potential. If the alveoli of the lungs are covered with fat and mucus, less oxygen is available to the higher cerebral centers, resulting in heaviness, dullness, and indecision. Colonic disorders, meanwhile, can lead to improper elimination of bodily wastes and toxins, producing corresponding mental and psychological blockages. Overactive or underactive kidneys produce feelings of insecurity that can find outlets in either aggressive or passive behavior. The foods we eat affect our metabolism, subtly influencing our mood and behavior.

DIET, CRIME, AND DELINQUENCY

In modern society, millions of schoolchildren suffer from chronically low blood sugar as a result of excessive consumption of sugar, soft drinks, desserts, fruits and juices, tropical foods, and other refined and chemicalized foods, together with overconsumption of poultry, eggs, cheese, and animal fat. They are often labeled "hyperactive," "learning disabled," or even "retarded." Millions of others suffer from some degree of poor coordination, speech disorders, perceptual-motor impairments, or low task performance. The problems of these children are often ascribed to familial, social, psychodynamic, or other causes; however, the underlying origin of their problem is usually dietary—an imbalance in blood

	TABLE 13.1 FOOD AND THE EMOTIONS.			
	HEALTHY FUNCTIONING		**UNHEALTHY FUNCTIONING**	
ORGANS	**PRODUCES**	**NOURISHED BY**	**PRODUCES**	**NOURISHED BY**
Liver, gallbladder	Patience Endurance Adventure Creativity	Whole grains Wheat and barley Leafy green vegetables Miso soup Pickles Sour foods Naturally fermented foods	Short temper Anger Violence Cruelty Stubbornness Narrowmindedness Rigidity	Meat Eggs Poultry Dairy White flour Fat and oil Sugar Sweets Alcohol
Heart, small intestine, brain	Gentleness Cooperation Tranquility Intuition Spiritual unity Merry, humorous expression	Whole grains (especially red millet and corn) Expanded leafy green vegetables Burdock Wakame Kombu Bitter foods	Separation Excitement Nervousness Agitation Excessive laughter or speech Impulsiveness Rigidity	Fat and cholesterol Sugar Sweets Excessive fruit and juice Tropical foods Coffee Refined oil Alcohol Chemicals
Stomach, spleen, pancreas	Sympathy Wisdom Consideration Understanding	Whole grains (especially yellow millet) Squash Onions Cabbage Round vegetables Naturally sweet foods	Irritability Criticism Skepticism Worry Jealousy Envy	Meat Eggs Butter Fat Cheese Milk Oil Sugar White rice Alcohol
Lungs, large intestine	Happiness Security Wholeness Unity	Whole grains (especially brown rice) Broccoli Cauliflower Lotus root Daikon Ginger Scallions Other pungent foods	Sadness Depression Indecision Fragmentation Overanalysis Confusion Weakness	Meat Eggs Poultry Dairy Oil White flour Spices Drugs Tobacco
Kidneys, bladder, reproductive organs	Confidence Courage Inspiration	Whole grains (especially buckwheat) Azuki and other beans Sea vegetables Spring water Unrefined sea salt Miso Naturally salty foods	Fear Defensiveness Hopelessness Low self-esteem Aloofness Coldness	Fats Oil Meat Dairy Poultry Sugar White flour Juice Excessive liquid Cold foods Refined salt and oil Drugs and medication

chemistry that directly affects their perception, understanding, attitude, and behavior. Millions of adults also suffer from hypoglycemia. Medical studies show that many of the mentally ill have chronically low blood sugar levels.

It used to be that medical doctors would treat hypoglycemia by advising their patients to eat sugar cubes, because sugar temporarily raised blood sugar levels. Physicians have since become aware that this only aggravates the problem and have generally advised those with this disorder to avoid or reduce sugar. Other therapists and nutritionists have treated this condition with vitamin and mineral supplements, as well as prescribed mental, emotional, and physical exercises to restore balance. While all of these steps will help erase symptoms of low blood sugar, from a macrobiotic point of view, the underlying cause of hypoglycemia is not sucrose and other simple sugars. Rather, it is the lack of stabilizing complex carbohydrates, particularly whole cereal grains, together with an overconsumption of more yang foods—eggs, meat, poultry, cheese, and others. To balance these more contracted foods, the body automatically seeks out sugar, sweets, alcohol, coffee, and other more yin foods. Simply eliminating the excessive yin items can often alleviate immediately obvious symptoms; but unless the underlying cause for the attraction to those items is eliminated, the hypoglycemia will continue to worsen and eventually express itself in other ways.

Alcohol and drug abuse are the most obvious consequences. Alcohol, marijuana, cocaine, hallucinogenic drugs, amphetamines, and other mood-altering drugs work to offset the effects of low blood glucose in the short run. However, in the long run, they badly destabilize glucose tolerance and weaken the entire organism.

Hypoglycemia itself creates a dim but pervasive feeling of desperation and urgency; depending upon the individual's particular dietary pattern, conditions of upbringing, social environment, and other factors, this may turn inwardly (creating a worsening self-image) or outwardly. In this case, the feelings of aggressiveness and general hostility can eventually erupt into a pattern of violent or criminal behavior. This outwardly-directed explosion of pent-up energies is caused by the expansive volatility of extremely yin foods like sugar, tropical fruits, alcohol, or drugs on top of extreme yang foods like meat, eggs, and poultry.

In the case of low blood sugar, the body's chronic lack of resources to meet immediate energy needs is experienced as lack of confidence in one's own abilities and as dependence on others. When basic vitality and faith in one's ability to keep up with the environment (including the household, school, or workplace) are absent, cheating or stealing from others or society is commonly the result. Imbalance takes a more aggressive form in direct proportion to the amount of animal food consumed. The liver, which governs the temporary storage and release of excessive blood sugar, can become inhibited by accumulations of fatty tissue, leading to the desire to be in complete control of the environment and explosive discharges of blocked energy. In some cases, imbalance can lead to fear and the belief that a gun, knife, or other weapon is needed to protect oneself from the environment. Studies have indicated that juvenile offenders or adult criminals have an abnormally high rate of hypoglycemia—about 80 to 85 percent.[2]

A change to a healthier way of eating can quickly restore blood sugar levels to normal, contributing to smooth mental and physical functions. Proper blood quality, including normal blood sugar levels, is essential to developing self-esteem and taking responsibility for one's conduct and behavior. A multitude of recent studies has demonstrated the effectiveness of a whole foods diet in modifying consciousness and improving behavior. Many of these studies have been carried out in prisons and other correctional institutions where violent and aggressive behavior is a way of life.

LOSS OF VISION AND DREAM

In modern society, the overwhelming majority of people experience some form of mental or psychological disorder. As our behavior becomes more destructive and self-destructive, our judgment and intuition deteriorate. Our vision of life and its possibilities dims, and we rely more and more on experts and authorities to tell us how to live. Our modern nutritional standards, for example, derive originally from laboratory studies of the amount of animal protein consumed by Prussian males in the nineteenth century—a diet that contributed to two devastating world wars. As this imbalanced way of eating continues, our vitality decreases and we rely increasingly on technology to perform simple tasks that we can no longer perform ourselves. Finally, we begin to look at the cosmos as a machine—impersonal, unfeeling, interchangeable. We see ourselves as victims or innocent bystanders in an alien world over which we have no control. We perceive that it is too difficult to understand the workings of our own bodies and too complex to solve the problems of war and peace. We take less and less responsibility for our personal sicknesses and the problems of society, leaving these to specialists, who are all too willing to assume control.

Instead of complex carbohydrates—whole cereal grains, vegetables, and fresh fruits—we consume the majority of our foods in the form of refined carbohydrates and hard, saturated fat. Today, petroleum—and its synthetic byproducts in food, medicine, clothing, transportation, building materials, and home furnishings—has become the modern staff of life. We have taken the germ out of the wheat and the rice, and the superstructure of modern civilization mirrors that separation and incompleteness. We no longer respect the integrity of what we eat nor the fruits of our own bodies. The low value we place on human life is a consequence of this biological decay. In the last half-century, the fertility of the land and the people has been severely depleted. As our ability to grow wholesome crops and give birth naturally declines, the only thing that keeps many of us going is the biological heritage of our ancestors. We are living off the fossil fuels, so to speak, stored in the DNA bequeathed to us by strong, hardworking parents and grandparents whose diet consisted of large amounts of whole grains and other fresh foods. That loss—the substitution of sugar and other refined carbohydrates for complex car-

Whole Foods and Criminal Offenders

The following stories are case studies that examined how adopting a diet based on whole grains and fresh foods affected the psychology of juvenile and adult criminal offenders.

1. Barbara Reed, chief probation officer of the Municipal Court in Cuyahoga Falls, Ohio, improved the quality of her own life by a change in diet. Recurring nightmares, mental lapses, fatigue, and violent mood swings disappeared as she eliminated sugar, sugary foods, white flour, and canned foods from her daily meals and began to eat more whole grains, vegetables, and fresh fruit. Ms. Reed introduced nutritional assessments in her court, designed to reveal possible dietary deficiencies and excesses, and began counseling probationers to eliminate refined sugar, white flour, and other deficient foods from their daily way of eating. Offenders reported feeling better, having more energy, and better control over their emotions by following her dietary recommendations. Over the years, Ms. Reed reported that over 1,000 ex-offenders had gone through her program, and of those who remained on the diet, 89 percent had not been rearrested in the next five years. Her recidivism rate was five times lower than the national average.[3]

2. At the U.S. Naval Correctional Center in Seattle, Washington, sugar, white flour, and other refined carbohydrates were reduced and replaced with more nutritious foods, including whole wheat. After a year, the prison administrator Chief Warrant Officer Gene Baker reported to U.S. Naval headquarters in Washington, D.C., that "since this time, the medical log shows that a definite decrease in the number of confinees at sick call and on medication has occurred, and that disciplinary reports for this year are down 12 percent from the same time frame of last year."[4]

3. Two criminologists identified excessive milk consumption as the primary factor distinguishing chronic juvenile delinquents from non-offenders in the same local school district under review.[5] The young offenders consumed, on an average, more than twice as much milk as the control group. Casein, the protein in milk, cheese, cream, butter, ice cream, and other dairy foods, cannot be assimilated by most people and begins to accumulate in the undigested state in the upper intestine and putrefy, producing mucus and toxins and leading to a weakening of the gastric, intestinal, pancreatic, and bile systems. This condition is known as lactose intolerance (lactose is the simple sugar in dairy foods). Other studies of juvenile offenders indicate that about 90 percent have a history of intolerance or allergy to milk, and eliminating milk from the diet can result in "markedly positive" behavior.[6]

bohydrates to stoke our inner fires—is the real energy crisis of our day, not the lack of petroleum or plutonium to fuel our unnatural lifestyle.

America

In the past, our ancestors dreamed of creating a healthy, peaceful society in harmony with their local environment or moving on to new settlements in quest of a secure and more joyful future. To realize their dream, they ate very simply, mostly grains and other complex carbohydrates, often sacrificing their material comfort and prosperity for the sake of the next generation. Today, that slow, gradual approach to life has largely been replaced by the rapid, instant ethic that emphasizes immediate gratification. Our attention span is measured in hours, minutes, and seconds rather than in epochs, years, and seasons. Instead of lifelong dreams and goals, we have short-term career objectives and an inventory of personal needs. Instead of values, we live by data. All of our modern escapes, addictions, and shortcuts to life—including compulsive television watching, use of social media, drug and alcohol abuse, gambling and playing the lottery, stock market and real estate speculation, psychological training seminars, and reliance on gurus—can be seen as essentially hypoglycemic reactions or other symptoms of underlying physical or emotional illness.

These addictions are destructive but generally nonviolent; however, sometimes the compulsive search for material or spiritual security takes a violent form, such as the behavior of extreme or exploitative national, political, and religious groups. Bloodshed and war are commonly the result. After chronic dietary and environmental abuse, our nervous systems become dulled and desensitized, requiring loud music, pornography, violent sex, and fanatical ideologies to stimulate us. We have become so separated from our true nature and eternal dream that we are now devoting most of our society's energy and resources to perfecting technologies that would destroy all life on earth.

From our understanding of food and energy, we know that a daily diet centered on meat and sugar leads to potentially violent, destructive behavior. Meat creates a rigid, inflexible, stubborn mentality, while sugar produces a scattered, confused way of thinking. Together they are a volatile, explosive combination. It is not surprising that nearly all of the early developers of the atom bomb were sugar addicts. Leo Szilard, the Hungarian-born physicist who came up with the original idea for harnessing nuclear energy, "preferred fatty or over-sweet delicatessen fare."[7] General Leslie Groves, head of the Manhattan Project, was also addicted to sweets. "Among the secrets in his office safe were pound boxes of chocolate creams and turtles which his staff was expected to keep replenished."[8] J. Robert Oppenheimer, director of the team of scientists at Los Alamos who actually constructed the first uranium and plutonium bombs, and Edward Teller, a physicist who later gained renown as the "Father of the Hydrogen Bomb," also had a craving for sweets. "Both were convivial, childishly impulsive, disdainful of detail, and they were insatiable sugarholics. Teller's addiction to chocolate was legendary."[9]

Japan

On the Japanese side, faulty diet also contributed to poor health and judgment, leading to the deaths of millions of people. In April 1941, the Tokyo government was divided about opening negotiations with the United States to avert a war in the Pacific. Prime Minister Konoe was supposed to ride with Foreign Minister Matsuoka, a leader of the war faction, from the airport to the Imperial Palace and brief him on peace efforts, but because of a bad case of piles, was unable to do so. When he arrived later, he found that Matsuoka had become irate about news he received in another car. The opportunity to defuse tensions between the two nations was lost, and the course leading to the attack on Pearl Harbor was set. "[I]t was not the first time this relatively minor ailment changed history," John Toland noted in *The Rising Sun: The Decline and Fall of the Japanese Empire, 1936–1945.* "Napoleon suffered intensely from hemorrhoids at Waterloo."[10]

Emperor Hirohito, Japan's guiding force before and during the war, embodied a tragic combination of extreme Eastern and Western values. For nearly a hundred years, Japan alone of the Asian countries had withstood efforts to become colonized by the West. Many leaders saw this as proof of Japan's racial purity and superiority.[11] Though steeped in Shinto tradition, Hirohito was trained as a marine biologist. Assuming power in the 1920s, he brought a thoroughly Darwinian worldview to the cause of ultra-nationalism.[12]

Like his father, the Emperor Taisho, and grandfather, the Emperor Meiji, Emperor Hirohito adopted a semi-modern diet and utilized modern techniques to carry out Japan's mission of conquering, unifying, and enlightening Asia by military force. For example, every day Hirohito had bacon and eggs for breakfast—two extremely yang foods that can produce an aggressive world view.[13] Fortunately, he also regularly ate oatmeal and toast in addition to some traditional Japanese foods, which moderated his thoughts and behavior. Following the atomic bombings of Hiroshima and Nagasaki, Hirohito had enough common sense to realize and admit that Japan had been defeated and—in the face of strong opposition to continue the war—prevailed upon the government and armed forces to surrender.

After the war, General Douglas MacArthur, the head of the U.S. Occupation, showed the Japanese people magnanimity in their hour of defeat. Sparing the Emperor's life and allowing him to retain symbolic power, MacArthur initiated democratic reforms. He wisely granted Japanese women the right to vote for the first time, explaining, "Women don't want war."[14] In the decades since then, Emperor Hirohito has seen Japan rise from the ashes and extend her influence internationally through culture, trade, and technological innovation. Unlike his father and grandfather (who died relatively young), he maintained his health in later years, observed a modest way of life, and lived to age eighty-seven.

The behavior of the Japanese expansionists and the American nuclear scientists a generation ago is not much different from the aggressive behavior or hypoglycemic reactions observed in millions of school children. Sugar, soft drinks, ice cream, and similar foods, in combination with meat, eggs, chicken, cheese, milk, and other animal products, create a dark, violent, vision of the future punctuated by brief flashes of light and energy. "The fate of a nation," Voltaire observed in another epoch, "has often depended on the good or bad digestion of a prime minister."[15] Today, the safety of the world depends not only on the health and judgment of a half-dozen world leaders entrusted with official command over nuclear weapons, but also upon the thousands of bomber pilots, missile silo operators, and submarine commanders who could launch World War III on their own. In the United States alone, a study showed that an estimated 100,000 military personnel have some form of access to, or responsibility for, nuclear weapons. Each year, about 4 percent of these people are removed from duty because of health problems, which in one year included 1,219 for mental disorders and emotional instability, 1,365 for drug abuse, and 256 for alcoholism.[16]

MECHANICAL THINKING: A CASE STUDY

Over the years, many people have come to me for way-of-life consultations. One of the most interesting cases took place in Belgium. A mother came to see me and brought along her grown son. He was very big in stature and about thirty years old. The mother was strong, small, and about sixty-five. She was crying. It turned out that her son could not speak or cope with practical matters but was a genius at figures and numbers. He was like a human computer. I asked him, "What day of the week was November 3, 1893?" He said, "Tuesday." He could also multiply two long numbers in his head and write down the answer in seconds. He had a really amazing intellectual capacity. Scientists had examined him, and he had been on TV and in the newspapers throughout Europe. Until age three, he had been normal, but after this time, he gradually became abnormal. He wanted to live a normal life and get married, but he could not convey anything. He made very simple sounds and was always smiling. He also had exceptional musical talent. Although he had not studied any music, when someone played him a Beethoven symphony, he could play it on the piano a half-hour later. Now some widow wanted to marry him, but the mother was worried about her intentions. When we talked about marriage, his eyes became bright, but he could not express his feelings.

Of course, over the years, his family had taken him to many specialists, but they all shook their heads and said there was nothing that could be done. The doctors and psychiatrists classified him as an "idiot savant"—a child prodigy who excelled in one area but was totally deficient in most other areas—and said the origin of his condition was an unfathomable mystery.

After meditating on the man's condition for a few minutes, I passed my hands over and around his head. Then I told the mother that there were three foods that she would have to discontinue feeding him if his mentality were to change to normal. The first was eggs, especially hard-boiled eggs. The second was cheese.

And the third was lemon. The mother jumped up out of her seat and explained that every morning from about the age of three, she had fed her son cheese and hard-boiled eggs with lemon juice squeezed on top. In amazement, she asked me how I knew what he had been eating. I noted that simple visual diagnostic techniques had been traditionally used in both East and West to evaluate a person's health and consciousness and see what they ate.

In her son's case, it was obvious that he was excessively yang. The man could hardly speak, his mentality was completely mechanical, and his face and features were very drawn—all contracted qualities characteristic of extreme yang. Moreover, one-half of his brain was overdeveloped and the other half totally underdeveloped. Figuring out things is mechanical judgment. I saw this right away. In traditional Oriental medicine and philosophy, it has been known that the right side of the brain governs more intuitive, aesthetic thought, while the left side governs more analytical, rational thinking. The front of the brain, meanwhile, governs the future, as well as more romantic, idealistic, visionary consciousness, while the back of the brain governs the past, memory, stability, and traditional values. Modern medical and psychological studies are beginning to confirm these elementary yin/yang polarities.

When I lightly touched his head, I could feel there was no energy radiating from the more artistic and intuitive portions while there was strong energy coming from the more analytical portions. What causes this kind of imbalance? From these signs, it was clear the boy was consuming almost exclusively animal-quality foods and very little vegetable-quality foods. Eggs—the most condensed food in the usual human diet—produce a very analytical mentality, as popularly recognized in the expression "egghead" for a scientific or mathematical genius. Eating eggs regularly also creates a shell of rigidity and stubbornness around a person, which other people find difficult to penetrate or which they themselves find hard to break out of. Cheese, meanwhile, produces overall stagnation in the digestive, circulatory, and nervous systems, impeding the smooth flow of electromagnetic energy through the body. In this case, mucus deposits were stored in and around various organs and functions, which prevented the circulation of upward, expanding energy from the earth from nourishing the yin half of the brain. This part of the brain governs artistic creativity, social relations, and language structure and sentence formation.

Since extreme yang naturally attracts extreme yin, I knew that the boy must be eating something very acidic to make balance. Also, while eggs create strong analytical capabilities, they do not in and of themselves produce the kind of mental acuity found in thinking of this kind. This kind of sharpness is produced by citrus fruit, especially lemon, which is the most acidic of the citrus fruits commonly eaten.

I told the mother that his condition could be improved by discontinuing these foods, as well as other articles in the modern diet, and by giving him foods that nourished the left side of the brain. For this, he needed whole cereal grains and—temporarily—raw, hard leafy green vegetables (as a rule, we minimize the use of raw vegetables in macrobiotic cooking, but in this case they were appropriate to use for medicinal purposes), not the lemon and animal-food extremes. The mother asked me how long it would take to return to normal. I told her it would be about four years. Blood quality takes about three to four months to change, after which organs and tissues start to change. Nervous system changes begin in about nine months and take several years to change, including restoration of full verbal abilities.

On my next trip to Europe, the mother came to see me. She said that her son had already changed dramatically on the new diet. He could communicate his feelings and had begun to play and mix with other people for the first time. His wonderful mathematical abilities had begun to disappear, however, and he could no longer be a perpetual calendar or play the *Moonlight Sonata* by ear.

I smiled and explained to her that human beings have the freedom to be and do whatever they want. Now that she knew the secret of food, it was entirely up to her what her son would become. He could become a well-rounded person with a balance of intuitive and analytical skills and a nice family, or he could become a great scientist, artist, or composer and live a lonely and probably tortured existence. Food is so powerful. If fully developed, the potential of the human brain is almost unlimited. Intuition, telepathic communication, knowledge of the distant past and far future, and other advanced capacities can be developed naturally through our day-to-day way of eating.

I mention this case history because it represents the extreme kind of mechanical thinking that is more and more prevalent in modern society, especially among the scientists, technicians, and politicians who are administrating the nuclear arms race. Of course, we are all eating in this direction, so it is not just the specialists who must change, but also the ordinary people of the world who rely on them. As our own health and judgment are restored, we naturally begin to take responsibility for our own lives, as well as the lives of everyone around us, including the scientists, doctors, and world leaders who are not eating well and are unable to envision a peaceful future.

SUMMARY

The healthy person takes responsibility for all mistakes and difficulties in his or her environment. The healthiest person takes responsibility for the entire world, future generations, and the human species as a whole: "Who is to blame for the threat of nuclear war? I am responsible. I was living upon the earth when these terrible weapons came out. It is up to me to change my way of life and way of eating. If I can change myself, then I can show other people how to change peacefully." This is the spirit that will guide us into a bright, peaceful new era.

PEACE PROMOTER

Kit Kitatani, United Nations

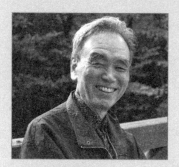

Kit Kitatani

In 1983, doctors in New York told Katsuhide Kitatani, a senior administrator at the United Nations for many years, that he had stomach cancer. After surgery, he was put on chemotherapy, but the cancer spread to the lymph system. After he was told that he had only six to twelve months to live, Mr. Kitatani started to wind up his affairs. Then one day at a party, he ran into a friend who had been suffering from lymph cancer. He noticed that all her hair, which had fallen out during medical treatment, had been restored. He asked her how she did it. She said, "I'm practicing macrobiotics." "What kind of economics is that?" he asked.

The friend gave him the name of a book to read, and in the fifth or sixth book store he looked, he finally found the book. It described how a medical doctor—the president of a large American hospital—whose body was riddled with tumors had healed his own terminal condition with the help of a macrobiotic dietary approach. "The diet looked very easy, very Japanese," Mr. Kitatani, who was born in Japan, reflected afterwards. "It included plenty of rice, wakame, and miso soup." After arranging a consultation with me in Boston, he started the diet. "I bought three macrobiotic cookbooks and asked my wife to start cooking. I was a very good supervisor." His wife started the diet immediately, but his twin sons were skeptical. Mr. Kitatani's friends were encouraging but also expected him to die shortly.

As his condition improved, Mr. Kitatani looked back on his own previous way of eating and the factors that had led to his illness: "I was fifteen when World War II ended. We were starving and had lost the will to produce. We received sugar from the American GIs. Soon I was crawling around on my hands and knees and developed skin disease, but I didn't associate it with what I was eating at the time." Hot springs helped his skin condition. In a U.S. occupation forces camp where he worked, Mr. Kitatani developed a liking for ketchup, ice cream, and many other highly processed foods. Later, he started working for the United Nations and over the next few decades, had been posted all over the world. "Wherever I went, the first question I would ask is, 'Where's the best restaurant?'" he said.

After nine months on his new diet, Mr. Kitatani's cancer went away completely, and he had the unexpected joy of having to replan the rest of his life. He decided that the best way he could help others would be to start a macrobiotic club at the United Nations. "The pace of life is getting quicker and quicker. All around the world, people now have access to modern supermarkets and industrially processed food. At the U.N., we arrange for fertilizers to be shipped, insecticides to be sprayed, and the symptoms of diseases to be eliminated without addressing their underlying causes. People talk till they're blue in the face, but don't seem to take action.

"All around the world, people are incapacitated and unproductive. U.N. debates are really selfish and guided by egocentric thinking. The U.N. has been successful on limited occasions in avoiding conflagrations. In the future, it seems to me that peace will come from individuals who are free of physical and spiritual diseases. Every one of us is an actual or potential peacemaker."

By the second year, the United Nations Macrobiotic Society had 180 members and sponsored a variety of lectures, dinners, and classes. A petition to begin serving macrobiotic food in the United Nations cafeteria garnered almost 1,000 signatures. A branch chapter opened at United Nations headquarters in Geneva, and there are plans to form other chapters at UNESCO headquarters in Paris and FAO central offices in Rome.

Mr. Kitatani's story is a wonderful example of the spirit of "one grain, ten thousand grains." Following the restoration of his own health, he began to endlessly distribute his knowledge to others. His whole family, including two grown sons, is now macrobiotic. After retiring from the United Nations, Mr. Kitatani and his wife, Akiko, went on to found 2050, a nonprofit organization in Asia devoted to health and community development. Gradually, the entire United Nations and NGO (nongovernmental organization) world community will be transformed into a truly healthy and peaceful forum for the spread of planetary family consciousness and the realization of One Peaceful World.

***

Source

Kitatani, Katsuhide. Speech at World Peace Symposium Summer Camp, Becket, MA, August 1985.

14.

Politics:
"Medicine Writ Large"

The diets of leaders, including emperors, prime ministers, and presidents, lead to an aggressive or a peaceful outlook, depending on what they eat and how they heal. Policies that are enacted often have a nutritional or medical dimension. Consider our discussion of the diets of the French and the Russians during the Napoleonic Wars in Chapter 8. While Napoleon and his men ate mostly white bread, meat, fruit, and alcohol, the Russians ate primarily grains and vegetable-quality foods. As a result, the Russians were more even-tempered and reasonable than the chaotic French. Diet and politics often intersect to shape the peacefulness or aggressiveness of a nation. As pharmaceutical companies become more powerful, medicine becomes an important participant in politics, often combining with technology to create larger-than-life solutions to illnesses that can more effectively be treated through diet. In this chapter, we examine how external war and internal war have come to be related to one another over time.

THE INNER WAR

In July 1945, President Harry Truman received an urgent cable in Potsdam: "Operated on this morning. Diagnosis not yet complete but results seem satisfactory and already exceed expectations."[1] The message referred to the explosion of the world's first atomic device in the New Mexico desert.

In the decades that followed, the cure for conventional warfare gave rise to an even more lethal disorder: the nuclear arms race. As the memorandum to Truman reveals, the way we approach disease and warfare is essentially the same. Whether the conflict is internal, as in an illness affecting the organs of the body, or external, as in disputes among nations, our posture is one of defensiveness. Rudolf Virchow, the nineteenth-century German scientist and founder of cellular pathology, originated this new way of thinking of disease as "a conflict of citizens in a cell state, brought about by external forces."[2]

In the modern view, disease is considered an abnormal or harmful condition caused primarily by microorganisms, parasites, or mutant cells. From an early age we are brought up to maintain vigilance against potentially harmful viruses, bacteria, and carcinogens that threaten to undermine our health and destroy our freedom of movement. These disease-causing agents are viewed largely of external origin and once they have invaded the body we feel that they need to be located, neutralized, and violently destroyed.

Military metaphors are now used routinely to describe bodily processes and to prescribe treatment. In "The Genetic Assault on Cancer," an article from the *New York Times Magazine,* we are informed:

> These researchers want to understand how the enemy [the cancer cell] masquerades as normal, slipping past the sentinels of the immune system undetected. . . . Antibodies that circulate through the bloodstream are on constant patrol. . . . The body is quickly alerted and dispatches special killer cells and a barrage of chemical artillery to dispose of the threat. . . . It is hoped that these 'poison-tagged' antibodies will act as miniature smart bombs, delivering their lethal payload to the diseased tissue—and nowhere else.[3]

Articles in *Science News,* the weekly digest of developments in different medical and scientific disciplines, voiced a similar theme:

> What do you do with a semi-powerful guided missile? Monoclonal antibodies, the proteins produced by immune system/cancer cell hybrids, have become important seek-and-bind weapons in diagnosing cancer and other illnesses. But the missiles are not as good at search-and-destroy missions—researchers have had only limited success in using monoclonal antibodies alone against cancer. Now, others are arming the antibodies with radioactivity, drugs, or toxins.[4]

In the article "The Human Body's 'Cell Wars' Defense," *Boston Globe* science columnist Professor Chet Raymo drew upon President Reagan's "star wars" space-based missile defense system for an analogy of how the body's strategic defenses operate:

> We live in a sea of alien viruses and microorganisms. Many are harmless. Some are deadly. The body is protected by a stupendous array of traps, triggers, walls, moats, and chemical alarms. Some of the body's cells act as patrols, sentries, infantry, and artillery to defend the integrity of the larger society. The 'cell wars' defense system never rests.[5]

Since the end of the Second World War, our approach to illness has been increasingly technological and combative. Though this is sometimes necessary—as in immediate life-threatening conditions or emergencies—by and large, it is less than adequate.

Each year, billions of dollars are funneled into the medical arms race to find the best and most effective defense against disease. The medical arsenal ranges from aspirin to antidepressants, from surgical incision to cobalt radiation. In the war against the natural functioning of our own bodies, over-the-counter preparations serve as the first line of defense. Pills are as common and accessible as bullets in modern society and come in all shapes, sizes, and strengths. Some, such as aspirin, are relatively weak and may be compared in strength to a pellet. Other tablets, such as sleeping pills, are more like rifle shots. Still others, including antihistamines, are more like mortar shells, whose explosive power disperses over a wider area.

The next line of defense is prescription drugs. Depending upon their charge, velocity, and fuse length, these capsules function like bombs. Tranquilizers and sedatives, for example, can knock out whole networks of cerebral functions. Anesthetics can immobilize entire divisions of pain.

The third and final line of defense is surgery, radiation therapy, and chemotherapy. These are the B-52s, Trident submarines, and MXs of the strategic medical command. The performance of this weaponry is sophisticated, accurate, and deadly. Some experimental treatments in which the body is subjected to radioactive bombardment or laser beam surgery can be compared to the use of ballistic missiles with multiple warheads homing in on their targets.

We are actually conducting a miniature arms race within ourselves. The U.S. Congress symbolically underscored this fact when it required that part of the money for the military's "Star Wars" laser missile defense established by Ronald Reagan in 1984 be applied to medical research. Physicians and nuclear scientists testified that the Free-Electron Laser, a beam weapon designed to shoot down Soviet missiles from space, may have had important medical uses such as treating tumors, improving surgery, and operating inside human cells.[6]

Over the last generation, presidents have "waged war" against disease. Richard Nixon famously declared war on cancer in 1971. In 2016, Barack Obama appointed his vice president, Joe Biden, to lead the latest onslaught against this scourge, making this war longer than the Vietnam War, both Gulf Wars, and the war in Afghanistan combined. Along with cancer, war was declared on AIDS, heart disease, diabetes, and other disorders. In the war on the Ebola virus (2013 to 2016), the U.S. even sent Marines to West Africa to aid in the construction of hospitals. In the war on the Zika virus (beginning in 2015), biotech companies began developing genetically modified mosquitoes to attack the disease.

Technological warfare waged on the body can result in debilitating injuries, ranging from impairment to paralysis and, frequently, death. As on the modern military battlefield, medical victories are elusive and armistices rarely last. The enemy forces usually regroup and pop up elsewhere, necessitating another round of radioactive bombardment, deployment of a sharper knife, or escalation in the dosage of the drug or genetically engineered pharmaceutical.

The campaign to repel bodily aggression is a protracted struggle. In the end, the individual has to recover not only from the original condition, but also from the side effects of the medical treatment, which weaken the entire system, making it more vulnerable to collapse.

As a result of our imbalanced way of eating, saturated fat, excess protein, and mucus deposits are proliferating in our blood and lymphatic systems, giving rise to stockpiles of arterial plaque, tumors, and toxic waste accumulations in and around vital organs. Without apparent warning, fat and cholesterol deposits may reach critical mass, setting off an uncontrolled chain reaction through the whole organism, resulting in a massive heart attack or stroke. Or, in the case of cancer, the malignancy will spread slowly, precipitating a widening conflict and making the body uninhabitable. To reverse this deadly spiral of escalating illness and treatment, we need a freeze on the use of chemical fertilizers, pesticides, and GMOs on the soil, and a moratorium or drastic reduction in the consumption of meat, poultry, dairy food, sugar, and refined carbohydrates. General and complete disarmament begins in our refrigerators and medicine cabinets. Mutual and balanced reductions in both the mega-dosage of drugs and medication and in the mega-tonnage of weapons are necessary for a peaceful world.

THE OUTER WAR

"Medicine is a social science, and politics is medicine writ large," Rudolf Virchow, the German pathologist, observed more than a century ago.[7] By this statement, he was asserting that the people and movements in politics are widely controlled by the goals of the pharmaceutical industry.

In medicine now, we are governed by modern concepts of cellular sovereignty—the notion that what happens in the cell or its nucleus is totally independent of the organism as a whole or its environment. Over the years, modern science has convinced us that disease is the result of external invasion or an aberration in an isolated gene, hormone, or other cellular component over which we have no voluntary control or moral responsibility. Scientists tend to assure us that if the specific factor that is causing the epidemic or abnormal cell growth can be pinpointed, a biochemical solution can be found to block its harmful effects. It almost never occurs to us that we have brought this pain and suffering upon ourselves because of a longtime imbalance in our way of eating, thinking, or living.

In the war on cancer, heart disease, diabetes, obesity, and other afflictions, as we have seen, treatments involve a variety of successively more violent means to protect healthy cells and conquer unhealthy ones. These methods are similar in design and execution to those implemented on a larger scale by military and political leaders to protect citizens from attack in the name of national sovereignty.

Our social ills follow a development similar to our personal ills. The pattern of progressive degeneration from less to more serious conflict can be seen in disputes between families, communities, states, and nations. These conflicts generally proceed from arguments and threats to violent outbursts and aggressive behavior, from confrontation and polarization to fighting and war. Disharmony is never the fault of only one side. Yet we act as if it were and adopt an adversarial, rather than a cooperative, attitude. Instead of seeking a peaceful solution that reconciles and takes into account the welfare and needs of all concerned, including the environment and the next generation, we take refuge in our own short-range goals.

Terrorism and revolt occur only in proportion to society's reliance on excessive military strength and neglect of underlying social factors that create disorder in the first place. The futility of suppressing revolution with force has been demonstrated in Southeast Asia, Afghanistan, Central America, the Middle East, and other areas of conflict.

At the global level, this antagonistic approach has led to the doctrine of national sovereignty. In order to halt the nuclear arms race, we must transcend our allegiance to individual nation-states. So long as countries see themselves as separate entities, they will retain the right to build and use nuclear weapons to protect their own national security. If all states banded together and formed a world federation, limiting their sovereignty, there would no longer be competing paramount national interests to defend. As presently structured, the United Nations lacks authority to intervene in the internal affairs of member states and is thus too weak to serve as the planet's system of natural immunity when conflict arises. A way needs to be found to unify the security forces of the world under a common jurisdiction, pending complete disarmament, while at the same time ensuring diverse political, economic, social, and cultural systems.

In all fields of life, the use or threat of excessive force proves counterproductive. The violent means with which we produce our foods, treat our bodies, and deal with conflicts must be replaced with peaceful and harmonious methods.

DUALISTIC THINKING

The further degeneration of the soil; the continuing spread of cancer, heart disease, and immunodeficiency diseases; and the outbreak of nuclear war are not inevitable. To stop or prevent such catastrophes, we must develop a new orientation toward life. Specifically, we must begin to seek out the most basic causes and implement the most basic solutions, rather than continue the present course of treating each problem separately in terms of its symptoms alone. Issues of war and peace, and sickness and health, affect us all in one way or another and in all domains of modern life. The responsibility of finding and implementing solutions should not be left to those within the government, the military, or the medical and scientific communities alone. Global health and security will emerge only through a cooperative effort involving people at all levels of society.

By orienting itself against rather than with nature, modern civilization has deprived itself of the capacity to evolve with the environment. Cancer, immunodeficiency diseases, nuclear war, and terrorism are only the most extreme manifestations of this adversarial orientation. Instead of considering the larger ecological, social, and biological causes of the breakdown of modern life, we have focused our attention until now in the opposite direction, viewing conflict mainly as an isolated disorder, affecting certain cells within the body, criminal elements within society, and terrorist networks and dissident factions within nation-states. The remedies we employ in our hospitals, legislatures, and world forums involve a cessation of hostilities and containment of the disruptive forces, all the while ignoring the overall conditions that caused the disorder to develop.

The modern way of thinking that has culminated in this dead end can be described as dualistic. Dualistic thinking divides good from bad, friend from enemy, and health from sickness, seeing the one as desirable and the other as undesirable. This divisive mode of thought actually underlies all of modern society, including education and religion, politics and economics, science and industry, communications and the arts. As long as our basic point of view is one-sided, it is impossible to cure fundamentally any sickness or put an end to family disputes, criminal activity, social unrest, or conflicts between nations.

From a larger perspective—such as that of the earth as a whole—we can see that no enemies really exist. On the contrary, all factors, however antagonistic to our own limited personal or national objectives, are complementary. All phenomena contain the seed of their polar opposite and are mutually influencing and changing into one another. By balancing extremes—reducing excesses, filling up empty spaces—nature makes for greater diversity and harmony as the spiral of life unfolds.

Sickness is a natural adjustment, the result of the wisdom of the body trying to keep us in natural balance. Degenerative disease is only the final stage in a sequence of events through which individuals in the modern world tend to pass because we fail to appreciate the beneficial nature of disease symptoms. In reality, disease is defending and protecting us by either eliminating or localizing undesirable factors from our body. It is a wonderful defense and adjustment mechanism that enables us to live one, two, five, or ten more years without changing our unnatural diet and artificial way of life. On the other hand, if we are willing to self-reflect, take responsibility for our sickness, and change our orientation, disease will cooperate with us and go away permanently if it has not yet reached the terminal stage.

As modern medicine is just beginning to discover, cancer and other serious illnesses can be prevented and, in many cases, relieved naturally, without violent treatments, by adopting a balanced diet centered around whole cereal grains and vegetables, together with other traditional basic supplemental foods, and administering safe, simple home cares. Thousands of people with cancer and heart disease, including many given up as terminal, have recovered their health and vitality by adopting natural, holistic approaches, including macrobiotics. Hundreds of thousands of others have prevented the onset of degenerative disease by changing their way of eating and living. Along with the change in diet, many patients have taken the initiative to apply traditional home remedies to reduce symptoms and discharge toxic material through the skin or urine. These medicinal drinks and external applications are safe, simple, and self-administered, and work by helping to activate circulation and by enabling the body's own electromagnetic, healing energy to flow smoothly to the affected region. These remedies include a drink made from umeboshi plums, shoyu, and kuzu root; a tea made from dried daikon; and a ginger compress that is applied to the kidneys, intestines, or other affected regions. In extreme emergency situations, when the person cannot eat at all or vital life functions are immediately threatened, surgery, radiation, or other conventional methods may need to be temporarily employed.

The natural macrobiotic approach to cooking and relief of illness is peaceful and gentle. All factors are considered to be complementary, and the emphasis is on restoring equilibrium. For thousands of years, humanity viewed life not as a battle in which enemies had to be violently subdued or destroyed, but as a game of limitless adventure and discovery in which opposites are gently harmonized. Health and peace will naturally follow from adopting this view.

SUMMARY

In recent years, medical doctors around the world have come together and taken the lead in alerting the world to the dangers of atomic and hydrogen weapons. This effort represents the true spirit of healing. Yet unless we change our basic orientation and end the war against the universe, nature, and our own bodies and minds, the nuclear arms race can never be reversed. To achieve lasting peace, we must not only beat our swords into plowshares, but also transform our scalpels and drugs into cooking utensils and natural foods.

PEACE PROMOTER

Masanobu Fukuoka, Africa

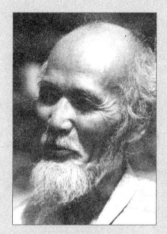

Masanobu Fukuoka

For over forty years, farmer and philosopher Masanobu Fukuoka had devoted himself to natural farming. His methods of raising crops without cultivation, chemical fertilizers and herbicides, and even organic compost resulted in amazingly high yields, fertile strains of seed, and an improved quality of the soil. His approach may have been very similar to that used by human communities around the world in the ancient spiritual and scientific world community.

Born in a small farming village in southern Japan, Mr. Fukuoka was trained as a plant pathologist. But as a young man, he questioned his scientific background and embarked on a rediscovery of traditional ways of farming that do not require human labor or toil. He believed that returning to a way of life in harmony with nature held the answer to the problems of modern civilization.

After World War II, Mr. Fukuoka turned his attention to the problems of reforming Japanese agriculture. After the publication of his book *The One-Straw Revolution* in 1975, Mr. Fukuoka increasingly devoted himself to global problems. In 1985, he visited Somalia, Ethiopia, and other drought-stricken areas of Africa. Environmentalists attributed widespread famine across much of the African continent to monocropping and other modern agricultural techniques—for example, desertification brought about from overgrazing by large animal herds, changing global weather patterns brought about by industrialization, and political and economic turmoil in the countries involved.

In Somalia, Mr. Fukuoka visited rural communities for forty days and discovered that the people there traditionally used natural farming methods, sowing mixed crops rather than single crops: "The people typically lived in circular village compounds with the houses inside, and the giraffes outside. They grew banana and papaya trees, vegetables grew in the shade under the fruit trees. Seeds were mixed together. I brought about one hundred kinds of seeds with me. I gave them to the children and they planted them together. Many types sprouted within a few days."

Mr. Fukuoka's experience demonstrated that after the seeds are scattered, crops will grow without cultivation, weeding, fertilizer, or pruning. Because different kinds of plants are mixed together, they do not attract the birds, insects, or other pests that commonly invade gardens and farms cultivated with only one variety. He also asserts that tractors and other heavy machinery that compact and harden the soil are a major cause of erosion and infertility. They destroy microorganisms and other small life that build up the tilth (physical condition) of the soil.

On a visit to the United States a few years earlier, Mr. Fukuoka began to think that natural farming could also be helpful in preventing desertification. In his 1975 book *The Natural Way of Farming*, he recalled, "While standing in an American desert, I suddenly realized that rain does not fall from the heavens; it issues forth from the ground. Deserts do not form because there is no rain; rather, rain ceases to fall because the vegetation has disappeared. Building a dam in the desert is an attempt to treat the symptoms of the disease but is not a strategy for increasing rainfall. First we have to learn how to restore the ancient forests."

To a macrobiotic gathering, he further noted, "Deserts do have water. It doesn't come up from below because there is no vegetation on the ground. The water will come up through plants. But no plants, no clouds. There are no clouds in the desert. Installing sprinklers is another poor method to irrigate the desert. Salt from underground comes up with the water and covers the ground. Also, underground water saved from the mountains for centuries is wasted. The best way to retain water and prevent erosion is to restore greenery."

To revegetate barren lands, Mr. Fukuoka proposed that the seeds of certain plants be sown over deserts in clay pellets. These pellets can be prepared by first mixing the seeds of green manure trees—such as acacia that grow in areas with an annual rainfall of less than two inches—and the seeds of clover, alfalfa with grain, and vegetable seeds. The mixture of seeds is coated first with a layer of soil, then one of clay, to form clay pellets containing microbes. These completed pellets could then be scattered over the deserts and savannahs.

"Once scattered, the seeds within the hard clay pellets will not sprout until rain has fallen and conditions are just right for germination," Mr. Fukuoka explained. "Nor will they be eaten by mice and birds. A year later, several of the plants will survive, giving a clue as to what is suited to the climate and land. In certain countries to the south, there are reported to be plants that grow on rocks and trees that store water. Anything will do, as long as we get the deserts blanketed rapidly with a green cover of grass. This will bring back the rains."

To restore green belts in Africa, Mr. Fukuoka proposed that seed mixtures be scattered from airplanes. If this method was proven successful, he would like to see the air forces of the world distribute seeds across desertified regions of the planet on a vast scale. In the developed countries, he would like to see seeds scattered by hand, by airplane, or from car windows to transform lawns, pastures, golf courses, and other denuded areas that are depleting the soil and reducing the formation of clouds into fruit and vegetable gardens. "Let's launch seeds from the air, not missiles. Freedom and peace with the land begin with natural farming methods. Grains and trees know no artificial boundaries."

Mr. Fukuoka estimated that one gram of soil from his own small farm in Japan contained about 100 million nitrogen-fixing bacteria and other soil-enriching microbes. He felt that enclosing these microorganisms and seeds in clay would be the spark that restored the life of the land.

"If a single head of rice were sent across the sea to countries where food is scarce and there sown over a ten-square-yard area, a single grain would yield 5,000 grains in one year's time," he said. "There would be grain enough to sow a half-acre the following year, fifty acres two years hence, and 7,000 acres in the fourth year. This could become the seed rice for an entire nation. This handful of grain could open up the road to independence for a starving people.

"But this seed rice must be delivered as soon as possible. Even one person can begin. I could be no happier than if my humble experience with natural farming were to be used toward this end."

Touring the vegetable garden that was cultivated based on his methods at the Kushi Institute in Becket, Massachusetts, Mr. Fukuoka concluded, "Everything starts from your family garden. Through natural farming, the destructive course of civilization can be changed. Once again, the earth can be transformed into a paradise of peace and happiness with enough food for everyone."

Source

Masanobu Fukuoka, *The Natural Way of Farming* (New York: Japan Publications, 1985) and lectures at Macrobiotic Summer Camp, Lenox and Becket, Massachusetts, August 28–30, 1986.

15.

The Spiral of Lasting Peace

The biological transformation of humanity is an entirely peaceful revolution, requiring no laws or doctrines, violence or mass movements. It is also the most universal revolution, able to prevail throughout the world, crossing over racial, cultural, religious, ideological, and national boundaries. It spreads from person to person, home to home, community to community, and country to country, beginning in every kitchen and ending in the realization of One Peaceful World.

CREATING A PEACEFUL MIND

The way to peace will develop naturally in a series of seven interrelated steps:

1. The recovery of our commonsense understanding of humanity; our origin and our future; and our place in and relation with the Order of the Universe, and its practical application to our daily lives.

2. The recovery of the wholesome quality of food through change toward a more natural and organic agriculture system and traditional food-processing methods.

3. Worldwide distribution of these food products, and their preparation according to principles of harmony and balance.

4. The gradual elimination of epidemic, degenerative, and immunodeficiency diseases through the spread of proper food and cooking methods.

5. The development of a new orientation of society toward education, medicine, economics, politics, and spirituality, in harmony with the natural environment.

6. The dissolution of unnecessary and destructive defensive and aggressive measures through a gradual and natural elevation of consciousness from the primitive stages of fear and insecurity.

7. The formation of one world society within which everyone is able to enjoy health, happiness, and freedom by the gradual elimination of all unnatural and artificial boundaries and by a more spiritual orientation.

In order to truly dissolve fear, hatred, and misunderstanding among individuals and groups, nations and international alliances, the means we employ must be peaceful ones. Otherwise, we will create just the opposite effect. Defensiveness only pours more energy into the opponent. Violent opposition only lends greater credence and power to an idea or a group. When a problem is suppressed, it inevitably pops up somewhere else in new guise. In macrobiotics, we use gentle, peaceful methods to dissolve and melt away physical blockages such as cysts and tumors without the need for artificial intervention. We need to find comparable mental and psychological methods to melt away the fears, grief, guilt, resentments, and negative memories of the past. Once these are dissolved, enormous positive energy is released.

Today, there is a trend toward verbalizing anger and other strong emotions, yet talking about a problem in this way usually makes it bigger. It is often better to forget the bad points and look at the good ones. Everyone has a front and a back. By appreciating a person's good qualities and letting them develop, the bad qualities will automatically disappear.

Through proper diet, our entire way of thinking can gradually be changed. By eating whole grains and vegetables, our thinking becomes oriented in a vertical direction, like growing plants, and the possibilities for our growth become unlimited. We develop spiritual energy and feel our unity with all other beings. In contrast, animal food produces a horizontal orientation. Like bulls and cows, tigers and lions, we adopt a territorial perspective. Material energy and power limits our horizon, since there is a limit to which we can expand horizontally. Animal food also creates a great attachment to the past. Meat, poultry, eggs, oily and greasy foods of all kinds, and especially dairy food, are the underlying biological cause of guilt and sinful feelings. Mucus, oil, saturated fat, and toxic protein wastes coat and clog the intestines, the bloodstream, and other bodily organs and functions, creating a sticky, stagnant internal environment. This creates sticky, stagnant thinking and behavior.

The macrobiotic approach to health and happiness is to balance the person's constitution (native strength and capacities) and condition (acquired strength and capacities) by applying the opposite predominant type of energy, e.g., yin to balance an overly yang condition and yang to compensate for an overly yin one. Traditionally, chanting, vibrations, and waves were used to control energy, making the mind and body more yin or yang, more passive or active, more mental or more physical. It is the same with breathing. There are many ways to control our thinking and metabolism through inhaling and exhaling. Breathing techniques form a part of most spiritual practices. Words also work to control energy and balance the mind, representing the spectrum of sounds from the condensed world to the realm of infinity. The Sanskrit syllable "Aum" (also spelled "Om") has been known for thousands of years as the universal sound because it unifies the relative and absolute worlds and activates the major energy centers in the mind and body. Lies, on the other hand, make for chaos. Curses make both sides unhappy. Waves and words influence us. Talking to plants and animals makes them stronger. We can influence the weather in the same way (by speaking, thinking, or visualization) in addition to our social and cultural environment. Through visualization, prayer, meditation, and song, we can begin to envision a world of lasting peace and then act on that vision.

We can begin by creating an image of the future world free from sickness, quarrelling, crime, and war. We will be surprised at what kind of society will result. Everyone will communicate very easily. If we are uncomfortable, we can't communicate with outside society. It's very easy to communicate once basic health and judgment are restored on whole, unprocessed foods. Group therapies, psychiatrists, and gurus would become unnecessary. When our health is recovered, we won't approach problems separately any more. We will understand that there is no such thing as a spiritually elevated person who is sick. The mind and body are one. Health and sickness proceed together as a whole. By projecting an image of world peace, even a few minutes a day, we can have a vibrational effect on others.

CREATING A PEACEFUL HOME

The family is the oldest and most natural human institution. It is, or should be, a microcosm of the Order of the Universe and nature. Evidence of family life has been found dating from the earliest prehistoric times. Long before the civilizations of Sumer, Egypt, China, the Indus Valley, and Mesoamerica flourished, the family provided the thread from which the fabric of human culture was woven.

The family has survived repeated challenges: ice ages, earthquakes, floods, famines, wars, plagues, and the rise and fall of civilizations. It is the most durable and long-lasting social organization. Strong and healthy families are the foundation of a healthy and prosperous society. When a family is strong, society is strong. When the family collapses, society collapses. Of all the challenges—both natural and human-made—creating and maintaining healthy families is the most difficult and the most urgent.

A healthy family is the greatest blessing. A sick family is the greatest tragedy. When one person becomes sick, the whole family suffers; and when one family suffers, the whole community becomes unstable. A family that has a sick person has been imbalanced for some time. A community that has many sick families has been disordered for a long period.

Above anything else, the orientation of family and community should be directed toward maintaining the best health of their members. To keep a family in healthy physical, mental, and spiritual condition, it is not necessary to have regular consultations or to receive any special treatment from a family doctor. The best traditional method is the common practice of gathering the family together regularly to eat meals that are prepared according to natural order and in a loving spirit. Usually, the center of the household is the mother, who is most mindful of everyone's daily health and well-being, including her own, though anyone who is physically and mentally mature can serve as the daily cook. Through her love and skill in the kitchen, the family is able to derive limitless benefits.

At the table, everyone's physical and mental conditions are periodically observed and discussed in a light, humorous spirit, and meals can be adjusted according to everyone's personal requirements with side dishes, condiments, garnishes, and seasonings. Special dishes may even be prepared for certain members of the family. During the meal, each member of the family exchanges daily thoughts and experiences in harmonious conversation, creating a spirit of fellowship and mutual respect. Naturally, as the family eats the same food together, a similar quality of blood—and consequently, thinking—develops. Over time, the family becomes one, with all members sharing the same dream and destiny in life.

Without eating whole, balanced meals together, there can be no biological, psychological, and social unity, which is the essence of the family. The home becomes only an impersonal living place. When family members eat in separate ways and at separate times, dissatisfaction and division spread. Personalities and opinions begin to differ and clash, eventually causing a lack of understanding and sympathy. Though there may be other contributing factors, the fundamental reason for the increase of conflicts, arguments, separation, and divorce among married people and the disintegration of the modern family is a decline of the home-cooked family meal shared together in a spirit of loving harmony.

Love and care for children are the strongest human instincts. They are even stronger than the instinct for self-preservation. These qualities develop quite naturally when we eat a well-balanced whole foods diet. Family unity occurs quite naturally among whole grain and vegetable eaters, while regular consumption of animal food in large volume produces separation. People who are isolated tend to see their world as separate and distinct from that of their children and neighbors.

Separation is the hallmark of our modern age: separation between mind and body, humanity and nature, married partners, parents and children, and neighbors living on the same street. If we are to continue on this planet in an age of nuclear weapons and biological degeneration, then separation, conflict, and isolation must be transformed into unity, harmony, and cooperation. Family health is the key to world peace.

CREATING A PEACEFUL WORLD

The nations of the world regard each other from different perspectives. Each judges the other according to its own point of view and is constantly shocked and angered. In cultural affairs, this chronic misunderstanding produces prejudice and discrimination. In foreign relations, one-sided thinking leads to direct military conflict. Unless these antagonistic points of view are understood to be complementary and part of a larger whole, there will be another world war.

One of the most basic divisions is between East and West. After centuries of separation, the two halves of the world are beginning to unite. The more analytical, materially-oriented West and North are irresistibly attracted to the more intuitive, aesthetic East and South, and vice versa. American truck drivers are practicing Transcendental Meditation, and Chinese farmers are watching color TV. European housewives are learning how to make sushi, and Arabic teenagers are dancing to popular music. Eventually the world will become one, but the process of integration includes stages of potential conflict. The competition for energy and natural resources, as well as the expansion of trade markets and extensions of ideological boundaries, can lead to harsh words, sanctions, and severed relations. Religious sensitivities, national honor, and cultural pride are easily wounded, and healing them usually takes much time and patience. It is up to us to see that the meeting between East and West, and with North and South, is a peaceful one. Ideally, the different halves of the globe will meet harmoniously, learn from each other, and form a new universal world culture synthesizing the material and the spiritual, the analytical and the intuitive, the pragmatic and the aesthetic.

However, national character and cultural differences still remain. Although the Cold War is over, tensions between America and Russia and between America and China remain. Table 15.1 on page 233 depicts some of these differences from an energetic perspective.

The relation among the three major world powers is like that between lovers. There is deep attraction and longing for union, but the courtship is fraught with obstacles and may be protracted. A beautiful marriage can result, enriching to both partners, but like the dance between the sexes, each side is moving in an opposite direction and will never fully understand the other. The relation between Russia and the U.S., for example, is more like that between two brothers or two sisters. They are basically united, but until they reach maturity, they are liable to quarrel, argue, and occasionally fight. Also, because their natures are similar, they tend to compete with and repulse each other slightly. Since they are moving in the same direction, they can easily unite and become one if inspired by a common goal.

The relation between China and the U.S. specifically is not so much between siblings as between father and eldest son or mother and eldest daughter. The older, wiser, more experienced parent and the younger, reckless, more immature offspring cannot always understand or appreciate the other's strengths and weaknesses. For a successful outcome, the older must make allowance for the younger's passion and idealism, while the younger must respect the knowledge and sacrifice of his or her elders. For world peace to come, the marriage of East and West must take place, and familial rivalries among the American, Russian, and Chinese blocs must be outgrown.

TABLE 15.1 AN ENERGETIC COMPARISON OF THE U.S., CHINA, AND RUSSIA.			
	UNITED STATES	**CHINA**	**RUSSIA**
Energy	Upward, warm, bright, more yin	Balanced, moderate, in between extremes of yin and yang	Downward, inward, cold, dark, more yang
Climate and environment	Varied, warmer	Temperate, milder	Rugged, cooler, vaster
Diet	Varied	Plant-based, increasing animal food	Animal food
Main foods	Wheat, beef, dairy, chicken, GMO soy and corn, sugar, beer, whiskey	Refined wheat and rice, fresh vegetables, fish, dairy, beer, millet wine	Buckwheat, sunflower oil, processed meats, sugar, vodka
National character	Idealistic, relaxed, expressive, casual, confrontational	Orderly, indirect, stable, reverent, unifying	Earthy, direct, materialist, soulful, fatalistic, generous
Mentality	Individual-oriented, up-front, optimistic, legalistic, messianic	Family-oriented, hard-working, values wisdom, education, seniority	Group-oriented, collectivist, egalitarian, pessimistic, secretive
Spirituality	Judeo-Christian, evangelistic	Maoist, Confucian, Buddhist, practical, tolerant	Orthodox, mystical, Marxist
Politics	Liberal, democratic	Hierarchal, imperial	Authoritarian, czarist
Economics	Multinational corporations	Central planning, markets	Oligopoly
Growth and development	Expands in a yin way by money and markets	Expands in a yin/yang way through foreign aid	Expands in a yang way by land and military force and threats
Strengths	Personal freedom, candidness, openness, innovation	Orderly, respectful, dignified, humble, practical	Hard-working, resilient, poetic, enduring, intuitive, ingenious
Weaknesses	Income disparity, unemployment, overconsumption, racial conflict	Lack of human rights, control of the press and Internet, treatment of minorities	Ruthlessness, concealing the truth, unrestrained ambition, holy foolishness

SUMMARY

To achieve our common goal of One Peaceful World, everybody must do his or her part. We must create a peaceful mind by developing peaceful solutions to our problems, whether that is through our words, our actions, or the approaches we take toward health. We must also create a peaceful family home through love and unity and by eating meals together. More widely, the societies of the East and West must put aside their differences and come to a harmonious understanding.

PEACE PROMOTER

Lidia Yamchuk, M.D., and
Hanif Shaimardanov, M.D., Soviet Union

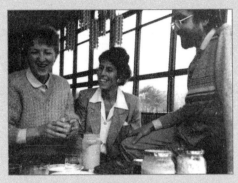

Lidia (left) and Hanif (right) with Cary Wolfe
(center), a Kushi Institute teacher, in Moscow

In 1985, Lidia Yamchuk and Hanif Shaimardanov, two young medical doctors in Chelyabinsk, Russia, organized Longevity, the first macrobiotic association in the Soviet Union. At their hospital in the central Ural Mountain city, where Longevity was located, they used dietary methods and acupuncture to treat many patients suffering from leukemia, lymphoma, and other disorders associated with exposure to nuclear radiation.

Since the early 1950s, radioactive and toxic waste from Soviet nuclear weapons production had been dumped into Karachay Lake in Chelyabinsk, an industrial city of one million people about 900 miles east of Moscow. The city was the center of atomic and hydrogen bomb production during the Cold War and, as a top-secret military city, did not appear on world maps. Only in the late 1980s was the city opened to the general public under Mikhail Gorbachev. Following the arrival of outside scientists, the United Nations declared Chelyabinsk the most polluted city on the planet.

Lidia and Hanif discovered macrobiotics when researching natural approaches to treating radiation sickness. They read about how after the Nagasaki atomic bombing, Dr. Akizuki saved all his staff and patients with brown rice, miso soup, and other strengthening foods. After attending a macrobiotic seminar in Germany, the physicians contacted the Kushi Institute in the United States and requested macrobiotic foods for their patients. At the Kushi Institute, general manager Alex Jack organized an airlift, and macrobiotic friends, families, and businesses from across the country donated to the cause. In the autumn of 1990, several thousand pounds of miso, seaweed, umeboshi plums, and other healing foods were collected and flown to Moscow courtesy of Aeroflot, the Soviet airline company.

Coincidentally, Alex and a contingent of other macrobiotic teachers were invited that fall to participate in a major environmental conference in Moscow. One hundred leading activists from America joined with a hundred of their Soviet counterparts in a weeklong gathering. Lidia and Hanif traveled to Moscow to participate in the conference and accept the shipment of foods from the United States. The American teachers also brought enough brown rice, miso, and other staples to cook for themselves in their hotel since the conference food was primarily cured meats, white bread, and sugary snacks and desserts (made from Cuban sugarcane). Fresh vegetables and fruits were purchased daily in street markets. In appreciation for the foods from America, Lidia and Hanif organized a banquet for their visitors featuring traditional Russian foods, including a variety of fermented oat and rye dishes.

Among the U.S. delegation was an elderly Native American, the spiritual leader of the Sioux Nation in South Dakota. He was extremely frail and spent most of his time resting. Bill Spear, a macrobiotic teacher from Connecticut, gave him a shiatsu massage and brought him meals prepared by Cary Wolfe, the main macrobiotic chef. One evening, the old man had a dream in which his ancestors came to him and said, "This is how we once lived, ate, and nourished each other. But now our people have forgotten the way of their forebears. Please listen to them."

Meanwhile, another delegation of physicians from Leningrad attended the conference. Yuri Stavitsky, a young pathologist and medical instructor, had volunteered as a radiologist in Chernobyl, Ukraine after its nuclear accident on April 26, 1986. Since then, like many disaster workers, he suffered symptoms associated with radiation disease, including tumors of the thyroid. He and his colleagues also requested macrobiotic foods, and a sizable amount of the airlifted foods was earmarked for the physicians from Leningrad. After the Moscow event, Alex Jack and the visiting teachers traveled to Leningrad, the Soviet Union's second largest city, to give lectures at the Cardiology Center, the Institute of Cytology (the main cancer research center), and the State Institute for the Continuing Education of Doctors. Zoya Tchoueva, a Leningrad psychiatrist and medical researcher, translated my book *The Cancer Prevention Diet* and other macrobiotic books into Russian.

In Pushkin, the former country estate of the Russian czars and a children's convalescent center, town officials and the Agricultural Institute of Leningrad invited the macrobiotic association to set up an ecological village and donated one hundred acres of land for organic production of grains and vegetables. Soviet medical and environmental groups, such as Union Chernobyl and Peace to the Children of the World, hoped to begin distributing miso, sea vegetables, and other macrobiotic-quality foods that would help to protect against the harmful effects of radiation.

In Chelyabinsk, Lidia and Hanif reported, "Miso is helping some of our patients with terminal cancer to survive. Their blood [and blood analysis] became better after they began to use miso in their daily food." Their center, Longevity, expanded its activities, including cultivation of brown rice and millet and production of tofu, tempeh, and other healthful foods. The macrobiotic physicians hosted a regular television program and helped many people recover.

Sources

Jack, Alex. "Soviets Embrace Macrobiotics." *One Peaceful World Newsletter,* Autumn/ Winter 1990.

Personal communication to Alex Jack, April 1991.

Personal communication to Michio Kushi, May 4, 1992.

16.

World Peace Through World Health

As the twenty-first century proceeds, we are at the threshold of an extraordinary period in human history, a time of great difficulties, great challenges, and even greater opportunities. Up until this time, humanity has, of course, encountered many difficult circumstances, and has undoubtedly realized great achievements. But what we are able to accomplish over the next few decades may deeply affect the course of civilization for thousands of years to come. The challenge we are now facing is nothing less than the culmination of civilization's suicidal course of development, from the dawn of recorded history up to the present time.

Beginning several thousand years ago, humanity based its entire concept of development and progress on mastery over nature rather than on harmony with nature. The essence of this concept is ultimately self-destructive. Over the centuries, this type of development has gradually spread and intensified; within the last 200 years, it has grown to encompass the entire world. And today, it has become so widespread and reached such a momentum that it could easily bring about the total annihilation of humanity through war, disease, or environmental destruction.

THE THREAT OF WAR

During the 1950s, this country was acutely aware of the possibility of nuclear war. Serious discussion of the dangers of nuclear attack, frequent civil-defense maneuvers, and other responses to this threat were common parts of daily life.

Recognizing the tremendous scale of destruction that newly developed atomic weaponry would wreak in an all-out world war, the leading intellectuals of the day began to organize an alternative system of world federal government in order to prevent the possibility of future international aggression. These people realized that another world war would very likely mean the extinction of the human race.

Today, I am constantly amazed to hear Americans speak so lightly about war. This is not the case in Europe, where many people are very concerned about this danger. But most people in the United States are too unrealistic to remember or imagine how truly horrible the reality of war, especially nuclear war, would be.

War means that you cannot survive unless you kill others and they cannot survive unless they kill you. So you do your very best to murder each other in any way possible, no matter how cruel and brutal. On a nuclear scale, this savage exchange would become unthinkably grotesque. Unless you have directly experienced the horror of war, it is impossible to imagine.

The Soviet Union collapsed, but the world is more divided than ever. Distinct blocs include the United States, NATO (North Atlantic Treaty Organization) members, and Japan; the Russian federation; China and its global economic network in Asia, Africa, and South America; rival Islamic sects, including terrorist offshoots; and nuclear states such as India, Pakistan, Israel, and North Korea that are strongly independent.

At the conclusion of World War II, a new national constitution was drafted for Japan. Article No. 9 of this constitution declared that Japan would permanently cease to wage war and would never again build up any military force on a large scale; it could, however, maintain a modest reserve for defense. Recently, in the early 2000s, the Japanese government has sought to abandon its post-war pacifism, create a standing army, and even develop as a nuclear power.

As the Crimea crisis in 2014 showed, the end of the Cold War has not necessarily removed the global thermonuclear threat. We must never forget the constant threat to peace. Twenty-four hours a day, just above our heads and off our shores, all around the world, nuclear-armed planes and submarines are running maneuvers that could at any time signal the end of the human race. Nuclear terrorism, including a "dirty bomb" that could destroy a city, is also an ever-present threat.

THE DECLINE OF EDUCATION AND SOCIAL VALUES

The third method of self-destruction, beyond degenerative disease and war, is more subtle and indirect in comparison with the first two; yet, it provides the basis for the continuing development of destructive farming, poor food, and military preparedness. Present-day society does not educate its young people in basic human matters, such as how to maintain health and order in daily life. It does not emphasize respect and love for others or teach how to develop harmonious friendships, personal relationships, families, and other social relations. Totally ignoring the spiritual nature of humanity, modern education fuels the profit motive in its students, giving them the necessary skills and attitudes to satisfy their desire to make money and consume ever more goods and services. This is done, of course, in the name of a "higher standard of living" for both individuals and society—but how is that standard judged? It is weighed exclusively in material terms, such as amount of money, variety of cars and credit cards, number of digital devices and greater bandwidth, and the amount of physical comfort.

Under the influence of this impelling material education and the narrow individualistic values it promotes, and already weakened by biological/biochemical degeneration, the modern family is naturally decomposing very rapidly. Parents are no longer true parents, taking responsibility for their children's diet, health, and well-being, and children are no longer true children, respecting and caring for their parents. The biological, social, and spiritual identity of the family is no longer passing smoothly from one generation to the next. This has signaled the end of human tradition.

I have often spoken with many young people who come from broken homes and can see how profoundly it has affected them and how difficult it is to make up for that loss. I also frequently talk with couples thinking of separation or divorce due to difficulties in maintaining their marriage. I ask them to reflect carefully on why they married in the first place; do they truly wish for their dream together to end now? Further, I ask them to think about their children and their future descendants; if they separate now, the children will be unable to carry on their parents' and ancestors' spirit and tradition.

Several hundred years ago, thousands of Africans were brought by force to this country to help develop a burgeoning plantation industry. When they arrived, husbands were separated from wives, children from parents; their names were changed and they were all sold and taken to different parts of the country. In this way, the new generation of African-Americans was totally cut off from its biological, cultural, and spiritual heritage. They no longer knew who their ancestors were or what they had accomplished, where they had lived or what sort of people they had been. In other words, they lost a large part of the meaning of their lives and could no longer pass on deep spiritual support to their own offspring. Weak, helpless, and dependent, they became spiritual orphans, sold into bondage.

This technique has been repeated countless times throughout history. Separation of tribes, clans, families, and individuals is a most effective way to bring about spiritual, intellectual, and moral decay and to create slaves. And today, we are voluntarily doing this to ourselves! Many of today's alienated youths wander around for years after leaving their families. Such people easily become the slaves of any religious cult or political ideology that comes their way. Or they become easy prey for recruiters from the armed forces, the universities, research and development labs, or multinational corporations, which resettle them far from home and offer them all the material comforts of life in return for their spiritual and intellectual submission.

The explosion of the Internet, smartphones, tablets, and e-readers have enriched our lives, making an unimaginable wealth of data and information, instant communication, and convenient online shopping available. At the same time, these marvelous advances have pulled people even further away from socializing in person. The oft-heralded environmental benefits of a paperless economy have also proved illusory, as the demand for digital bandwidth and cloud computing has skyrocketed, requiring accelerating amounts of coal, nuclear, and other harmful energies to operate. Computers, cell phones, and other electronics also require rare earth metals and conflict minerals to manufacture, while most large paper mills today manage sustainable forests.

THE SPREAD OF ARROGANCE

The fourth avenue to self-destruction is the most subtle, yet it underlies and perpetuates the other three; it is perhaps the most difficult to change. It is very similar to arrogance, which George Ohsawa called the most terrible disease—arrogance, or willful ignorance of the truth.

Our society is riddled with so many conceptual, theoretical delusions that insulate people from reality. We can find these delusions everywhere in conventional modern thinking—in books; in the media and on the Internet; in legal, economic, and social institutions; in religions; and even in some teachings of the New Age, ecology, and peace movements.

Let's look at an example: Suppose some poor country is suddenly plagued with a terrible famine. Our response as a nation is to send the country's inhabitants plenty of food, including sugar and refined flour; an ample amount of new farming technology, including pesticides and chemical fertilizers; and perhaps money that they can use to help their farm industries to recover. This is well-intentioned, of course, but so deluded—we don't see beyond our superstitious faith in money and modern technology to realize that modern farm practice and technology may have played a part in causing the famine! The refined foods we send this country may cause the very diseases that the medical aid we are sending is supposed to prevent or treat, but we don't see the connection because of our blind faith in modern food and modern medicine as necessary parts of living in the world.

Or, to take another example: Many people concerned about the threat of nuclear war feel that we should protest the construction of nuclear power plants. The radiation from these plants, we are told, poses a health hazard to the community; the plutonium they create can be used in the manufacture of atomic and hydrogenous weapons. These concerns are quite valid, but a confrontational approach is very dualistic and impractical. It is based on fear—the fear of personal or family injury. And it would only erase symptoms—eliminate nuclear energy, and scientists and engineers are forced to develop even more dangerous forms of energy to meet society's energy needs.

In order to offset this problem, we first need to study the subject of energy very thoroughly. Why do we require such enormous sources of power? Of course, there are various economic interests involved, together with society's delusions of safety and confidence in modern technology. But essentially, the original impetus behind this movement is the lack of sufficient industrial energy to meet the demands of modern civilization. We need tremendous amounts of energy to maintain our present standard of life—automobile manufacturing, consumer goods, food processing, central heating, air conditioning, high-speed information networks, and many other facets of modern life, including chemical farming.

Such demand for energy is usually overlooked. For example, a *Boston Globe* article described a victory barbeque held by members of a New Hampshire anti-nuclear group when the federal government agreed temporarily to strike their state off a list of sites under consideration for a nuclear waste dumpsite:

> Munching hot dogs and watermelon, about 75 New Hampshire residents quietly celebrated a temporary victory yesterday but vowed to continue battling a federally proposed nuclear waste dump. . . . 'We have every right in the world to eat hot dogs . . . and whoop it up today,' said [the spokesperson for] the Hillsboro-based People of New Hampshire Against the Nuclear Dump.[1]

The irony of this quote is that the anti-nuclear group supporters were eating hot dogs. According to a study by the American Association for the Advancement of Science, the processing, production, and preparation of animal foods takes up 14 percent of the national energy budget and accounts for "more than twice the energy supplied by all our nuclear power plants." To further back this up, in the book *Ecological Cooking*, Joanne Stepaniak and Kathy Hecker reported that animal food production uses more than one-third of all raw materials and fossil fuels consumed in the United States. Producing a single hamburger uses enough fuel to drive twenty miles and causes the loss of five times its weight in topsoil, according to John Robbins in *The Food Revolution*.

So long as people continue to eat hamburgers, hotdogs, and other energy-intensive foods, nuclear energy will be necessary. Of course, no one wants a nuclear dump in their backyard, but if it is not built in New Hampshire, it will be built somewhere else. Protests like these are based on a very superficial understanding.

Interestingly, the law preventing the nuclear waste from being stored onsite was quietly repealed in 2011. In 2015, state representative Renny Cushing—a co-founder of the anti-nuclear Clamshell Alliance in 1976—reactivated the law and established a fee for storing nuclear waste onsite. The ongoing dilemma, however, is figuring out what to do with the nuclear waste.

One way to solve the energy problem is to reduce demands for it in the first place by emphasizing a simpler, more natural way of life, including less animal-quality and more vegetable-quality food in our diets. This we are already doing, of course, but it will take some time to fully accomplish. Meanwhile, society will still have considerable demands for energy production on a fairly large scale.

Secondly, we need to come up with a viable alternative—a simpler, safer, and more economical method for producing industrial energy, a method which is at least as effective as and preferable to nuclear energy. Whenever we approach government, scientists, or other officials, we must first study the subject well and prepare an alternative plan. In the case of nuclear energy and environmental pollution, we do not yet have a viable plan to present. There have been some important advances in solar energy, wind energy, and other renewable resources, and many families and small businesses are using these methods successfully. However, many other households have abandoned these technologies after a few years because they are not really sustainable or perfected yet. All across the world, there are protests against wind farms and other renewable technologies that turned out to be as destructive as the fossil fuel-based approaches they replaced. In China—the world's leading solar energy manufacturer—the production of solar panels has polluted neighboring rice farms and provoked citizen protests. Organic farming on a corporate scale also has a strong downside. In South America, entire tracts of the Amazon jungle have been turned into organic soy and maize plantations, largely for export to Europe. Quinoa, the native grain of the Andes, is now prohibitively expensive for most people in Peru and Bolivia because its popularity in affluent societies has priced it out of reach. According to NPR, the price of quinoa tripled between 2006 and 2013.

The growing popularity of quinoa has both its benefits and its drawbacks. Because quinoa is a very healthy and filling grain, we celebrate its rising consumption in all parts of the world. However, trouble lies ahead. The higher prices do not necessarily close the wage gap between the working-class growers and the upper class—and in fact, the Peru National Household Survey showed that people who eat but do not grow quinoa "are roughly twice as well-off as those who grow it." As more countries hop aboard the growing and exportation train, the growers in quinoa's native land—the Andes region in South America— receive less of the market share, and therefore less of the profit. As for the environment, degradation has fast become a problem. This is because land that had once been allowed to rest started to be used year-round to meet demand; additionally, farmers have reduced their cattle herds, resulting in less manure (natural fertilizer) for the soil. As only a few of the thousands of varieties of quinoa are in demand, crop diversity has shrunk. A lack of diversity leads to recurring pests, which are then contained with harmful fertilizers. To meet demand, farmers have begun to use fertilizers to increase their crop yields. The challenge of creating simple, practical methods for energy and food production is just one of the several examples of the new frontiers we will face over the next decades.

We must begin to approach the problems of the modern world from a larger, more comprehensive view. Until now, we have entirely overlooked the underlying cause of our problems, seeking only to eradicate their symptoms by some harmful technique or conventional palliative. We never proceed to address our challenges through self-reflection or a basic change in our way of life, way of eating, or way of thinking. And by acting on the basis of fragmentary or destructive theories such as waging war on nature, disease, or even war itself, we are every day further crippling our bodies, our families, our earth, and our future as a species.

THE DEGENERATION OF HUMAN JUDGMENT

These four tendencies (degenerative disease, the threat of war, the decline of education and social values, and the spread of arrogance) have been accelerating over the last several hundred years, but as we move through the twenty-first century, the situation has become critical. With the acceleration of delusions and conceptual thinking, we are now reaching the point where human judgment has become so clouded as to be practically irremediable.

At this time, for example, many people have come to the Kushi Institute and macrobiotic centers around the world for dietary advice. By understanding the Order of the Universe and its application to food and health, tens of thousands of these people have been able to heal themselves, and millions have prevented chronic diseases from arising. National and international dietary guidelines are now oriented in a plant-centered way of eating. But still there are many people who are already so weakened physically, and so confused mentally, that they cannot grasp this information and cannot learn to cook or eat properly. Practically speaking, the time left for these people to change and recover their natural human condition is about ten to twenty years. After that, it will be very, very difficult.

Throughout life, our ability to judge—to see yin and yang or complementary and antagonistic tendencies in the things and events around us—is constantly growing and developing. As an infant, we develop our mechanical reflexes and the use of our discriminating senses. During childhood, we explore our likes and dislikes, our emotions and sentiments, and our intellectual curiosity. During adulthood, we extend this curiosity to the realm of society and further into the realm of philosophy or spirituality, where we explore the principles of nature and of the universal change underlying all phenomena. If we are able to master all these realms of exploration—so that we can see front and back and the spiral pattern of growth and decay in all realms—our understanding reaches the universal or supreme level, where we live with a constant, direct sense of infinite justice and harmony. The seven levels of consciousness may be summarized as follows:

1. Mechanical or reflexive awareness

2. Sensory awareness

3. Emotional or aesthetic awareness

4. Intellectual awareness

5. Social awareness

6. Philosophical or spiritual awareness

7. Universal or supreme awareness

For health and peace to spread, we must refine our expression and way of presenting the laws and principles of harmony and change. To reach as many people as possible, we need to first make some kind of evaluation or assessment of the group we are approaching, according to their level of awareness and to their various merits and limitations. Let's look at a few examples.

The youth subculture is often termed a "social movement," but its basic tenets are actually contrary to the strong development of the family, which is the center and base of society. The popular music world, as well as the drug subculture, are more oriented toward the exclusive freedom of the individual. The level of judgment is generally sensory or emotional.

Business operations generally are conducted on a sensory level. The global economy is based on material gain and comfort—sensory gratification, as well as bigger, better, and faster. Intellectual, social, environmental, and spiritual considerations are all subservient to the profit motive. Even emotional and aesthetic awareness plays little role in business decisions.

Among political revolutionaries, we need to distinguish between the original thinkers and philosophers of such movements and the movements themselves, as presently practiced. Karl Marx, for example, never intended to create a violent society with his ideas; dictatorship is actually contradictory to the original idea of communism. Marx's judgment was on the more intellectual or social levels. The young Mao Tse-tung's judgment was also far higher than most of his followers. But he turned into a tyrant, and tens of millions of Chinese perished in his social experiments.

Within traditional religions, again we must distinguish between the original prophets and leaders and present-day followers. Buddha, Lao Tzu, Confucius, Abraham, Jesus, Muhammad, and other great spiritual and religious leaders had spiritual or universal consciousness. At the present time, however, as well as historically, most of the churches, temples, and mosques that grew up around their teachings have declined and appeal to the level of emotional awareness. There are individuals who intuitively attain glimpses of a much larger view of reality while practicing these religions, but they are seldom able to understand these visions or apply them to other areas of life. As a whole, formal religious practices are mechanical: They are the blind practice of ancient traditions.

New Age movements are also, by and large, appealing to the level of emotion. A new era without war and with unlimited freedom is a very idealistic goal, but how should we practically go about achieving it? How do we prevent chronic disease? What role does the family play? These groups are beginning to experiment with some valuable holistic techniques, but as a whole, their thought patterns are based on emotional likes and dislikes.

Some scientists and physicians are working at the emotional level, some with intellectuality, but present science is primarily based on the data of microscopes, telescopes, MRIs, and other scanning devices that mechanically extend our senses. Science and medicine tend to be very intellectual, but the basic level of contemporary understanding is actually more sensory and mechanical. There is very little social responsibility or environmental consciousness, and for the most part the world of vibration and spirit (which is infinitely larger than the sensory detectable world and which was the concern of natural philosophers in past ages) remains wholly unexplored and unknown by present-day scientists and doctors.

Like members of many groups and movements, peace activists have very noble and idealistic motives. They usually have little practical understanding, however, of how to attain their goals and lack a substantial alternative solution that can be proposed and implemented. Protests often increase polarity between sides, harden and supply energy to the antagonist, and make an overall solution more difficult. Peace activists include people who rarely see the whole view—the back and front to all phenomena, including atomic energy—or their own responsibility for world chaos. So long as we are eating foods grown with chemical fertilizers, pesticides, and GMOs; drive cars using Middle Eastern oil; rely on energy derived from fracking; consume hamburgers, fried chicken, and ice cream that take away grain from direct human consumption; and eat bananas and other tropical fruits, coffee, tea, and other imported foods, world poverty, hunger, and competition for scarce resources will continue. Occasionally, someone like George Ohsawa, Albert Einstein, Albert Schweitzer, Pope John Paul II, the Dalai Lama, or Nelson Mandela comes along and makes deep self-reflection, confesses his own complicity in the arms race and injustice, and proposes positive initiatives (on the behalf of humanity as a whole) that do not set one group against another. These efforts arise out of social or philosophical judgment and, while not producing immediate results, have a profound and lasting impact on society and future generations.

Among soldiers, a small number—including some commanders such as Robert E. Lee, Ulysses Grant, General Nogi Maresuke (of the Russo-Japanese War of 1905), and Douglas MacArthur—demonstrated highly evolved social judgment, taking responsibility for the lives and actions of millions of human beings and showing compassion to the vanquished. Even at the lowest levels, many ordinary soldiers are motivated by a desire to serve society and realize a more peaceful world. However, in actual practice, the armed forces operate mechanically and reflexively. Interestingly, as Harvard psychologist Steven Pinker observed in *The Better Angels of Our Nature* (2011), contemporary studies show that only about 10 to 15 percent of men in combat will fire their rifles to kill. The vast majority aim to miss. But it is the rare soldier who refuses to carry out an inhumane or unjust order that is directly given by a superior.

MACROBIOTIC JUDGMENT

The majority of today's population is generally functioning at the first three levels of mechanical, sensory, and emotional consciousness, so all of these movements and groups naturally appeal to many people. Now, at what level is our way ideally operating? Our way should always be trying to see from the eyes of infinity; to see, for example, that all antagonisms are actually arising from the same source and complementing each other. When we see the oneness of fortune and misfortune, prosperity and decline, communism and capitalism, or peace marchers and soldiers, we are seeing from the supreme level of understanding; then, we use the philosophical level of yin and yang (the most simplified, universal way to distinguish phenomena) to explain or interpret that supreme vision.

From there come various social, intellectual, emotional, sensory, and mechanical applications. Once one understands the Order of the Universe, one can easily become a great social prophet; a great intellectual leader; a guide for relationships and other emotional matters; or a wizard of sensory, technical, and mechanical problems. We are free to play at will on all levels. This way always proceeds from the eyes of infinite, supreme understanding. All it requires is to constantly see everything in terms of yin and yang, and to always remember that "all antagonisms are complementary," "what has a front has a back," and the other principles and theorems of yin and yang. This intuitive, commonsense wisdom is the birthright of us all. It is not the monopoly of any one country, culture, religion, class, race, sex, or institution—including macrobiotic organizations. It is life itself, and can never be artificially or exclusively controlled.

THE WAY OF APPROACH

Instead of rejecting or judging other people, we have to embrace them as our friends. Viewing them from the eyes of infinity, we can see that everyone is here for a reason; we need to go to them, understand them, and take them fully into our heart. Then, we can work together to become freer from various limitations and misconceptions and become free to truly accomplish what we would like to do.

It is important to always tell people two things; first is the Order of the Universe. Explain yin and yang in their terms, in a way they can easily see and appreciate. Let them see that there is an invincible order going on. Secondly, we can always introduce good food and good health. No matter what their interest is, it will certainly benefit from better health; even if they are not interested in physical health, we can show them that it is beneficial for emotional, intellectual, or spiritual health. Then, by improving their quality of blood, they themselves will begin to change and eventually see a larger view. They will no longer have any interest in an extreme way or approach to change. Whatever one's interest may be doesn't matter. What matters are the Order of the Universe and food. With these two things, eventually everyone's exclusive thinking will diminish and we will all become brothers and sisters.

SUMMARY

The macrobiotic movement has now reached the point where it can contribute to the changing of the course of our civilization and to the firm establishment of world health and world peace. To meet these challenges, we must create a virtually new species of humanity composed of people who can keep their health and vitality and who can develop their happiness and their offspring's happiness. Members of this new planetary species will have no exclusive identification with a certain nationality, race, religious institution, or sectarian belief. The peaceful reconstruction of humanity is available to all: The new species will be one of universal people, with a comprehensive way of eating, thinking, and living, with the ability to spread their own health and happiness to all surrounding people, families, communities, and countries. It is up to each of us to take the initiative and help create this planetary family.

PEACE PROMOTER

Edward Esko, The Northeast

The problem is how to keep radioactive waste in storage until it decays after hundreds of thousands of years. The geologic deposit must be absolutely reliable as the quantities of poison are tremendous. It is very difficult to satisfy these requirements for the simple reason that we have had no practical experience with such a long-term project.
— Hannes Alfven, Nobel laureate in physics

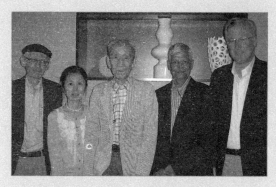

Edward Esko (right) with Alex Jack, Midori Kushi, Michio Kushi, and Mahadeva Srinivasan, a founder of atomic energy in India.

Once each season for several years during the early 2000s, the Quantum Rabbit LLC research team, including members Edward Esko, Alex Jack, and Woody Johnson, would meet at the Moore Mill building in Bellows Falls, Vermont, to conduct tabletop carbon-arc experiments. Bellows Falls is on the Connecticut River. Thirty miles downriver, in the town of Vernon, was the Vermont Yankee Nuclear Power Plant, which operated from 1972 to 2014.

Vermont Yankee epitomized the chaotic state of affairs within the nuclear industry. The amount of radioactive waste stored at Vermont Yankee was substantial. It exceeded that of all four damaged reactors at Fukushima in Japan. The used fuel rods at Vermont Yankee were about one million times more radioactive than they were before being used in the reactor. The rods were hot enough to catch fire if they were not stored under water. Five hundred tons of spent fuel is now being stored in pools of water seven stories above ground. Even after the plant's closing, the nuclear residue will have to be stored there or elsewhere for millennia to come.

Following decades of conflict with local residents and with the state of Vermont, Vermont Yankee announced it would close in 2014. The Yankee plant went on line in 1972 and has the same General Electric boiling water system as the failed nuclear reactors at Fukushima. Following the disaster at Fukushima, Entergy (the owner of Vermont Yankee) was being pressured to make expensive modifications to improve safety. Financial experts point to low natural gas prices as another factor in the closure of the plant, explaining that competition from cheap natural gas-fired electric plants severely limited Vermont Yankee's margins.

The Problem of Nuclear Waste

The closing of the plant meant that Vermont Yankee would no longer be producing radioactive waste. However, still unresolved is what will happen with the tons of highly radioactive spent fuel rods stored at the site. On a planetary scale, there are more than 430 locations around the world where nuclear waste continues to accumulate. Most is stored at individual reactor sites. Nuclear reactors on planet Earth create about 10,000 metric tons of spent nuclear fuel each year. Thus, the problem gets worse with each passing day. The shutdown and decommission of nuclear power plants solves only the problem of *new* nuclear waste. It does nothing to solve the problem of already existing waste. Moreover, the process of cleaning up the existing waste is expensive (between $300 million to $5.6 billion per unit), time-consuming, and hazardous to workers and the natural environment. It opens a window for disaster caused by human error, accident, or sabotage.

In the U.S., there are thirteen reactors that have shut down and are in the process of decommissioning (as of 2016). None have fully completed the process, which can last as long as 100 years. The timeframes when dealing with nuclear waste disposal are enormous; they range from 10,000 years to millions of years. Storage of nuclear waste, whether "temporary" or "permanent," does not solve the problem. It simply passes it on to future generations. The very existence of nuclear waste is itself the problem. For the sake of future generations, we need to seriously investigate promising ideas not just for storing nuclear waste, but also for *getting rid* of it.

Quantum Conversion

Toward that end, Quantum Rabbit LLC, a small macrobiotic company, started conducting tabletop research on quantum conversion in 2004. *Quantum conversion* is defined as transforming one atom into another by changing its nuclear structure. Until now, this has been done primarily by high-energy nuclear processes and is extremely costly and dangerous, and generates radioactivity and atomic waste.

Quantum conversion attempts to achieve this with simple tabletop equipment, using electric power from car batteries, solar panels on a HUBERT generator, or the wall socket, all under relatively low temperatures and low pressures in the open air or in glass vacuum tubes. It is inexpensive and safe. This is in contrast to the high temperatures, energies, and pressures necessary for so-called "hot" fusion—the next generation of nuclear reactors.

The Quantum Rabbit experiments are based on the work of George Ohsawa, the Japanese philosopher and educator, who, together with French biochemist Louis Kervran, developed the theory of biological and elemental transformation. In 1964, Ohsawa claimed to have converted sodium into potassium in a tabletop experiment conducted in Tokyo. Ohsawa believed that this change took place through a process of low energy fusion in which two lighter elements, sodium and oxygen, fused to form the heavier element potassium.

Sodium has the atomic number 11 and the atomic weight 23. Oxygen has the atomic number 8 and the atomic weight 16. If we add the atomic number and weight of sodium with the atomic number and weight of oxygen, we get the atomic number (19) and weight (39) of potassium. The formula is written as follows, with the plus sign (+) indicating a fusion reaction and the arrow ($\longrightarrow$) indicating the fusion product:

$$^{11}Na_{23} + {}^{8}O_{16} \longrightarrow {}^{19}K_{39}$$

Following this initial experiment, Ohsawa began researching the conversion of carbon into iron, with the addition of oxygen. In Cambridge, Massachusetts, I joined Ohsawa in performing experiments in which carbon and oxygen were apparently fused to form iron. The year was 1965. The carbon into iron experiment was done in the open air and is another example of low energy fusion. Graphite (carbon) powder was placed on a copper plate. A graphite rod was connected to several car batteries. An electrical arc was struck when the rod was placed near the graphite powder. The arc sucked in oxygen from the surrounding air. The process was repeated and the remaining powder was found to be magnetic and to contain trace amounts of iron. The low energy fusion formula can be written as follows:

$$2(^{6}C_{12} + {}^{8}O_{16}) \longrightarrow {}^{26}Fe_{56} + {}^{2\,protons}$$

In the past, many scientists have pursued similar goals. For example, only recently did I learn that Professor Hantaro Nagaoka of Tokyo Imperial University, my alma mater, conducted studies in 1924, two years before I was born, in which isotopes of mercury and bismuth yielded platinum and other precious metals.

New Research

Forty years after the experiments Ohsawa and I began, Edward Esko, Alex Jack, and Woody Johnson—three of my students—formed Quantum Rabbit, LLC (QR), a Massachusetts company, in 2004 to develop our ideas and address the contemporary problems of society. Edward served as vice president of the East West Foundation, our original education organization in Boston, and a senior teacher and counselor at Kushi Institute. Alex had managed the Kushi Institute. and written many books with me and my wife Aveline. Woody founded Woodland Energy Company. They established a small lab in Nashua, New Hampshire to begin experiments on quantum conversion using custom designed glass vacuum tubes. Carbon arc experiments were also started at the Woodland Energy Company in Bellows Falls, Vermont. In 2009, the vacuum lab moved to Owls Head, Maine.

TABLE 16.1 RESULTS OF CARBON ARC EXPERIMENTS.			
ELEMENT	CONCENTRATION*	ELEMENT	CONCENTRATION*
Silicon	10,500	Titanium	440
Magnesium	1,800	Scandium	35
Iron	4,700	Cobalt	160
Aluminum	7,800	Nickel	1,120

*parts per million

As with the experiments conducted forty years earlier, in these experiments, carbon displayed magnetic activity when subjected to the arcing process. Placing the treated graphite powder on white paper and waving a neodymium magnet underneath it repeatedly confirmed magnetic properties. Not only was the graphite magnetic, but also when analyzed independently, it showed traces of elements such as silicon, iron, and aluminum—the elements shown in Table 16.1 on page 249. Quantum conversion formulas help the team to understand the presence of anomalous elements in treated graphite.

After publishing articles in *Infinite Energy,* a leading new science journal, Quantum Rabbit began to spark the interest of other researchers. The macrobiotic researchers were approached by Continuum Energy Technologies. This is a large innovative corporation founded by John Preston, who served as director of technology development and licensing at MIT, where he was responsible for the commercialization of intellectual property developed at MIT. Edward, Alex, and Woody began experiments at their facility in Fall River, Massachusetts. Also joining in the testing was David Pelly, an MIT graduate, a Harvard MBA, and CEO of Stealth Energy Technology. In carbon arc experiments, David verified that the Quantum Rabbit researchers had produced iron, nickel, vanadium, titanium, and silver. In a subsequent tungsten experiment, holmium and samarium, both rare earth metals, appeared. On the basis of Artax spectrometer analysis, David concluded that the "signal" (meaningful data) compared to "noise" (background data) was highly significant.

Nuclear Remediation

Over the years, the U.S. Department of Defense has expressed interest in low-energy nuclear conversion. In 1978, military scientists verified some of the original tests of Kervran. At a presentation to the American Chemical Society in 2002, Pamela Mosier-Boss, a scientist with the U.S. Space and Naval Warfare Systems Center (San Diego), reported: "We have compelling evidence that fusion reactions are occurring" at room temperature. The results are "the first scientific report of highly energetic neutrons from low-energy nuclear reactions," she explained.

In 2005, Edward developed preliminary formulas for the low energy fission of heavy elements. Low energy fission is the opposite of low energy fusion. In low energy fission, a heavy element, such as lead or bismuth, splits into two lighter elements. The Quantum Rabbit team began to speculate about the possibility of using low energy nuclear reactions (LENR) to convert the radioactive isotopes (forms of the same element) found in nuclear waste into stable non-radioactive elements. In theory, the process of subtracting lithium or another light element from super-heavy elements could be used to condense the decay cycle of radioactive elements such as uranium-235 and plutonium-239 from thousands or millions of years to a few years at most (see Figure 16.1 on page 251.) On a parallel track, low energy fusion could also be deployed to instantly convert radioactive fission products like iodine-129, technetium-99, and cesium-137 into useful elements like barium, palladium, and neodymium.

In 2011, Dr. Mahadeva Srinivasan met with me, Edward, and Alex in the Boston

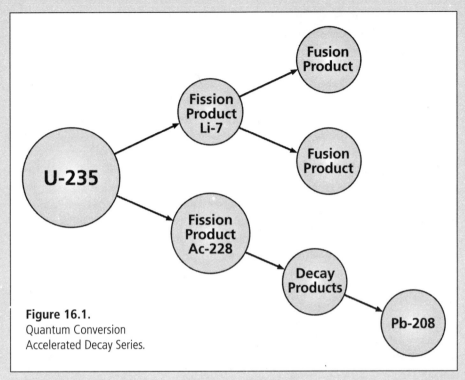

Figure 16.1.
Quantum Conversion
Accelerated Decay Series.

The illustration shows uranium (U-235) changing into lead (Pb-208). Uranium fissions into lithium (Li-7) and actinium (Ac-228), setting in motion an accelerated decay cycle lasting 1.9 years instead of millions of years.

area to discuss the possibility of converting radioactive waste into harmless, stable elements. Dr. Srinivasan, who recently retired from the Bhabha Atomic Research Centre in Mumbai, was one of the fathers of nuclear energy in India. Over the years, he had encouraged his colleagues to verify the original Ohsawa experiments. They were also replicated by an associate at Texas A&M University and published in the peer-reviewed journal *Fusion Technology* in 1994. Dr. Srinivasan described the Quantum Rabbit project as "farsighted," and in the foreword to Edward and Alex's book *Cool Fusion,* observed: "Their motivation in undertaking such experimental investigations was to pave the way in establishing a technology, which can be relied upon to hopefully come to the rescue of mankind when it runs out of precious heavy element metals. An added incentive is the potential application . . . to convert radioactive waste left behind by the nuclear fission power industry into more benign stable elements."

On April 10, 2013, Quantum Rabbit conducted the first of a series of preliminary tests on the remediation of nuclear waste. The test involved the conversion of stable iodine-127 into barium-134 through a simple low energy fusion reaction. Radioactive iodine-129 is created by the fission of uranium and plutonium in nuclear reactors. With a half-life of 15.7 million years, iodine-129 poses a significant threat to human health and the environment. Successful conversion of stable iodine-127 could provide a pathway for research on converting radioactive iodine-129 into non-radioactive barium.

As predicted, barium appeared in all three test samples, ranging as high as 463 ppm from a starting concentration (in the iodine used in the test) of 0.43 ppm, more than a thousand-fold increase. Moreover, the distribution of isotopes (forms of the same element) in the treated sample varied considerably from the distribution of isotopes found in nature. Novel isotope distribution is considered the gold standard for ruling out contamination and proving quantum conversion.

A Reverse Manhattan Project

Clearly, much work needs to be done. Quantum Rabbit has continued experiments at its small lab in Maine and at CET in Fall River, but with limited time and resources, the work remains preliminary, like that of Apple's Steve Jobs and Steve Wozniak in their garage in Silicon Valley or the Wright Brothers in their bicycle shop in Ohio. The researchers' hope is to eventually partner with established labs or universities to take the preliminary work to the next level. The Ceramic Cement Corporation, which stores waste for the Nuclear Regulatory Commission at Idaho National Labs, has expressed interest in collaborating with Quantum Rabbit on remediation.

"Nuclear energy was unleashed seventy years ago with the Manhattan Project," Edward explained. "In today's dollars, the creation of nuclear power cost about $26 billion. With research and development in thirty locations, the project employed 130,000 people. That was the effort required to let the nuclear genie out of the bottle. It may require an even greater effort from now on to put the nuclear genie back into the bottle, with researchers around the globe all working toward that one goal. The entire planet may need to unite behind the goal of eliminating nuclear waste. All promising proposals, no matter how far out of the mainstream, should be considered. We owe it to ourselves and to future generations to act now."

Quantum conversion is still in its infancy. However, as it develops, practical ways may be found to make scarce, valuable industrial metals from common, ordinary elements like silicon (beach sand). In addition to reducing toxicity (from biological, chemical, and nuclear pollution), this would gradually reduce the need for costly, dangerous, and environmentally destructive mining, smelting, and other technologies. In turn, territorial claims for precious resources (as in the Congo over conflict metals) are a major cause of violence and war. Along with a balanced plant-based diet, quantum conversion is a key to creating a healthy, peaceful world.

Sources

Esko, Edward, and Alex Jack. *Cool Fusion*. Becket, Massachusetts: Amberwaves Press, 2011.

Esko, Edward, and Alex Jack. *Corking the Nuclear Genie*. Becket, Massachusetts: Amberwaves Press, 2014.

Various articles, *Infinite Energy*, 2005–2016.

17.

The Government of the Future

World peace is the eternal dream of humanity. In ancient Greece, the well-spring of Western civilization, Plato's *Republic* discussed a proposal for a new world political structure, governed by universal law as interpreted by a "philosopher king," rather than by artificial law and material power. Other writers and thinkers have presented various proposals in works such as *Utopia* by Sir Thomas More, *The City of the Sun* by Tommaso Campanella, and *The Discourse of Eternal Peace* by Immanuel Kant. St. Augustine proposed a global nation of God—a world society managed according to Catholic principles. Marx and Engels envisioned a classless society in which human beings were no longer alienated from each other and governed peacefully.

None of these visions or proposals, however, has been realized or fulfilled. In fact, sickness, war, hostility, and conflict have only continued to escalate with the advent of modern technology. To address this problem, the League of Nations was formed after World War I as an attempt to unite the world. The United States actually initiated this action, but didn't join. While President Woodrow Wilson was in favor of participation, the Senate did not want to approve it, so the headquarters was moved to Switzerland. Then, because of differences of opinion, various countries dropped out, including Germany and Japan. The League of Nations became virtually meaningless.

After World War II, a second attempt was made; the United Nations was formed to prevent another world war from arising and to secure world peace for the future. The United Nations, however, is in fact powerless to do so. It is not a world government, but only an association of independent sovereign nations. If one country opposes the others, little can really be done.

THE WORLD FEDERALIST MOVEMENT

In light of such problems, a worldwide movement arose after World War II, proposing a single world federal government. Many leading intellectuals of the day joined this movement between 1945 and 1960, including such notables as Albert Einstein, Thomas Mann, Upton Sinclair, Norman Cousins, Mahatma Gandhi, and Jawaharlal Nehru. Many members of the United States Congress also presented resolutions to direct U.S. foreign policy toward the establishment of one world federation.

At the close of the war, some World Federalists formed a committee to draw up a preliminary draft of the new Earth Constitution, with the University of Chicago as their base of operations. Quite a few scientists and scholars participated, and after years of work, they produced a very substantial document. They also published a study journal, *Common Cause.*

The preliminary draft of the Earth Constitution outlined a world governmental structure modeled after the United States. They proposed a World Executive Office, with the hope of electing Gandhi as the first World President, and a World Parliament, divided into a World Senate and a World House of Representatives. World Senators were to be elected from among each individual country's government, and one World Representative was to be elected for every one million people in a country. The World Federalist movement also proposed a World Supreme Court, forming three independent powers—much like the United States federal government.

At that time, the World Federalist movement had two general ideas. One was to amend the existing charter of the United Nations to gradually bring it more toward an active world governing body; this approach was the main current in the U.S. In Europe, a more radical approach was favored: Europeans felt that changing the U.N. would be very difficult, and proposed instead that the World Federalists organize themselves and create a World People's Convention to institute their preliminary draft of the new Earth Constitution themselves.

Then, the Cold War set in between Russia and the United States. As the Soviets began to try and exert more influence on the People's Convention approach, the movement became more sharply divided into conservative and radical camps. The Cold War intensified, and gradually people forgot about the World Federalist movement altogether. Since then, the idea of a world federation or world government has almost disappeared from public view. The fear of global dictatorship, mirrored in George Orwell's *1984* and other dystopian novels, heavy-handed vaccination campaigns by the World Health Organization (WHO), and environmentally destructive policies of the World Trade Organization (WTO), have fueled widespread fear of world government and planetary federation.

AN ANCIENT PROPOSAL FOR WORLD GOVERNMENT

Let's take another example, further back in history. About 2,600 years ago in ancient feudalistic China, in the small kingdom of Lu, a giant thinker was born. His name was Qiu; later in life, he became known as Confucius. Confucius spent years studying human relations and the problems of society and came to the conclusion that the various kingdoms of China were all governed by powers and laws, each conflicting with the other. He concluded that government should be changed to operate according to *Jing Gi,* meaning "Virtue and Righteousness."

He carefully worked out what those qualities would entail. Unless the kingships manifested and advocated these principles, Confucius believed, the people would continue to be unhappy, and local wars and conflicts would wage interminably.

Confucius began to teach these conclusions. Many students came to him, and he taught them continuously: how to govern society, how to create future governments, and how future leaders should be the masters of virtue and righteousness. Then he began to travel from kingdom to kingdom, meeting with kings, princes, princesses, and lords, urging them to promote the study of arts and the classics and to develop the principles of *Jing* and *Gi* in themselves and in their societies.

They all received him politely and treated him with great respect, but very few actually listened to him or tried to implement his ideas. At that time, according to a story in *The Book of Soshi*, Confucius went to visit Lao Tzu, the great Taoist philosopher. When he returned to his disciples, he could not speak for three days. Finally, his disciples asked him what had happened, and he told them:

> I have met kings and lords of all kinds, but now I have finally met a man who carried within him the energy of the infinite universe itself. When I opened my mouth to speak to him, I couldn't speak for several minutes.
>
> Finally I said to him, "From a young age I have studied day and night, mastering the arts of music, poetry, literature, courtesy, manners, the law of change, history, and more. I have learned far beyond many other people, and believe that I well understand what these books have told me. Now I want to spread the way of virtue and righteousness among the leaders of all countries; so I visited seventy-two kings, lords, and princes. I have presented to them the secrets of the wonderful way the ancient kings and lords managed their countries and their people. But not one of them accepted my words. . . . It seems to be very difficult to bring the way of peace to the world!"
>
> And Lao Tzu replied, "It is so fortunate for you that nobody listened! You are so lucky that nobody wants to follow your way of achieving peace! All those studies you learned were just ideas; those many books are nothing but the footprints of great men. The important thing is not their books or their ideas, but their actual doings and conduct; and these cannot be repeated.
>
> "Time changes, circumstances change, and the way to achieve peace must also change. The spirit and the principle does not change, but the expression and the realization may change very much. It is foolish to try and recover the ancient ways exactly as they were practiced; and it is very fortunate they didn't understand you. It could only make things worse!"

Three months later Confucius again visited Lao Tzu and said, "I now understand. When parents love their children that is natural. When birds sing in the spring that is also natural. Naturally, they make love and have children, following the Order of the Universe and the laws of yin and yang. All animals, plants, and all the phenomena of the universe follow that natural way, including humanity. If we try to change it by our artificial intentions, it cannot help. So we must first truly understand the workings of the Order of the Universe and can then inspire people themselves to change in a natural way, without special goals or intentions." And Lao Tzu replied, "Wonderful. You understand."

The compass of yin and yang will help us recover our native, intuitive memory and understanding of the infinite Order of the Universe, its mechanism of change, and its manifestation in our human life and daily activities.

In order to release ourselves from sickness, anxiety, fantasy, and violence, and to change our deluded conceptions of health and happiness, we must first apply our understanding of yin and yang to our daily dietary practice—how to choose, prepare, and take our food and drink. Through proper eating, our blood and body will become sound and whole. Mental and spiritual well-being will naturally follow. Without any special preventive measures other than diet, we are able to maintain our physical health, suffering no serious sickness or disability. Without any other additional mental or psychological training, we are able to establish a calm, peaceful mind, experiencing no delusions or other mental disorders. Without any extraordinary efforts other than the simple compass of yin and yang, we are able to understand with ease any subject that we desire to learn. Without any special education, we are naturally able to develop a spirit of love for other people and of harmony with our environment. Without imposing any restrictions upon ourselves, we are able to resolve disagreements and conflicts peacefully by coming up with a solution that will benefit the whole rather than just one side. Without any special experience, we are naturally inspired with the spirit of perseverance and endless aspiration, enduring any hardship with gratitude. Without any other training, we are able to experience our oneness with every being and all phenomena surrounding us.

THE BIOLOGICAL FOUNDATION OF SELF-GOVERNMENT

We can divide all world peoples throughout history into two basic dietary groups: agricultural and nomadic peoples. Warfare has, of course, been common to nearly all societies, particularly during the last eight to ten thousand years; but historically, there has been far less war among those societies practicing an agricultural way of life. If we can adjust world dietary patterns to follow the harvest rather than livestock breeding, to rely on grains, beans, and vegetables far more than on animal foods, the spirit of all the world peoples will automatically, biologically begin to change—not by laws ("You must be peaceful or else") or by education and morals ("You ought to become more peaceful if you want to be a good person"), but by Lao Tzu and Confucius's way of natural change. This peaceful spirit will naturally come from within the people themselves, as part of their own growth and self-development.

For example, I was brought up in a semi-macrobiotic way, eating grains and vegetables, but still influenced somewhat by modern thinking. While our diet was normally pretty good, we were occasionally eating eggs and perhaps a small piece of meat once a month. My elder brother and I would generally get along very well; but every now and then, we would argue and begin to fight—really serious fighting. Of course, it wouldn't last long, and this only happened about once a month; but it would happen regardless.

Now, I'm amazed to see macrobiotic families (including my own children and grandchildren) who are really eating well; they play around and push each other, but they never fight. It's so amazing. In the rest of the world (especially in the bigger cities), even in kindergarten and grammar schools, children are always fighting and yelling at each other—they even fight their teachers. Many high school teachers now need to carry weapons with them to school for self-defense! But it seems that macrobiotic children, without being taught in any special way, or without being disciplined, never fight.

Through the natural foods of the earth, we are creating a new race of people who are naturally peace-loving, without needing any special, artificial teachings, laws, codes, or enforcement. If all people began to eat this way, we would become a peace-loving society. Before we can really develop a practical world governmental structure, in other words, we need to further society's natural evolution, to create a biological, spiritual base for a new type of civilization. This is the ultimate purpose behind our macrobiotic movement, which has already begun to significantly change society's dietary habits and conventional views toward food and health.

BIOLOGICAL ORGANIZATION OF SOCIETY

We have seen many attempts to discover the ideal way of organizing society; every method involves the polarization of society into two complementary groups—the "governing" and the "governed." For example, monarchy and feudalism, in which individuals govern larger masses of people, have often been followed by various forms of democracy, in which the majority prevails over the minority, and socialism and communism, in which certain classes or political parties dominate other classes or parties. Modern nations see their own political forms as unique. But most nations today are actually governed largely by some version of bureaucracy, in which small groups of people (bureaus) govern the rest, as in the United States, Russia, China, and Japan.

What is the most natural social organization? The family. The family is the natural, time-tested, self-governing unit within all human society. Order is very easily and naturally established in the family: Parents guide their children, because they have more experience, and therefore more understanding and higher judgment; and parents automatically love and care for their children. When a child becomes sick, his or her parents can't sleep. They stay up all night at the foot of the child's bed, worrying, watching—selflessly caring for the child. This is very natural.

Today, of course, this natural structure is collapsing everywhere; families are disintegrating, and people are saying that this type of structure is arbitrary or obsolete and can't work anymore. Why? Of course, there are many factors involved, but there is one central issue in the family that has gone awry. After a hard day's work, everyone returns home in the evening to eat. Of course, sex is there, too, but food is more urgent; everyone needs to eat every day. As long as everyone is eating together, the basis for family unity is established; if that collapses, the family will collapse. Eating together establishes a similar quality of blood, consciousness, and dream.

Suppose everyone eats at different restaurants and then comes home to sleep. This is not a family, it is simply a hotel. Even when the whole family eats together, if the food is not selected and prepared with a thorough and balanced understanding of its effects on health and peace of mind, troubles will begin. The family may stay together physically, since they are still eating together, but they will argue and fight constantly. Or, they will gradually fall apart because of their degenerating health.

To maintain a unified, happy, peaceful family, there must be some central person providing all family members with the correct biological foundation for their own health and happiness. Then, naturally, all family members will orient themselves around that person; naturally, the children's love and respect will be there, without being artificially taught; and naturally, the parents will want to love and care for their children. When families eat this way, and then communities and nations as a whole begin to eat this way, the world will begin to think in family terms—family communities, family societies, one planetary family.

GOVERNMENT BY NATURAL ORDER

The approach of modern government is from the front: power and law. Our approach is from behind; changing people's quality. Along the way, almost any type of government is fine, but the ultimate goal is non-government. This is not to be confused with anarchy or with chaos. Our way is not human government, but the Order of the Universe. In the *Tao Te Ching*, Lao Tzu says that ruling a state is ideally like cooking a small fish: the less interference, the better. Table 17.1 on page 259 illustrates the major approaches to government as represented by the three major types of civilization.

In a family-based society, government would not need to enforce certain behavior through codes, laws, and military and police power, as we presently do. This government would be less a power or police organization and more of a service or educational organization. This government would provide the people

TABLE 17.1 THREE TYPES OF CIVILIZATION.		
	SPIRITUAL AND AESTHETIC	**MATERIAL AND SOCIAL**	**COMPREHENSIVE**
Ruled by	Idea	Law	Understanding
Backed by	Truth	Power	Love
Authority	Moral code	Constitution	Natural order
Food	Vegetable quality	Animal quality	Balance
Environment	Rural	Urban	Natural
Lifestyle	Agricultural	Industrial	Holistic
Orientation	Spirit intuition	Matter analysis	Energy synthesis
Center	Church	State	Family
Social unit	Tribe/clan	Nation	Geographic, climatic, ecological region planet
Occupation	Rest	Work	Play
Direction	East; South	West; North	Global

with information about how to manage agriculture, industries, education, and energy, and consider solutions to any problems that might arise.

Suppose, for example, some people propose to create an enterprise to refine and distribute sugar. Under our present government, as long as the structure of this business proposition is in order, and the right amount of money goes to taxes, that plan is fine. Government, of course, is incapable of evaluating the effects this industry will have on human health; for that, medical specialists are consulted, but with few exceptions they testify that sugar is harmless. Some environmental questions are raised about the new factory, but because of the sagging economy, these are waived in favor of putting more people to work. From society's point of view, the company can start distributing sugar. Everything is quite legal.

From the perspective of the Order of the Universe, however, this business is highly illegal, so nature's judiciary system issues a sentence of punishment: Everybody who foolishly eats sugar excessively gets sick. Then, the government proposes a new method of health insurance, whereby people can go to the doctors and receive medications (that will eventually make them worse) without depleting their household budget so severely that they cannot continue buying this quite legal product. Then suppose some of our sugar buyers—instead of getting headaches, tooth decay, stomach ulcers, or cancer—get high blood pressure, various nervous disorders, and go on to become criminals. They go out and steal or commit armed assault and sooner or later are caught by the government's police.

In court, they are found guilty and sentenced to prison. This is considered a very reasonable, sensible way to retaliate for the person's bad behavior. While in prison, these people are fed more sugar, together with meat, dairy, and very fatty, poor-quality foods; naturally, they come out worse than when they went in! And meanwhile, nature's laws are being violated again and again, by everyone involved.

A world service educational institution would see the initial proposal and immediately say: No, better not set up a sugar industry; it would make people sick. Instead, why don't you use that machinery to make a good-quality miso or process kuzu roots into kuzu powder that people can use as natural home medicine when they get sick from eating too much sugar? As for prisons, we should transform them into educational places where criminals are fed the best-quality natural and organic foods, properly selected and prepared, and where every day they can study the laws of the universe and the dreams and aspirations of humankind. Then, six months later (or a year, two years, or more in some cases), after a change of blood quality and consciousness, they will come out, clean and healthy, ready to inspire people and really help society.

The people who would be able to make such evaluations and educate in such a way do not exist in our present-day governments. This is why "politics" has earned such a low reputation. We should eventually replace this type of government by power with a governing body which has the capacity to evaluate or judge things with respect to the natural order. In other words, we need a new type of world leader.

Who should be the new world leaders? Who are the most respected people? In a natural family, the oldest members are the wisest and most respected. Today, of course, many old people become very weak or sick; but regardless, they have more life experience than we do. If we could begin to recover our natural sense of respect for elders—giving them our seats in the subway or bus, offering them assistance in the grocery store, or asking for their advice or opinion in making difficult decisions—this alone would greatly change our present society. And if our elders were nourished with a better diet, then their judgment would become even sharper, clearer, and wiser.

To manage the affairs of our world family society, we need to discover law— not artificial, arbitrary human laws, but real law: natural, absolute law that is invincible, immutable, and universal. That law is, of course, the law of change, the eternal principle by which all phenomena are created, animated, and finally dissolved. This law is expressed in abstract form in the seven principles and twelve theorems (see Appendix B, page 322). However, our world government service organization must be able to apply these abstract principles efficiently and accurately to any situation. Practically speaking, we would need an interpreter of the Order of the Universe and its manifold applications and appearances in all society's affairs.

For this interpreting function, ancient societies automatically created a council of elders, a gathering of the wisest people among them, people with ideological or supreme judgment. In our terms, we need to have some kind of World Congress, composed of friends who have deeply studied and mastered the principles of yin and yang in many different fields and areas of life. This Congress would serve to evaluate, judge, educate, and guide all local, regional, and worldwide enterprises and activities—not as a legislative instrument, but more as a universally respected educational advisory board.

THE GOVERNMENT OF THE FUTURE

The day may not be far off when world government by such a gathering of people may become a reality. Accordingly, our macrobiotic movement has also begun to prepare for this development, along with spreading sound, sensible, natural, and organic ways of eating. We have begun to introduce and explore the workings of yin and yang and the Order of the Universe in many domains and applications—health and healing, family life, spirituality, art, architecture, language, history, science, cosmology, industry, and many others.

We have also begun to hold our regional congresses, such as the annual North American Macrobiotic Congress, the European Macrobiotic Congress, the Caribbean Macrobiotic Congress, and the Middle Eastern Macrobiotic Congress. Additional congresses will be initiated in other regions, including the Far East, South America, and Africa; and in the future, we hope to assemble for our first joint World Macrobiotic Congress. The congresses' role will be to bring representatives of the macrobiotic community together to address global problems and solutions.

These are very small beginnings, of course. Most of our friends are not actually elders at all, but are still quite young and very inexperienced in the practical realities of managing society's affairs. It will take time—but it is definitely humanity's last hope and last chance of survival.

"Law" won't work; teaching ethics, morality, and virtue won't work; school education, religions, psychological teachings, technology, governmental measures—none of these methods will work, as history has shown us. After thousands of years, billions of dollars spent, and vast numbers of people killed, we have learned that all these attempts are futile. The only way is to recover the human way of life in accord with nature and the universe—and to reestablish our biological identity as humans, beginning within the family.

Our way to relieve cancer or heart disease is not a nutritional or dietary technique. We can offer nutritional or dietetic explanations as to why or how illness develops, but it is not a fix or magic bullet. It is simply a return to the human way of life, and nothing else. Gradually all sickness, disorders, and personal troubles disappear.

In the same way, when all people return to the human way of life, all family troubles and all society's troubles would disappear. We can explain this with various social, political, or economic explanations, but it is actually simplicity itself.

SUMMARY

The government of the future—or what we might call a planetary common-wealth—will not be created through any secret, complicated teaching; through any specialized education or any political theory; or through any party, sect, or elite. These things are useless. The government of the future is being created right now, through our daily practice of eating good food, our study of yin and yang, our respect for our elders and love for our juniors, and through the growing happiness and health of our families. From these simple beginnings, we can definitely realize humanity's long-cherished dream of one happy, peaceful world.

PART IV

Practical Steps

International and national congresses for peace resemble the fabled congress of the rats and mice that were united by fear of a large cat. They manifested highly against the cat and showed themselves courageous. But unfortunately, they were not able to imagine a practical idea, as for example a bell, and still less were they able to find someone who could attach it to the cat's neck.

—George Ohsawa

18.

Qualifications
of a Peace Promoter

The greatest of all the social problems facing us today is world war. Until now, modern civilization has been unable to come up with a cure or remedy for this illness.

The common dream of humanity—the goal of all philosophies, religions, and traditional ways of life—is to develop a peaceful and harmonious human society and create one home, or one family, on this planet. Since the 1960s, the macrobiotic community has begun to secure good-quality food and agriculture, changing patterns of modern food consumption to a more natural and organic direction. We also have demonstrated how to approach degenerative diseases in a peaceful way without further injuring people. Medicine has been symptomatic rather than preventive in orientation; thus, troubles constantly recur. Today, we are educating people to understand that they can heal themselves of many degenerative diseases and other physical and psychological disorders with peaceful methods of self-recovery. Everything we have done so far is only a prelude. Ultimately, we have to eliminate world war. To this end, we must begin to take responsibility for our social health and security as well as our personal health and well-being.

Up until now, most approaches to world peace have been partial. They didn't deal with peace as a problem of persons as a whole. The approaches have dealt with peace as a moral problem, a political problem, an organizational problem, or a military problem. Past and present approaches have not considered sickness, appetite, crime, and desire for material wealth and safety as factors in the conversation about world peace. What is humanity as a whole? What is health, crime, and mental illness? We cannot separate world peace from agriculture, from eating, from day-to-day relationships, from psychological and spiritual consciousness, from driving the car to work or the market, from paying taxes, and from many other ordinary, everyday concerns.

THE IMPORTANCE OF UNITY

At the present time, all aspects of modern life are separated from each other. In the field of medicine, we look only at the symptoms of disease, not the underlying cause of the disorder. This separation is one of the big troubles in modern society.

We have different doctors for different diseases. For cancer, we go to an oncologist, not to a psychiatrist, dentist, or gynecologist. It is the same with education; for poetry, we must take a literature class, not geology, mathematics, or physics. This causes divisions and separations. Yet, the fact is, we live one life. We eat a certain way. We breathe a certain way. We live in a certain place. The seasons change. All of these and other factors are part of our life and are inseparable from our condition, sickness, and destiny.

This concept also has relevance to the issue of world peace. We can't separate peace from our day-to-day life. Separation is the problem. Future peacemakers will not be specialists, but will have a general and comprehensive understanding of life. We may call such a person a life teacher, one who can guide others to health and happiness. In traditional Eastern and Western thought, the lowest grade of doctor or teacher is one who takes care of physical or psychological symptoms. The middle grade of healer, counselor, or educator deals with the cause of illness and unhappiness and advises a change in diet, environment, consciousness, or lifestyle. The highest physician or philosopher can cure the sickness of the nation and bring peace to the world as a whole.

The greatest minds of modern times have been unable to solve personal and social problems because of the dualistic mentality that prevails. Descartes introduced the idea that mind and body are entirely separate. Darwin popularized the idea of the survival of the fittest among different species. Marx applied a similar reasoning to human society and saw life as perpetual conflict between different social classes. Malthus taught that war and hunger are necessary to keep the population in check in a world chronically short of food. Today, many government officials, soldiers, and peace activists believe in "fighting for peace."

As we have seen, it is a delusion to think that life is a battle or war. We think we need to defend ourselves. We carry a ring full of keys, memorize electronic passwords, and utilize other security devices wherever we go. We establish a police force and a military system. We set up a vast defense system all around us, beginning with the pills, medications, vitamins, and supplements that we take at home. The social welfare system, retirement system, insurance system, and medical system are all part of this defense network. We are everywhere and always on guard. When fear and mistrust govern, everyone thinks, "They may attack first. I have to defend and attack back." When I first came to this country, I was shocked to discover that lawyers wrote up marriage contracts. Marriage is not a contract or business. It is a spiritual, emotional, and physical union based on unconditional love and trust.

In reality, there are no enemies. Everything is in harmony with the natural environment. We have grown so out of touch with our own minds and bodies, however, that we no longer understand the beneficial nature of disease and difficulties. The makers of the modern world all saw nightmares and experienced life as a struggle. But what they were seeing was not the world as it is, but their own internal condition. Darwin was an invalid for most of his life while writing *The Origin of Species.* Marx was unable to finish *Das Kapital* because of chronic lung problems. Freud had mouth cancer that interfered with his writing and counseling. Each of these thinkers devised elaborate theories of conflict to explain the world. Each failed to understand that sickness—of body, mind, spirit, or society—is a wonderful adjustment mechanism working to keep us alive, despite our violation of natural order. Each failed to understand that we create our own destiny. We produce our own happiness or misery. In short, each shaped his or her world concept in his own image.

Macrobiotics does not necessarily protect you from sickness. Indeed, I have come down with chronic disease, as have a number of my family members, students, and associates. In today's modern world, it is very difficult to eat in a naturally balanced way. We are living in two worlds to begin with, and even good-quality organic foods are increasingly contaminated by pollution, GMOs, artificial EMFs (electromagnetic fields), and other influences. However, when we get sick, we can analyze our condition using the compass of yin and yang and, in most cases, confidently change direction and find a safe, affordable, and effective natural way to heal and recover.

War is a collective human sickness. We must deal with it using the same principles that have proved effective in dealing with heart disease, mental illness, and other contemporary disorders. We need a total view, a unified view, a peaceful view. We need to understand human beings as they are. We need to understand their joys and sorrows, their successes and failures, their dreams and aspirations. This is the first step. To do this, we need to observe people and understand what is humanity. Proposed constitutions for world peace and order never discuss how we should be eating, or ethics, family life, and other practical problems—but they should.

Observing people working, walking, talking, eating, and playing will enable us to understand life as a whole. Gradually, we will see underlying patterns to behavior and thinking, and we will be able to understand the past and present as well as the future. These insights and understandings naturally come with deep observation, a peaceful mind, and a simple, harmonious way of life. On this basis, we formulate our vision of the world. We begin with an understanding of the Order of the Universe and the environment in which we live and act, not with political manifestos, economic theories, or religious codes. We must begin to see the secret melody of life. Actually, however, there are no secrets; the answer is always right in front of us. However, many people cannot see it. For centuries, we didn't notice that what we eat every day affects our health and consciousness. A few people, such as Samuel Butler, Edward Carpenter, George Bernard Shaw, and other English naturalists, noticed and turned to whole, mostly vegetable-quality food and lived to an advanced age and understanding. But the majority didn't notice, including most of modern society's great scientists, philosophers, artists, and social leaders. They became seriously sick and died prematurely and unhappily. They did not understand that they had created their own illness through improper diet and lifestyle. Instead, they saw their sickness and unhappiness as the result of external forces for which they were not responsible. They were casualties of a war against nature—a war against themselves.

OUR COSMOLOGICAL CONSTITUTION

At the present time, we view everything in the world as different and unrelated. We have many different sciences, different arts, and different professions. Modern education is compartmentalized into many departments, courses, and degrees, and we naturally grow up looking at life in fragments and parts rather than as a whole. Different names give the appearance of differences to things. We think that China and Russia are different from the United States. We think that blacks are different from whites. We think that Arabs are different from Jews. We don't see the similarities or our sameness as human beings.

Emphasizing our differences leads to comparison and competition. This is followed by fear, mistrust, and confrontation. Today, conflict has spread all over the world. Individuals are struggling with one another, families are divided, companies are engaged in fierce trade wars and corporate takeovers, nations are aligned in blocs and alliances against other nations. Ultimately, war breaks out and everything is destroyed.

Because the modern way of thinking emphasizes differences, not similarities, we have conflicts and wars. As Chinese, Arabs, Jews, Latinos, Anglo-Saxons, Native Americans, Catholics, and Buddhists, we have to see the similarities that unite us rather than the differences that divide us. Everything is moving. Everything is changing. Nothing is excepted. If we understand the laws of harmony and change, we can understand why things appear and disappear, how history unfolds, and what the future holds. Just as the earth, solar system, and galaxy are constantly changing, our mind too is undergoing continuous change and development. If we understand this process, we understand everything—day and night, birth and death, health and sickness, peace and war.

All phenomena are composed of antagonistic and complementary structures. These include front and back, up and down, right and left, surface and interior, roots and growing parts, center and periphery, soft and hard, high speed versus low speed, high temperature versus low temperature, and many others. The spiral—the universal form of nature and the cosmos—is the key to unifying differences; while these phenomena may seem to be completely different, in actuality, all share a common origin and destiny. They are all spirallic in nature and pass through the same phases of energetic change.

The spiral, moreover, is the only symbol or model that unifies different ways of thinking and human behavior. At first it may appear that all these people are moving in different directions, but when we enlarge our view, we see that everyone is part of the same spiral and in reality, there is no conflict.

The logarithmic spiral is the common, universal constitution of the whole world, even if we migrate to another planet. The future world must build upon this cosmological constitution instead of upon conceptual differences. To the Order of the Infinite Universe or the Order of God, everything is part of one unity. As peacemakers, we must use the unifying principle of yin and yang to harmonize our differences.

OUR SPIRITUAL CONSTITUTION

Our body appears as solid matter, but in actuality, it is energy. Our body is composed of trillions of atoms. These are sensitive to changes in atmospheric pressure, light, heat, sound, and other stimuli from the environment. When we are in good health, the energy flows smoothly between our internal and external environment. However, when we are sick, energy blockages occur. Energy accumulates and stagnates. Coronary heart disease, for example, is a more condensed state in which energy gathers in the form of obstructions that localize the spread of toxins, protein wastes, excess fat and cholesterol, and other dietary excess throughout the body. All sicknesses can be understood through the concept of energy. Plants also are governed by energy. Depending on their seed quality, exposure to the sun, climate zone, and other factors, some plants are oriented more in an upward and outward direction, while others are oriented more in a downward and inward direction. Winds and tides are also energy. Everything in the world is energy.

If we understand how energy changes, we can understand life as a whole. Everything is both visible and invisible. At death, our energy—especially the energy of our consciousness—separates and we enter the world of vibration. The physical body, which is composed of slower, denser energy, returns to the soil, while consciousness, which is composed of faster, more refined energy, continues to grow and develop in the world of electromagnetic vibration. The world of spirit and death is still energy. Every person is a spiritual, energy manifestation. The future world constitution must be built on an understanding of vibration, energy, and spirit.

OUR BIOLOGICAL CONSTITUTION

Nomadic people are more warlike than agriculturalists, as we discussed in Chapter 9. The frequency of war and the methods of war are much less violent among agricultural communities. The relation between a simple, wholesome diet and a peaceful mind and society was recognized in all traditional cultures and preserved in all ancient teachings. The best biological way to secure a peaceful mind and peaceful energy is a diet centered on whole cereal grains and vegetables. The modern diet, high in animal food, sugar, and processed, mass-produced commercial food, is the underlying cause of most of the violence, fear, anger, mistrust, and aggression in the world today.

OUR PSYCHOLOGICAL CONSTITUTION

In all cases of disease or disharmony—including AIDS, cancer, heart disease, family unrest, and social disorder—we are responsible for our own suffering. If we made the sickness, we can unmake it. In all cases, it is we ourselves who are the source of our unhappiness. In some cases, the immune system may be weak, in others the liver may be troubled, or the blood pressure may be high. But each of these conditions, as well as many others, can cause anger and other imbalanced emotions. The people we are angry against are not the cause of our difficulties. People who accuse others are worse than those they accuse. The person who accuses is already sick—he is suffering from a dualistic mentality.

The same thing is true with war. The White House or another country's leader, parliament, or other governmental structure or function is not the real cause of war, though they are directly handling international affairs. As long as we are angry, hateful, and regard others—viruses, crop pests, protesters, minority group members, revolutionaries, capitalists, migrants, refugees, or terrorists—as our enemy, our daily life is a battlefield. The actions of the chief executive and legislature just represent our tight livers, our weak intestines, our overactive kidneys. Governments will not change their view until we change our view. In reality, there are no enemies in this life. The earth is a happy, peaceful world. When difficulties or conflicts arise, we must admit that we were wrong, we were arrogant, and viruses or terrorists appeared because of a serious imbalance in our way of life. If we eat simply, maintain a clear, calm mind, cultivate a grateful, humble, and modest spirit, and express a sincere willingness to change our own orientation and behavior, violence and bloodshed can be avoided. Modern society is living in hell. If we concentrate on the mistakes of others, we are already at war. We must change our thinking. To change our brain chemistry, we need good blood circulation, and for that, whole foods (especially whole cereal grains) are essential. This is the psychological foundation on which the future world depends.

OUR SOCIAL CONSTITUTION

Over the next several centuries, social institutions will change fundamentally if human life continues to evolve and develop on this planet. The present-day prison system, for example, is barbaric. We segregate and punish offenders. We suppress symptoms but don't understand the underlying causes. Modern society does not really investigate why crime exists. Take a typical bank robber. Why did he, out of money, turn to crime? What is his biological and psychological condition? What environmental and dietary factors caused him to become overly aggressive? If we understand his mentality and physical condition, we can easily help him change his thinking and behavior. Through proper dietary guidance, we can transform the bank robber into a saint, or at least a clear-minded, healthy individual who will take responsibility for his life. In the future, prisons will become more like health care centers, helping people to restore physical and psychological balance.

Likewise, in the era to come, education will become less compartmentalized and analytical. Schools will become schools of life. Cooking classes will be taught alongside the usual subjects, but all subjects will be more integrated and the emphasis will be on originality and cooperation, rather than on repetition and competition. Medicine, too, will undergo a major transformation. The emphasis will be on prevention rather than cure. Doctors will provide life guidance and their husbands or wives will give cooking classes and show people how to pressure-cook grains, peel onions, and brew medicinal teas. Surgery and other advanced technology will still be available, but they will be used only in emergencies or in life-threatening situations.

OUR MATERIAL CONSTITUTION

Without food, clothing, shelter, and the other basics of material life, human culture and civilization would not exist. Today we have many economic systems, including communism, capitalism, and socialism. There are also revised capitalist systems, revised socialist systems, and several other ways to handle our material desires and needs. Until a new planetary system is developed, based on principles of environmental balance and dietary harmony, the old economic systems will have to exist side-by-side. Creating a new world economy is essential if we are to realize a peaceful world. Who should take the initiative—families, consumers, manufacturers, governments, world government? In the years to come, we need to study this problem and find the proper way to fulfill humanity's material needs.

BECOMING A PEACE PROMOTER

Over the next several hundred years, One Peaceful World will be built on the principles discussed earlier in this chapter. People who are expressing these principles in their daily life are true peace promoters. Their qualifications can be summarized under ten headings:

1. *They know that life is immortal.* We all came from One Infinity. Our life originated before the material universe was born. Each of us has journeyed through seven stages of the spiral of life. First, we manifested as primordial energy—yin and yang, then as light and vibration, and then as matter and elements. As minerals, we were absorbed by the plants, and then as plants we were transmuted into the animal kingdom. Eventually, we manifested as human beings. Then, after our life here in the air world, we shall all die, evolve to the next level, and return to the world of spirit. Our life is immortal and endless. A person who understands our place in the cosmos sees that the earth is our temporary home. He or she knows there is no reason to fight and kill each other. We are all brothers and sisters, sharing the same origin and destiny. People who think that this planet or this life is all that there is are willing to kill or be killed for territory, money, or power.

2. *They know that all antagonisms are complementary.* When capitalism developed in the nineteenth century, socialism and communism developed as its natural counterbalance. Their relationship is that of yin and yang, front and back. Capitalism is oriented more toward people's individual and material needs, while socialism and communism are directed more toward group and social needs. Similarly, when high ideals come out in society, low ideals soon come out to make balance. When spiritual teachings develop, vulgar teachings also develop. That is the Order of the Universe. One extreme produces its opposite. And opposites are always changing, transforming into each other. Night and day, winter and summer, man and woman, and countless other opposites in the natural world are supporting each other. Capitalism and socialism and communism, too, are supporting each other. The modern mind sees opposites as enemies to be destroyed rather than as complements to be harmonized. Peacemakers have no such hostile feelings. They understand that all of these different social, ideological, and cultural expressions emerged to create harmony. They see everything in terms of front and back, yin and yang, and are able to resolve conflicts peacefully by embracing all sides as part of a larger whole.

3. *They can change enemies into friends.* When we criticize or attack other people, we are actually making them stronger and contributing to their resistance and expansion. Instead, we must develop our attitude, expression, and approach so that others will understand us. For this, we need to eat well and refine our physical, mental, and spiritual conditions. Otherwise, we can never make peace. For example, Jesus didn't complain when he was crucified. He prayed for his accusers. His spirit moved the world after his death, and his teachings of peace spread around the world. He loved all people, even those who killed him, and wanted to help them. That is the spirit we need.

4. *They eat in a macrobiotic way.* A simple, natural way of eating is essential to spreading calm and tranquility, much like the diets of Jesus, Mary, Buddha, Lao Tzu, Confucius, Abraham, Sarah, Muhammad, and other men and women of peace demonstrate. As we have seen, meat, sugar, refined and chemically artificialized foods, and foods grown out of season or imported from different climates are the cause of much of the conflict in the modern world. Eating whole cereal grains, cooked vegetables, and other whole unprocessed foods will provide the day-to-day health, vitality, will, and endurance necessary to devote ourselves to creating world peace.

5. *They are responsible for their family and their life.* Divorce, nursing homes, family violence, family custody battles, disputes between men and women, and other manifestations of family disorder are epidemic. The decline of the family is a grave illness. Parents must learn to love and care for their children unconditionally, and when children grow up, they must learn to love and take care of their

parents without reservation, even at the sacrifice of their own happiness. Unless we respect our parents and ancestors, we cannot respect our origin—food, the earth, the universe, God. People whose home life is in disorder—who are arguing, quarreling, and fighting with their husbands or wives, parents, or children—cannot speak about peace. They are mentally and emotionally imbalanced. The way to peace leads through family harmony and is inseparable from it.

6. *They nourish, help, and develop others.* Many in the modern world try to take advantage of others. For example, 70 to 80 percent of surgery today is regarded as unnecessary. The same tendency is found with pharmaceuticals, insurance, and many consumer goods. In all areas of life, people are fooling each other and being fooled. The natural foods movement is not exempt. When we first introduced whole, unprocessed foods on a small scale, the quality was very high. We made foods available in bulk at an affordable price and educated consumers about proper diet and nutrition. Natural, organic foods is now a big industry. Many items have declined in quality, packaging has become a primary focus, and the profit motive has replaced education as the driving force. Our first goal should always be to help people and perform justice for the whole world.

7. *They respect different ideas, traditions, cultures, and customs.* If we are Christian, we should sometimes visit a Jewish synagogue or an Islamic mosque and pray there. If we are Hindu, we should respect Buddhist teachings. If we are followers of Lao Tzu, we should understand the principles of Confucius. If we think our religion is the only valid one, then we are prejudiced and exclusive. We must respect everyone and go forward together.

When I was young, I studied Shinto and went to the shrine. At the same time, my family had been Zen Buddhist for several hundred years and, before that, had observed other Buddhist teachings. About age thirteen, I read the Bible and began teaching it along with nuns at the Roman Catholic high school for women where my mother taught. I later belonged to the Japanese Protestant Christian Association. In the United States, at age twenty-three, I joined the Baptist Church and the Quaker Wider Fellowship. I also studied the Jewish prophets, the wonderful teachings of the Mormons (especially their dietary laws), and the Quran, which is very inspiring in many aspects. To be peacemakers, we must see the unity of the world's faiths and cultures. We should feel at home kneeling down and praying everywhere on our beautiful planet—in a church, synagogue, or mosque, as well as in the woods, the seashore, and fields of ripening grain.

8. *They take responsibility for what others do.* As parents, we must take responsibility for our children. All too often, however, we think a problem is theirs alone and we don't want to be involved. Jesus took responsibility for others, as did other great teachers and guides. That means really loving people and taking responsibility for what they did or are doing. If the results are bad, we should always

think, "This is my fault. I will try to change." If the results are good, we can think, "They did it." But we also rejoice and share in their success. For example, after World War II, who took responsibility? War crimes tribunals were held, and a few top military and civilian leaders were pronounced guilty. Everyone else washed their hands of responsibility, and in the future we will repeat the mistakes of that war on an even larger scale. What we have to do instead, as fellow human beings, is to take responsibility for whatever happens during our life together on this planet.

9. *They are first to grieve and last to rejoice.* This quality, too, is an expression of our love for other people and taking responsibility for their happiness or unhappiness. We are always the first to sympathize with others' troubles and the last to rejoice in times of general happiness. This latter habit is a traditional expression of humility and represents the virtue of not putting oneself before others.

10. *They marvel at nature, the universe, and their being alive here and now.* When we see plants, we naturally marvel that such wonderful forms appeared on this planet at the same time that we appeared. The stars, the oceans, clouds, water, small flowers, and countless other forms all move us to wonder. The bright moon overhead, the insects and birds singing to each other, the buds blossoming in spring, the snow falling in winter—these are our companions and teachers, guiding us to greater harmony and awareness. Appreciating the whole spiral of life is happiness. Let us think, "I am here now on this beautiful planet surrounded by beautiful things. Despite all our mistakes, isn't life wonderful?" This is the spirit of the peacemaker.

If we don't have these ten qualities, let us develop them. They are the natural birthright of us all and naturally follow from living in harmony with our environment and eating simple, whole meals in a spirit of thankfulness.

SUMMARY

The ideal approach to world peace is not one based on any individual considerations. It is instead based around people and nature as a whole. Our daily lives and every aspect of them should be carried out with the idea of peace in mind. To unify our differences, we must acknowledge complementary antagonisms. Our cosmological, spiritual, biological, psychological, social, and material constitutions work in harmony to produce a mind, spirit, and energy that contribute to One Peaceful World.

PEACE PROMOTER

Dennis Kucinich, Washington, D.C.

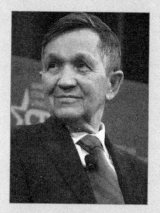

Dennis Kucinich, a Congressman from Ohio and onetime Democratic presidential candidate, first came to public attention in 1977 when, at age thirty-one, he won the election for mayor of Cleveland. As mayor, he stood up to the banks, utility companies, and other special interests and won a reputation as a champion of the people. In 1997, he was elected to Congress for the first time and was reelected every two years until 2013, when his district was redrawn and he lost a runoff election.

"There is another way. It is time to reject the politics and the policies of fear, suspicion, and preemptive war which, if left unchecked, will lead to the demise of our nation," asserted Kucinich. "It is time to jettison our illusions and fears and to transform age-old challenges with new thinking. We must dedicate ourselves to peaceful coexistence, consensus building, disarmament, and respect for international treaties."

"Violence and war are not inevitable," Kucinich went on. "We must call on our higher capacities for communication, dialogue and compassion. We are in a new era where we must understand the fundamental truth of our time is human unity. The world is interconnected and interdependent. We are all one. Acting from that thinking we can pursue the science of human relations to determine ways to settle conflict without violence. We must develop the capacity for nonviolent conflict resolution or risk being engulfed by an ever-widening circle of violence."

In Congress, Kucinich focused on foreign policy and took the initiative to promote peace and reconciliation. Several months before 9/11, he introduced legislation to create a Department of Peace. The proposal to create a cabinet-level department as part of the executive branch of the government went back to Dr. Benjamin Rush, a Founding Father, who first introduced the idea in 1793. It has periodically been resurrected throughout the years since then. In the post-Cold War era and time of rising terrorism, Kucinich revived the proposal. Under his proposal, the Department of Peace (DOP) would provide violence prevention, conflict resolution skills, and mediation to American schoolchildren in classrooms as an elective or requirement, providing them with the communication tools they need to express themselves beginning in elementary through high school.

The DOP would provide support and grants for violence prevention programs, including programs against domestic violence, gang violence, drug- and alcohol-related violence. The department would also introduce peacemaking among conflicting cultures and rehabilitation programs among the prison population. The DOP would support the military with complementary approaches to ending violence and monitor domestic arms production (including conventional military weapons, nonmilitary weapons, and weapons of mass destruction).

The DOP would make expert recommendations to the president on the latest techniques for diplomacy, mediation, and conflict resolution. It would take a proactive level of involvement in the establishment of international dialogues for international conflict resolution. It would establish a U.S. Peace Academy, monitor human rights progress, and consult with the Secretaries of State and Defense prior to any engagement of U.S. troops. The DOP would establish a national Peace Day, participate in meetings of the National Security Council, and expand the national Sister City program.

In the early 1990s, Kucinich came to the Kushi Institute to attend the Way to Health Program and has been eating in a macrobiotic way ever since. He credits diet with helping him recover naturally from Crohn's disease. He has worked with Alex Jack and Edward Esko, founders of Amberwaves, a grassroots network to protect whole grains from genetic engineering, and in 2000 he wrote the foreword to Alex Jack's book, *Imagine a World Without Monarch Butterflies*. He met with me and other macrobiotic leaders on many occasions.

In Congress, he served as leader of the campaign for mandatory labeling of genetically modified (GMO) foods and was in the vanguard of elected officials seeking to end the wars in Iraq and Afghanistan. In 2004 and 2008 he ran for president, but lost the Democratic nominations to John Kerry and Barack Obama. Kucinich is the recipient of the Gandhi Peace Award and since leaving Congress, he has continued his health and peace activism as a speaker, writer, and television commentator for Fox News. Dennis is the most energetic, eloquent, and engaged statesman and public servant of our time and has contributed immeasurably to creating one healthy, peaceful world.

See Appendix F for the complete text of Dennis's proposal for the Department of Peace. Following Michio Kushi's death, Dennis gave a tribute at the memorial service at the Arlington Street Church in Boston on January 31, 2015.

19.

Nourishing a World View

Food is creating us. If the nourishment we receive is proper, we are naturally more energized physically, more comfortable emotionally, and more elevated spiritually than when our way of eating is imbalanced and disorderly. If our daily food is improper, our health declines, our emotions are disturbed, and our spirit becomes chaotic. Personal feelings, social relations, and our approach to any problems are influenced by what we eat. When we feel any frustration and disturbance, when we meet any difficulty and hardship, when we experience violence and opposition, we should first reflect upon what we have been eating. Our physical and mental habits, as well as tendencies in our thinking and capacities of our consciousness, all depend upon what we have been eating, from the embryonic stage through childhood up to adulthood and old age.

Babies and children ordinarily do not experience the physical and psychological disorders, including feelings of separation, common to adults. Their physical condition is still generally soft, clean, and flexible. They are usually receptive to their environment and keep active mentally and physically. A flexible mind and body are associated with positive attributes such as imagination, creativity, playfulness, optimism, curiosity, and honesty. Children are not normally isolated from their surroundings, but feel very much a part of what is happening around them.

As we grow older, however, our physical condition becomes more rigid on the modern diet, and our thinking and outlook begin to change. Imitation replaces creativity, and instead of being open-minded and curious, we become narrow and closed to new ideas. Pessimism replaces optimism, and instead of intuitively trusting ourselves and other people, we become doubtful and suspicious. The natural love and warmth that we experienced as children give way to coldness and detachment by adolescence and early adulthood.

As our physical and mental condition becomes harder and more inflexible, our expressions become increasingly harsh and critical. Even when we wish to express love or affection, it comes out in the form of criticism, scolding, or other form of negativity. Frustration builds as we lose the ability to express ourselves freely through words, actions, movement, creative work, or play. Frustrations can only be withheld for so long before erupting violently, especially when they are fueled by an imbalanced diet. All too often, the family dinner table, traditionally a place of love and harmony, becomes a modern battlefield, with loud and abusive behavior being the main course. This can change with some adjustments in way of thinking, the cooking process, and in the type of food that is served.

THREE REQUIREMENTS OF A KITCHEN

The first requirement of a kitchen that nourishes a world view is that whole, unrefined grains comprise the staple food of every meal. These include brown rice, barley, millet, whole wheat berries, rye, oats, maize, and quinoa. The most ideal grain for intuitive, comprehensive vision is brown rice, the most recent grain biologically to develop and the grain with the most balanced energy and nutrients. Cracked grains, refined grains, or flour products such as bread and noodles are more conducive to divided, analytical thinking. They may be used occasionally. To supplement whole grains, a wide variety of other foods can be used, including vegetables of many kinds, beans and bean products, sea vegetables, seeds and nuts, locally grown fruit, and a small to moderate amount of animal food, especially white meat fish and seafood.

The second requirement of the kitchen of world peace is that the major portion of foods are cooked; for grains, cooking with a heavy lid or pressure-cooking with a pinch of sea salt is the most universal method. This makes the food more digestible and contributes to smooth, even absorption of nutrients into the blood. The use of fire in cooking created homo sapiens: The transformation of raw rice, millet, wheat, or barley by heat, pressure, water, and sea salt heightened the charge of ki, or electromagnetic energy, in our food, and added a dimension of universality to humanity's peaceful, holistic consciousness. This was the development that created our first full vision of one unified, peaceful worldwide civilization.

The third requirement of the kitchen that nourishes world vision is for the cook to be calm, peaceful, happy, and healthy, especially during the preparation and serving of the food. The meal she or he prepares is literally a model of the future world. The cook's energy, as well as the food's, helps form the thoughts, words, and deeds of the entire family, as well as others who dine at the table. From the cook's image, ultimately, we will finally realize our universal image of world peace.

STANDARD DIETARY RECOMMENDATIONS

To secure the basic health and vitality of individuals, families, and communities, the following macrobiotic dietary guidelines have been formulated for temperate regions of the world (see Figure 19.1 on page 279). These guidelines also take into account harmony with evolutionary order, universal dietary traditions in East and West, the changing seasons, and individual conditions and needs. They have been further modified with a view to enjoying, within moderation, the benefits and conveniences of modern civilization.

Macrobiotic Dietary Guidelines
for Temperate Regions

including North America, Europe, Russia, China, East Asia, and Moderate Regions
in Southern Africa, South America, Australia, and New Zealand

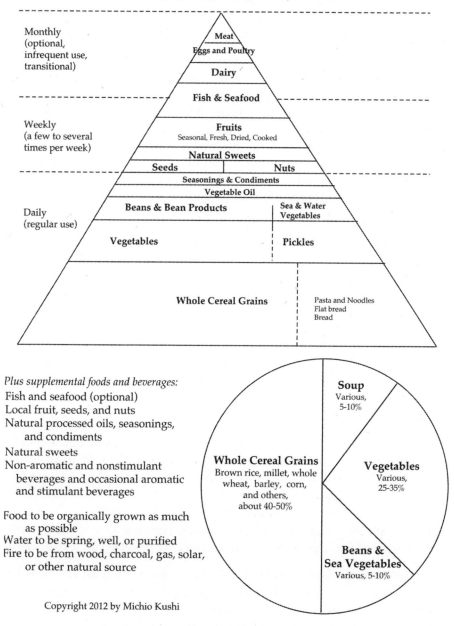

Figure 19.1. The Standard Macrobiotic Diet.

1. *Whole Cereal Grains:* The principal food of each meal is whole cereal grain. It should make up about 40 to 50 percent of the total weight of the meal. Whole grains are high in complex carbohydrates, fiber, minerals, and some vitamins and enzymes, and include brown rice, whole wheat berries, barley, millet, and rye, as well as maize, quinoa, and other cereal plants. From time to time, whole grain products such as cracked wheat, rolled oats, noodles, pasta, bread, baked goods, and other flour products may be served as part of this volume of principal food.

2. *Soup.* One to two small bowls of soup, making up about 5 to 10 percent of daily food intake, are consumed each day. The soup broth is made frequently with miso or shoyu, which are prepared from naturally fermented soybeans, sea salt, and grains. Several varieties of land and sea vegetables (especially wakame or kombu) and other vegetables such as carrots, onions, cabbage, Chinese cabbage, daikon greens and root may be added during cooking. The taste of miso or shoyu broth soup should be mild, not too salty nor too bland. Soups made with grains, beans, vegetables, and occasionally a little fish or seafood may also be prepared frequently as part of this category.

3. *Vegetables.* About 25 to 35 percent of daily food includes fresh vegetables—high in fiber, carbohydrates, minerals, and vitamins—prepared in a variety of ways, including steaming, baking, sautéing, and boiling, and as in salads or pickling. The vegetables include a variety of root vegetables (such as carrots, burdock, and daikon radish), ground vegetables (such as cabbage, onions, fall- and winter-season squashes, and cucumbers), and leafy green vegetables (such as kale, collard greens, broccoli, daikon greens, turnip greens, mustard greens, and watercress). The selection will vary with the region, season, availability, personal health, and other factors. Usually more than two-thirds of the vegetables are served cooked, and up to one-third may be prepared in the form of fresh salad or pickles. Vegetables that historically originated in the tropics, such as tomato and potato, are avoided or minimized.

4. *Beans and Bean Products.* A small portion—up to 10 percent by volume—of daily food intake includes cooked beans or bean products such as tofu, tempeh, and natto. This food, which is high in protein, fat, and some minerals and vitamins, may be prepared separately or cooked together with grains, vegetables, or sea vegetables, as well as served in the form of soup. Though all dried and fresh beans are suitable for consumption, the smaller varieties such as azuki beans, lentils, and chickpeas contain less fat and oil and are preferred for regular use.

5. *Seaweed.* Sea vegetables, rich in minerals and vitamins, are eaten daily in small volume, about 2 to 3 percent or less of food eaten daily. Common varieties include kombu, wakame, nori, dulse, hiziki, and arame. They may be included in soups, cooked with vegetables or beans, or prepared as a side dish. They are usually seasoned with a moderate amount of shoyu, sea salt, or brown rice vinegar.

6. *Animal Food.* A small volume of fish or seafood may be eaten a few times per week by those in good health, if desired. White-meat fish generally contain less fat and oil than red-meat fish or blue-skin varieties. Saltwater fish also usually contain fewer pollutants than freshwater types. To help detoxify the body from the effects of fish and seafood, a small volume of grated daikon, horseradish, ginger, or mustard is usually consumed with the meal as a condiment. Other animal-quality food, including meat, poultry, eggs, and dairy food, are usually avoided, with the exception of infrequent cases in which they may be recommended temporarily for medicinal purposes.

7. *Seeds and Nuts.* Seeds and nuts, lightly roasted and salted with sea salt or seasoned with shoyu, may be enjoyed as occasional snacks. It is preferable not to excessively consume nuts and nut butters, as they are difficult to digest and are high in fats.

8. *Fruit.* Fruit (preferably cooked or naturally dried) is eaten by those in normal health a few times a week as a snack or dessert, provided the fruit grows in the local climate zone. Raw fruit can also be consumed in moderate volume, preferably during its growing season. Fruit juice is generally too concentrated for regular use, although occasional consumption in hot weather is enjoyable and relaxing, as is cider in the autumn. Most temperate-climate fruits are suitable for occasional use. These include apples, pears, peaches, apricots, grapes, berries, and melons. Tropical fruits such as grapefruit, pineapple, mango, and others are preferably avoided in a temperate climate.

9. *Desserts.* Dessert is eaten in moderate volume two or three times a week by those in good health and may consist of cookies, pudding, cake, pie, and other sweet dishes. Naturally sweet foods such as apples, fall and winter squashes, azuki beans, or dried fruit can often be used in dessert recipes without additional sweetening. To provide a stronger sweet taste, a natural grain-based sweetener, such as rice syrup, barley malt, or amasake—all of which are high in complex sugars—may be used. Simple sugars, such as sugar, honey, molasses, and other sweeteners that are highly refined, extremely strong, or of tropical origin, are avoided. A delicious seaweed gelatin called kanten, which is made from agar-agar and often supplemented with fruit, nuts, or beans, is a very popular dessert dish.

10. *Seasoning, Thickeners, and Garnishes.* Naturally processed, mineral-rich sea salt and traditional, nonchemicalized miso and shoyu are used in seasoning to give a salty taste. Food should not have an overly salty flavor; seasonings should generally be added during cooking. Occasionally, personal adjustments may need to be made at the table, in which case a moderate amount of seasoning may be added. Other commonly-used seasonings include brown rice vinegar, sweet brown rice vinegar, umeboshi vinegar, umeboshi plums, and grated gingerroot.

The frequent use of spices, herbs, and other stimulant or aromatic substances is generally avoided or minimized. For sauces, gravies, and thickeners, kuzu root powder or arrowroot flour are preferred over other vegetable-quality starches. Sliced scallions, parsley sprigs, nori squares or strips, fresh grated gingerroot, and other ingredients are commonly used as garnishes to provide color, balance taste, stimulate the appetite, and facilitate digestion.

11. *Cooking Oil.* For daily cooking, naturally processed, unrefined vegetable-quality oil is recommended. Dark sesame oil is used most commonly, though light sesame oil, olive oil, and corn oil are also suitable. Other unrefined vegetable-quality oils such as safflower oil, mustard seed oil, and walnut oil may be used less frequently or for special occasions. Although coconut oil is a popular choice, it is more appropriate for use in the environments in which it is grown (such as the South Seas), not temperate, four-season environments. Generally, fried rice, fried noodles, or sautéed vegetables are prepared several times a week using a moderate amount of oil. Occasionally, oil may also be used for preparing tempura, deep-frying grains, vegetables, fish, and seafood, or for use in salad dressings and sauces.

12. *Condiments.* A small amount of condiments may be used on grains, beans, or vegetables at the table to provide variety, stimulate the appetite, and balance the various tastes of the meal. Regular condiments include gomashio (roasted sesame salt), roasted seaweed powders, umeboshi plums, tekka root vegetable condiment, and many others.

13. *Pickles.* A small volume of homemade pickles is eaten each day to aid in digestion of grains and vegetables. Traditionally, pickles are made with a variety of root and round vegetables such as daikon, turnips, cabbage, carrots, and cauliflower and are aged in sea salt, rice or wheat bran, shoyu, umeboshi plums, shiso leaves, or miso.

14. *Beverages.* Spring, well, or filtered water is used for drinking, preparing tea and other beverages, and for general cooking. Bancha twig tea (also known as kukicha) is the most commonly served beverage, though roasted barley tea, roasted brown-rice tea, and other grain- based teas or traditional, nonstimulant herbal teas are also used frequently. Grain coffee, umeboshi tea, mu tea, and dandelion tea are prepared occasionally. Less frequently, green tea, fruit juice, vegetable juice, soymilk, beer, wine, sake, and other grain, bean, vegetable, and herbal beverages are served. The consumption of chemically-treated black tea, coffee, herb teas that have stimulant or aromatic effects, distilled water, soft drinks, milk and dairy beverages, and hard liquor is normally avoided.

The standard macrobiotic diet is not limited to the above examples. An almost infinite variety of meals can be created from the standard suggestions. The amount, volume, and proportion of food in each category may also be adjusted slightly for each person or family member depending upon changing environmental conditions such as climate and weather, as well as upon age, sex, ethnic background, constitution and condition of health, and social and personal needs. The guidelines presented above are generally for persons in sound health. Persons with more serious conditions may need to temporarily adopt a more limited form of the diet, preferably under the guidance of a qualified macrobiotic counselor or a medical professional trained in this approach. The macrobiotic dietary approach is very flexible, always looking at the needs of the individual or family as a whole. The development of intuition is essential to balanced cooking and food preparation.

The way of cooking these foods should be spiritually very refined and peaceful, and all energies should be very well balanced. Our health and happiness depend upon our practical understanding and application of the principle of balance and harmony, namely yin and yang. Beyond modern nutritional considerations, it is important to understand the vibratory quality of different foods. For this we need to study color and form, manner of cutting and stirring, proper use of fire and water, pressure and time, and quality of cookware. The macrobiotic cookbooks listed in the recommended reading list, which begins on page 345, are very helpful in getting started. We also encourage all family members to take introductory macrobiotic cooking classes in order to sample the foods prepared and have a standard against which to measure their own.

SUMMARY

Peace begins at the dinner table. There are three values that should be demonstrated in every kitchen: whole, unrefined grains should comprise the center of the meal; the majority of the food should be cooked to ease digestion; and the cook must have a positive and peaceful attitude that radiates into the food. The components of a standard macrobiotic diet were outlined in this chapter, but this lifestyle is certainly not limited to just these foods. Your personal condition will determine what is best for you.

PEACE PROMOTER

Baydaa Laylaa, Syria

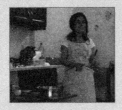

Baydaa Laylaa

Baydaa Laylaa comes from Lattakia, a Syrian city on the Mediterranean Sea. She grew up in the countryside, close to nature, and was one of four girls. Her family followed the Alawite form of Islam, which is a mixture of Islam, Christianity, and Confucianism. For example, it believes in reincarnation. "It was very easy for me to become macrobiotic," she recalled. "The orientation was so similar. It answered my questions."

Growing up, Baydaa ate many grains, lots of vegetables, beans, and very little meat and dairy. But sugar was a challenge. She ended up overindulging and developed an eating disorder. She was also depressed and couldn't concentrate. Her field was English literature, and after becoming macrobiotic, she could focus better.

In Lattakia, there was a macrobiotic group. The woman who headed it introduced Baydaa to the standard macrobiotic diet, and she learned how to cook in this way. The group also had a book club, discussed many topics, and encouraged meditation. Baydaa's moodiness gradually went away, and soon she was full of energy.

Baydaa met her future husband, Hussain Muhammad, through Miriam Nour (see page 28), the leading macrobiotic teacher in the Middle East. Miriam gave a seminar which both Baydaa and Hussain attended. Hussain came from Kuwait, where Baydaa had already applied to teach English to schoolchildren. In Kuwait, she was shocked to see how poor the kids' health was compared to the kids in Syria. In the entire Persian Gulf area, except for much of Syria, the modern way of eating had spread. McDonald's and pizza parlors were very common, along with asthma, diabetes, and other chronic diseases.

In Kuwait, a private food company delivered lunchboxes to the school. These lunchboxes included ingredients with up to 50 percent sugar. After the midday meal, Baydaa couldn't control her students. They would kick, stick each other with pencils, and engage in other violence. She also noticed they were very itchy and always scratching—symptoms that come from taking too much sugar.

In Syria, the food situation was much better. Mothers cooked at home for their children. Flat bread was still the staple and made without milk or sugar. "In Lattakia, we have an organic market," Baydaa reported. "The coastal area where I live is very peaceful. When the violence first started in Syria in 2011, most violent parts of the country were in the interior, more of a desert climate, where people used to keep flocks of sheep and cattle and consumed large amounts of meat, dairy, and other animal food."

In her grandmother's village, there was only one cow. Country people ate beef only once a year. Meat was expensive and rarely consumed. Today in the Middle East, many cows have been imported from Holland and Scandinavia.

Baydaa's religion observed the lunar calendar. During the full moon, practitioners customarily fast. Iman Ali, the cousin of the Prophet Muhammad and a spiritual master himself, taught dietary and lifestyle practices: "Don't let your stomach became a cemetery for animals." He advised people to eat to only 80 percent of capacity. He also practiced a type of Feng Shui and other very precise, scientific disciplines.

The war in Syria has been fueled by global politics. "On one side is the U.S., Europe, Saudi Arabia, and Israel, and on the other is Russia, China, and Iran," Baydaa pointed out. "Weapons have been smuggled into Syria from Turkey and other neighboring countries. Syria has been caught in the middle."

"The Western media has exaggerated and distorted the conflict," she continues. "In recent years, Syria has been a force for peace in the region. The Alawite form of Islam that governs the country is secular and moderate. Unlike most of the Gulf region and North Africa, Syria has resisted Westernization. People still honor their traditional cuisine, family relations are strong, and divorce is rare. No woman in my family is divorced," she noted. "I never met a girl who was raped or attacked."

Crime in Syria is traditionally one of the lowest in the world. According to Interpol, until the current civil/regional war, Syria and Japan had the lowest rates of murder, rape, robbery, and assault in the world. By contrast, America has the highest. The rate for all violent offenses combined was indexed at 29 for Syria, compared to 1,709 for Japan and 4,123 for the U.S. "It is very sad and painful to see the outside world export its drugs and weapons to my country," Baydaa said.

"We are worried that an extreme form of Islam will emerge if the conflict escalates. Right now, I don't have to wear a veil or fuss about Ramadan. But in some places, I might be executed," Baydaa said. "Syria suffered under Ottoman occupation for many years. We all know about the Armenian genocide, the horrors of the Holocaust, and other crimes committed against humanity. I fervently hope that a peace settlement can be achieved."

After marrying Hussain, Baydaa returned to Kuwait with her husband. In the future, they would like to start an organic farm. "There is no organic farming in Kuwait now," she said. "Organic produce is imported, but it is expensive, and the Ki energy is depleted. We also want to start a macrobiotic kitchen and introduce a healthier way of eating to children, parents, and the general public." Throughout the Gulf region and in Kuwait, most women no longer cook. Petrodollars (money earned from the export of petroleum) have made everyone wealthy, and the cooking is done mostly by Filipinos and other women brought in from other countries in Asia.

In nearby Saudi Arabia, there is a mountainous area that is very temperate. It grows abundant organic crops under cultivation, and Baydaa and Hussain hope to bring them to Kuwait. The Suaedaa region of Syria, near the Israeli border, is similar. It has strong, volcanic soil, like Hokkaido in Japan, and produces excellent grains and vegetables.

The whole mountainous area in Syria is a traditional pilgrimage spot and abode of spiritual teachers.

Damascus, the capital of Syria (where Saint Paul had his famous conversion experience) is located in the center of the country in a hilly, temperate region. For thousands of years, Damascus and Aleppo, a city to the northwest, have been beacons of learning, culture, and peace. "My ultimate goal is to grow brown rice in Syria," Baydaa says. "Right now, all the rice is imported from Italy. Wheat and barley are traditionally eaten in the Middle East. They create health, prosperity, and in the form of bread, give a strong, analytic mind. Rice contributes to spiritual development and insight. I believe it could help bring peace to Syria and the entire region. That is our ultimate dream."

As the war in Syria entered its fourth year, America and Russia initiated air strikes against ISIS, the terrorist group that established a Caliphate in the region, and millions of refugees fled the country. After graduating from the Kushi Institute in the United States, Baydaa returned to her homeland to give macrobiotic cooking classes.

Because of the war, the price of meat increased, so people have reduced their consumption. Because of sanctions, some pharmacies offer whole foods instead of drugs. Sanctions have also reduced the availability of macrobiotic specialty foods. Fighting has disrupted organic farming, so vegetables have been in short supply. However, Baydaa is hopeful that sanctions will ease and fighting will cease so that organic foods will once again become widely available in the future.

Source

"Bringing Brown Rice and Peace to Syria." *Amberwaves*, Summer 2012.

20.

Visions of a New World

It may appear that the biological process of elevating humanity through proper diet would be too slow and gradual to have an impact on the critical world situation. But we must realize that so far, all other solutions—however well-meaning—have failed to slow down or reverse the nuclear arms race, or promote friendly feelings among the peoples of the world. If biological improvement through proper diet is ignored, world peace will remain an illusory and elusive goal. Only if we are physically and mentally healthy shall we have the strength, vitality, and will to obtain our goal. For this, correct food is essential.

Most of today's leaders and populations of the world are physically unhealthy to the extent that they cannot envision peaceful reconciliations of our present conflicts. Without a clear vision of a peaceful world, there can be only war. Intuitively, we know that if we go on creating nuclear weapons, it is inevitable that they will be used in war.

Each day, we materialize our vision of the future. Every morning, each of us awakes at a certain hour and keeps certain appointments that are important to us. We have a vision of doing certain things, and we materialize parts of that vision. In this way we are constantly creating the day-to-day world by realizing our vision of life.

Why do some people see war in the future, while others see peace? Why are some people successful in achieving their vision, while others are too weak to realize what they would like the future to be? As we have seen, our vision of life is largely the result of our physical and mental conditions. The food our mothers ate during pregnancy and the food we eat every day are playing the most essential part. This food gives rise to a certain type of vision—violent for some, peaceful for others—and also makes us either strong enough to pursue our dream or too weak to accomplish things in life.

Those who are sick can see only a sick vision of the future. The vision of those who are perpetuating the arms race is a destructive vision. We are now witnessing the materialization of that vision. Due to their own chaotic health, many leaders—as well as many ordinary people—can only envision the chaotic end of the entire world.

If individual families around the world become healthier physically and mentally through proper lifestyle, including proper diet—namely, macrobiotics—peaceful visions of the future will prevail. Families will begin to meet in assemblies or in congresses to support and encourage one another beyond any differences in belief, race, age, sex, or economic class. Regardless of how many there are, these first families will constitute the sprout of a giant tree that will blossom centuries later when a peaceful world is fully realized.

THE TRANSFORMATION OF SOCIETY

Our small macrobiotic movement has far to go before we can realize the beginning of a new era. Let us take a closer look at the challenges ahead of us. Dividing the 120 years from 1980 to 2100 into six twenty-year periods, we can trace the age of transition (see Figure 20.1, below) in more detail. Let us look first, however, at the first twenty-year period.

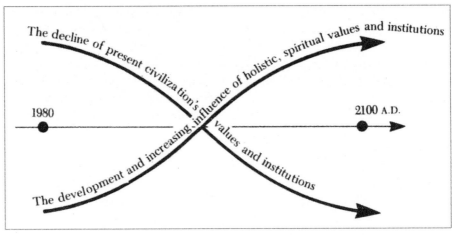

Figure 20.1. The Age of Transition.

Foundation (1960–1980): Groundwork

Spearheaded by Lima, Muso, Chico-San, Erewhon, Mitoku, Eden Foods, and other macrobiotic food distributors that began in the late 1950s and early 1960s, millions of families around the world changed their way of eating to whole, unprocessed foods, naturally and organically grown. Schools, hospitals, restaurants, businesses, prisons, and other institutions began to serve healthier food. By the mid-1970s, government and medical associations began to issue national dietary guidelines calling for drastic reductions in fat, sugar, and refined food consumption and substantial increases in whole grains, vegetables, and fresh fruits. Research studies focusing on macrobiotic people at the leading medical schools in the United States and Europe helped establish diet as the leading cause of heart and blood vessel disease—the major cause of death in modern society. By 1980, the macrobiotic approach to cancer had also begun to be studied and implemented in scientific and medical circles.

Period 1 (1980–2000): World Health

As the influence of our present movement spread, it began to have a profound effect on agriculture, the food processing industry, and medicine. Introduced in 1992, the U.S. Government's Food Guide Pyramid set the stage for a revolutionary transition in modern society from a diet centered on animal food to one based on plant food. Grains formed the foundation of the Pyramid, followed by vegetables and fruits, high-protein foods (including meat, beans, seeds and nuts), and small amounts of sugar and other refined sweeteners. It replaced the Four Food Groups, which included about 50 percent meat, poultry, and dairy foods, supplemented by fruits, vegetables, cereals, and breads.

During this period, other degenerative conditions, including Alzheimer's disease, multiple sclerosis, arthritis, and diabetes, began to be treated with dietary adjustments and environmental modifications. Many doctors, nurses, and other health care professionals became involved in complementary alternative medicine, including macrobiotics, as scientific studies (including case-control studies) continued, demonstrating the efficacy of our dietary and environmental approach. Meanwhile, macrobiotic education began to focus in a more social direction, turning its attention to the problems of society and the development of consciousness, especially peace and world order.

Period 2 (2000–2020): World Economy and Social Structure

With the development of agriculture and medicine in a more natural direction, the holistic movement, including macrobiotics, began to have more social influence, as the nature of the family and other social structures—and of the world economy as a whole—began to change. The rights of women, children, homosexuals, and other minorities or long-abused groups in society strengthened. The Internet and social media put people in closer touch with each other, breaking down old prejudices and stereotypes and fostering multicultural tolerance and unity. Proper nutrition and diet began to be seen as a key element in creating and sustaining healthy relationships, families, and communities. Sustainable practices spread to all domains of life as consciousness of preserving the environment heightened.

Period 3 (2020–2040): World Science and Industry

Unlimited energy and natural resources will become available through the introduction of transmutation—the synthesis of necessary but unavailable chemical elements out of simpler, available ones. For example, iron can be made from manganese, while silica can be transformed into calcium. Early experiments by macrobiotic educator George Ohsawa and French scientist Louis Kervran that transmuted one element into another peacefully, without smashing the atom, have been furthered by Quantum Rabbit LLC, a small energy and materials company started by my students. In the early twenty-first century, practical applications will be developed to implement transmutation, (also called quantum conversion or cool fusion) on a worldwide scale. For example, titanium, palladium, and other industrially important elements—a principal reason for competition among global powers today—may become readily available from common, inexpensive elements such as silicon (found in beach sand). Similarly, this new science may be applied to rendering harmless nuclear wastes, toxic spills, and other chronic environmental hazards. This Third Industrial Revolution will completely revolutionize the world of science and further change existing forms of economy and improve the quality of life.

Period 4 (2040–2060): World Philosophy and Religion

New developments in astronomy, history, and cosmology, coupled with social and economic changes, will usher in a new conception of universal origin and spirit. Refined on a social level, this universal metaphysical sense will dissolve the barriers of traditional cultural and religious separation, creating one world language and one general sense of universal spirituality. Religion, as we now know it, will begin to disappear.

Period 5 (2060–2080): World Travel and Politics

With the development of natural transmutation, natural energy, and other scientific advances, together with the advent of the new cosmology and spiritual insight, active worldwide transportation and space travel will commence. Together with the new world language mentioned in the previous section, this will finally dissolve all barriers of national sovereignty, ushering in a totally new conception of politics. Passports and visas, as well as armies and weapons, will finally become things of the past.

Period 6 (2080–2100): World Government

As we can see, the first five periods alternate from times of more yang (physical and structural) change, to times of more yin (metaphysical or spiritual) change. During this last period, all these developments will merge together, further refining and unifying all our new discoveries. Humanity will begin to experience the realities of its new civilization and as we pass through the final maturing process, we will learn to maintain and administer this civilization through a new world government.

END OF THE SPIRAL OF HISTORY

And God gave Noah the rainbow sign,
No more water but fire next time.

—AFRICAN-AMERICAN SPIRITUAL

As we have seen, universal will (or, we may say, the consciousness of God) travels with infinite speed, differentiating into yin and yang, time and space, life and breath. As this movement begins, a curving vibration is produced, and the relative world, including stars and planets, elements and compounds, plants and animals, and human beings, appears. Infinite consciousness manifests in a wavelike motion, creating at first simple spirals, then more complex spirals, and finally spirals within spirals. These spirals manifest as atoms and particles, stars and solar systems, galaxies and clusters of galaxies, body and mind, male and female, nature and history.

The Spiral of History is now rapidly moving toward its climax. In the early twenty-first century, the pace of life is accelerating, traditional structures and boundaries are dissolving, and personal and planetary challenges are converging. Under high pressure, temperature, and other forms of stress, there is a danger that human culture and society will end violently.

As material civilization declines, we are quickly running out of key minerals that have formed the foundation of technology for thousands of years (see Figure 20.2, below). Virtually all major industrial minerals, precious metals, rare earth metals, and other elements that constitute the backbone of industrialization and the modern economy, especially computers, cell phones, and other communications, will run out in the next generation.

Millions of species of plants and animals are threatened by globalization, envi-

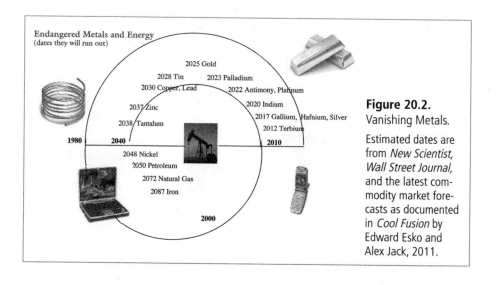

Figure 20.2.

Vanishing Metals.

Estimated dates are from *New Scientist, Wall Street Journal,* and the latest commodity market forecasts as documented in *Cool Fusion* by Edward Esko and Alex Jack, 2011.

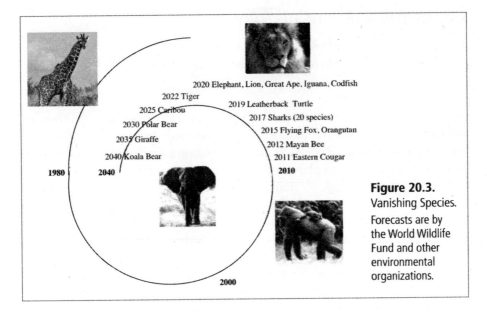

Figure 20.3.
Vanishing Species.
Forecasts are by the World Wildlife Fund and other environmental organizations.

ronmental destruction, and climate change. Between one-third and two-thirds of all plants and animals are currently endangered by globalization, climate change, and other threats. Figure 20.3, above, illustrates when several iconic species are expected to become extinct in the wild.

Even the nutrients we eat in our daily food are vanishing as chemical fertilizers, pesticides, GMOs, and other harmful materials degrade the topsoil, pollute the air, and contaminate the water (see Figure 20.4, below).

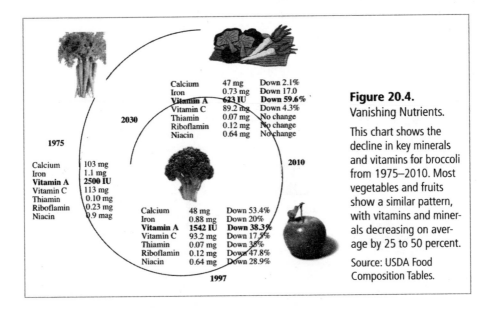

Figure 20.4.
Vanishing Nutrients.

This chart shows the decline in key minerals and vitamins for broccoli from 1975–2010. Most vegetables and fruits show a similar pattern, with vitamins and minerals decreasing on average by 25 to 50 percent.

Source: USDA Food Composition Tables.

The worlds of minerals, animals, and plants—the realm of nature—are in profound crisis and will peak about 2030–2040. This coincides, incidentally, with the current 81-year Nine Star Ki cycle that is governed by 9 Fire and ends in 2036 (recall the atmospheric energy cycle from Chapter 8). The 81-year cycle governs world ages and generational change. The current 81-year cycle began in 1955. It represents an age of climactic, fire-like energy. Fire energy governs petroleum, coal, and other fossil fuels, as well as nuclear energy. It is also characterized by high-energy food, fast transportation, rapid industrialization, the spread of epidemic disease, global warming, and other explosive, rapidly expanding technologies and environmental influences.

The 81-year Fire cycle coincides with the end of the Spiral of History and the end of the 26,000-year Vega/Polaris cycle. The Great Year, as the latter is also known, may end with destruction by fire, just as the world experienced a megaflood or series of floods about 13,000 years ago (halfway back in the cycle). The fire challenges today, of course, are nuclear war and energy, industrialization, petroleum and other fossil fuels, chemical agriculture, artificial electromagnetic radiation, global warming and climate change, and new viral epidemics—all volatile, fire-like phenomena that can spread quickly and destroy the planet.

However, the most challenging threat we face as a species may not be a global conflagration but a slow, steady path to destruction through improper cooking. The quality of the fire used for food preparation and processing has changed dramatically in recent years. For most of its existence, humanity utilized wood, charcoal, and other natural fuels for cooking and technology. Then in the early modern era, coal started to be mined from underground, spurring the Industrial Revolution. Then petroleum replaced coal as the chief energy source and natural gas became the chief cooking fuel. In the twentieth century, electricity and the microwave started to displace gas. As we have seen, these forms of fire are inherently unstable, unhealthy, and give rise to artificial electromagnetic fields. Quite apart from declining food quality, the use of these extreme forms of fire for cooking may mark the end of humankind—constituting the ultimate Fire destruction—just as mastery of cooking with wood, flint, and other natural means signaled its origin.

As the historical spiral of materialization ends, a new centrifugal spiral will begin and continue for thousands of years, culminating in the construction of a new golden age. It will be based on more comprehensive values, unifying spiritual, holistic, and energetic approaches with a peaceful, sustainable foundation of natural abundance. Transmutation of elements, or cool fusion, will play a central role in this momentous shift in personal and planetary consciousness, leading to the creation of a world of enduring health and peace.

The contours of the new logarithmic spiral are already apparent, in the emergence of the natural foods and organic farming movement, alternative and complementary medicine, intentional communities (those with a common purpose or utopian mission, like an ashram, kibbutz, or ecovillage), and nonviolent peace activism around the planet. It will probably take another 81-year cycle (2036–2117) under the influence of Soil 8—the energy governing deepest night and leading to revolutionary change—for the old orientation to fade away and for the earth as a whole to begin to purify and regenerate itself. Figure 20.5, below, illustrates twelve key milestones in the final orbit of the Spiral of History and the transition to the new era. The entire new orientation will last for about 13,000 years and reach a zenith in about seven or eight thousand years, when the center of the Milky Way once again comes overhead.

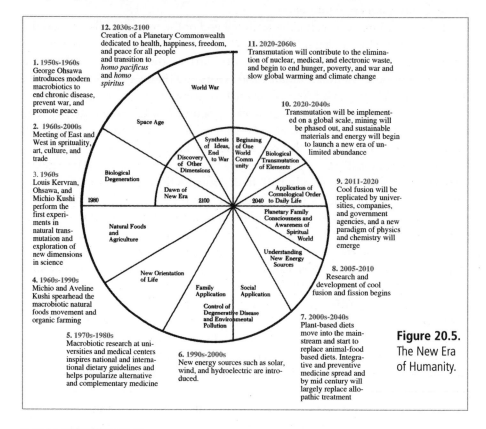

Figure 20.5. The New Era of Humanity.

THE NEW WORLD

When we finally arrive at the dawn of a new world, coinciding with the rise of the North Star directly overhead at the beginning of the twenty-second century, all the people of the world may celebrate this happy occasion with the introduction of a new world calendar. This calendar will start anew, with Year One, the first year of the era of One World. This calendar will reflect all the great traditions of cosmological understanding, composed from our new world cosmology and written in the new world language.

Like Stonehenge, the *I Ching*, or the Aztec and Mayan calendars, the new calendar will provide astronomical and meteorological information for our planting and harvests; it will gauge periods of change and of rest, of physical progress and inward reflection. Charting the turning of the cosmos and the stirrings of the earth, the new world calendar will assist us as we create, change, and recreate the affairs of humanity, playing day and night as one peaceful world family within this infinite universe.

Nothing is guaranteed in the above scenario. It is just one of many that may play out. But it is one that accords with natural order, if we live in a more natural way, including adopting a more balanced way of eating. Of course, it will not be easy to create such a world. It is the natural course of events for this to happen, according to the Order of the Universe or, we may say, according to the will of God—but it will not happen automatically. It certainly won't happen by our eating natural nondairy ice cream and organic apple pie while lying on the couch and daydreaming or watching TV.

Already, millions of human lives have been sacrificed on our circuitous road to a peaceful world. And for it to be finally realized, now that the time is historically ripe, it will still take the endless dedication and efforts of many, many people.

Actually, once a peaceful world government is established, things will not be so interesting. This present time, by contrast, is full of degeneration, greed, and hostility, with many modern institutions collapsing and many disagreements about what to do to save them. Americans are practicing yoga and the martial arts. The Chinese are watching TV and drinking Coca-Cola. It's a very exciting period of history. Such thrilling adventures as we are now having will not come again on earth for perhaps another 10,000 years.

There will be great adventures. Our peaceful civilization will become enormous and probably spread to other planets to grow on a solar system-wide scale. And we will create many technological, intellectual, and social miracles. But in comparison, the present time is much more interesting and challenging.

MENTAL AND PHYSICAL ACTIVITY

In addition to our dietary practice, there are a variety of activities that can help us to create a more peaceful mind, home, and world community. These include self-reflection, meditation, prayer, visualization, chanting, and singing. As a complement to our daily way of eating, these measures will help us recover and develop our physical, mental, and spiritual health, as well as build community and feelings of peace and harmony among all people.

Self-Reflection

To develop our intuition and understanding, we can spend a part of each day—as little as five or ten minutes—alone in self-reflection. This involves reviewing the events of the day, including our thoughts, feelings, actions, and relations with other people, and our overall purpose and direction in life. During this period of quiet, meditation, or prayer, we can contemplate reorienting our way of life in the following ways:

• Are we pursuing only sensory pleasure and emotional comfort, forgetting our native potential for greater happiness and higher freedom?

• Are our meals really balanced to produce the best quality of blood and cells, as well as to secure the best mental and spiritual conditions?

• Is our respect and love for our parents, family, friends, and other people really dedicated from the heart and is our behavior toward them really serving for their health and happiness?

• Are we really building a society, culture, and civilization in harmony with the order of nature or are we ignoring the larger, natural environment, of which we are a small part?

• Finally, do we really know where we have come from and where we are going in this infinite universe?

Visualization

The world of the future is created by our thoughts, feelings, perceptions, and dreams. Each of us can visualize the ideal society that we would like to build. By projecting positive and peaceful thoughts, we are directly contributing to the creation of a positive and peaceful world.

By imagining the world as we would like it to be and projecting that image daily, we are giving that vision life and strength. Devoting a few moments each day—for example, during early morning or late evening or before our meals—to visualizing One Peaceful World will immeasurably strengthen our will and perseverance.

We may also frequently visualize our long journey from One Infinity or God through the different stages of biological evolution to our present life as human beings and the return journey to our source and our realization of freedom and peace.

When our physical, psychological, and spiritual health is sound, our energy overflows, spilling out into the world around us, contributing to the vitality and confidence of our family, society, and ultimately to the world as a whole. This creative energy can then be used on any level we choose to further harmony and peace.

Visualization is especially recommended for children, parents, government officials, and peace leaders who have nightmares about nuclear war or feel helpless about bringing about change.

Prayer and Meditation

Prayer and meditation will also help us keep a peaceful mind, a grateful heart, and a sound body. The prayers in this section are just a few of the many used by macrobiotic families around the world. Please feel free to recite or observe any traditional prayers or meditations, as well as create your own and share them with others.

Meditation on Food and Destiny

> *The foundation of the world is the nation.*
> *The foundation of the nation is the home.*
> *The foundation of the home is the body.*
> *The foundation of the body is the spirit.*
> *The foundation of spirit is food.*

> —SAGEN ISHIZUKA

One Peaceful World Proclamation

1. I trust in the endless order of the universe that manifests in the stars, planets, trees, flowers, and other phenomena of the natural world in addition to the life of humanity and the development of society on this planet.

2. I consider that all humankind are brothers and sisters of one planetary family, sharing the same origin, home, and destiny—returning to God or the infinite universe.

3. I believe that our proper ways of eating, breathing, thinking, and behavior in a healthy, natural environment—the macrobiotic way of life—are the biological, psychological, and spiritual foundations of human health, social well-being, and world peace.

4. I know that our respect for parents, ancestors, and elders, as well as love and care of children and offspring, are essential for the well-being of human society on this planet.

5. I am convinced that our respect for the diverse spirits, beliefs, traditions, customs, lifestyles, and other heritages and expressions of humankind is essential for One Peaceful World.

6. I realize that our universal love, daily dedication, patience and perseverance, and selfless assistance extended to one another are essential for a healthy, peaceful world.

7. I recognize that all human life and affairs on this planet are temporary, transitory, and infinitesimal manifestations of one endless, universal, immortal, permanent being that is forever in harmony and peace.

One Peaceful World Prayer

Having come from, being within, and going toward infinity, may our endless dream be eternally realized upon this earth.

May our unconditional dedication perpetually serve for the creation of love and peace.

May our heartfelt thankfulness be devoted universally upon everyone, everything, and every being.

Daily Dedication for One Peaceful World

When we eat, let us reflect that we have come from food that has come from nature by the Order of the Infinite Universe, and let us be grateful for all that we have been given.

When we meet people, let us see them as brothers and sisters and remember that we have all come from the infinite universe through our parents and ancestors, and let us pray as one with all of humanity for universal love and peace on earth.

When we see the sun and moon, the sky and stars, mountains and rivers, seas and forests, fields and valleys, birds and animals, and all the wonders of nature, let us remember that we have come with them all from the infinite universe. Let us be thankful for our environment on earth and live in harmony with all that surrounds us.

When we see farms and villages, towns and cities, arts and cultures, societies and civilizations, and all the works of humanity, let us recall that our creativity has come from the infinite universe and has passed from generation to generation and spread over the entire earth. Let us be grateful for our birth on this beautiful planet with intelligence and wisdom, and let us vow with all to realize endlessly our eternal dream of One Peaceful World through health, freedom, love, and justice.

Meditation for Inner and Outer Peace

The exercise represented in Figure 20.6 on page 299 may be performed at any time to generate harmonious feelings, lessen international tensions, and contribute to building a world of enduring peace.

Sitting on the ground or floor, or in a chair, and holding the hands in the prayer position on the lap (Position 1), begin to breathe deeply through the slightly opened mouth with the eyes either fully closed or half closed, seeing far, without focusing upon any particular object. The duration of exhaling should be four to seven times that of inhaling.

During the exhalation, pronounce naturally the sound Su ("su—u—u"), the sound of peace and harmony, as long as possible. It is not necessary to make the sound loudly, but it is necessary to make the sound peacefully. At that time, let the sound echo, spreading its vibration through the inner regions of the chest, throat, and face. (Instead of Su, we may use the words Aum, Amen, Allah, One, Peace, Shalom, Shanti, or any other harmonious syllable, if we like.)

While inhaling, intensively imagine that we are inhaling the whole universe deeply into us, and that it is being distributed into all the billions of cells, organs and functions, meridians and chakras, and to all corners of our body, mind, and spirit. While exhaling, imagine that we are distributing the inner universe toward the boundless space of the outer universe.

Repeat this breathing with the sound of peace and harmony (e.g., Su) four to eight times, in order to harmonize with all environmental conditions including the people and human affairs that are surrounding us.

Keeping the peaceful state of mind in the meditating posture, we slowly raise the hands to the level of the heart in the prayer position (Position 2), and then again raise them slowly to the level of the mouth (Position 3). Then gradually we extend both arms forward with the palms naturally opened toward the front, in order to send out peaceful waves of energy through the palms, especially from the centers of the palms (Position 4).

Making one long sound of peace and harmony (e.g., Su), while concentrating on the image of sending peace to all beings and to the world, gradually we open the arms, moving them horizontally until they make a straight line with the shoulders (Position 5).

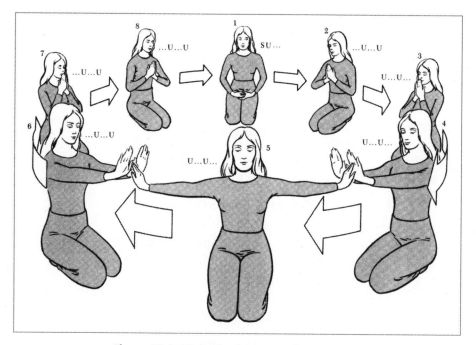

Figure 20.6. Meditation for Inner and Outer Peace.

Then, with the next long sound of peace and harmony, we gradually move the arms back to the outstretched center position, continuously concentrating on the image of radiating waves of peace and harmony in all directions (Position 6).

Upon the completion of this practice, we slowly bend the arms back to the mouth-level prayer position (Position 7), then down to the ordinary prayer position (Position 8). Then, placing our arms and hands back in the meditation form (Position 1), we return to normal and natural breathing. This exercise may be repeated slowly several times.

One Peaceful World Songs

Through singing, dancing, and playing music, we can also strengthen ourselves at all levels. The following songs of peace and harmony have grown out of the modern macrobiotic way of life. Along with similar traditional and modern compositions, they can help us envision a bright, cheerful future and spread feelings of being brothers and sisters in one common home and one world.

Additional Verses for "One Peaceful World"

To the sun that shines above us.
To the earth that lies below.
To the universal spirit,
Our thankfulness shall go.
And the light will shine upon us,
Every single day.
When dreaming of tomorrow.
This is what we say.

Oh-Oh one peaceful world
Oh-Oh one peaceful world.

(Chorus)

In the east the sun is rising.
In the west it's going down.
And the two will join together.
In the new world comin' round.
Where unity will guide us.
In everything we do.
And dawn will soon be breakin'
On a world that's fresh and new.

(Chorus)

Some are white and some are yellow.
Skins of black and skins of brown
When we listen to our hearts beat.
They all make the same pure sound.

(*Chorus*)

All the boundaries of the nations
Can't be seen from outer space.
It is all just land and ocean,
A beautiful home for the human race.

(*Chorus*)

From Atlantic to Pacific,
From Suez to the North Sea,
From Tierra del Fuego,
To wherever you may be.

(*Chorus*)

From Jesus to Zoroaster,
From Moses to Mahavir,
From Buddha to Muhammad,
There is truth for us to hear.

(*Chorus*)

From Boston to Buenos Aires,
From Moscow to Tokyo,
The same sun shines upon us,
And around it we all go.

(*Chorus*)

From Sudan to Australia,
From Cape Can'veral to the Great Wall,
From Stonehenge to Mt. Fuji,
From the Rockies to the Taj Mahal.

(*Chorus*)

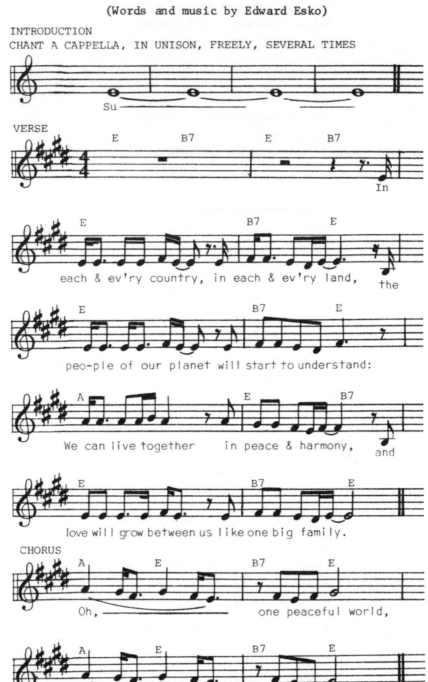

Way-of-Life Suggestions

For a more orderly and peaceful life, the following way-of-life suggestions are recommended:

• Live each day happily without being preoccupied with your health; try to keep mentally and physically active.

• View everything and everyone you meet with gratitude, particularly offering thanks before and after every meal.

• Prepare or eat at least one (ideally two or more) fresh home-cooked meal each day.

• Chew your food very well, at least fifty times per mouthful, or until it becomes liquid in form.

• Retire before midnight and get up early every morning.

• Avoid wearing synthetic or woolen clothing directly next to the skin. As much as possible, wear (non-GMO) cotton, especially for undergarments. Avoid excessive metallic accessories on the fingers, wrists, or neck. Keep such ornaments simple and graceful.

• If your health permits, go outdoors in simple clothing.

• Walk on the grass, beach, or soil for up to thirty minutes every day.

• Keep your home in good order, from the kitchen, bathroom, bedroom, and living rooms, to every corner of the house.

• Initiate and maintain an active correspondence, extending your best wishes to parents, children, brothers and sisters, teachers, and friends.

• Avoid taking long, hot baths or showers—unless you have been consuming too much salt or animal food—as they deplete the body of minerals.

• Scrub your entire body with a hot, damp towel until the skin becomes red every morning or every night before retiring. If that is not possible, at least scrub your hands, fingers, feet, and toes.

• Avoid chemically perfumed cosmetics. For care of the teeth, brush with natural preparations or sea salt.

• If your health permits, exercise regularly as part of daily life, including activities like scrubbing floors, cleaning windows, and washing clothes. You may also participate in exercise programs such as yoga, martial arts, dance, or sports.

• Avoid using electric cooking devices (ovens and ranges) or microwave. Convert to a gas or wood stove at the earliest opportunity.

- It is best to minimize the frequent use of television, computers, smart phones, and other electronics and digital devices that emit artificial electromagnetic fields.

- Include some large green plants in your house to freshen and enrich the oxygen content of the air of your home.

- Start a garden, make your own tofu, tempeh, or other naturally processed foods, and use locally grown foods as much as possible.

- Make your own clothes or purchase naturally made products from free-trade, indigenous, or home-made craftspeople or collectives.

- Sing a merry song each day.

A BRIGHT NEW WORLD

Balanced dietary practice, grounding physical activity and exercise, and uplifting mental and spiritual activity are the three pillars of *macrobios*—living a long, happy life. By developing and centering ourselves, we create a spiral of health and peace that radiates out to our family, friends, neighbors, and eventually the entire world. Each of us carries the seeds of a bright new world—the world of peace and prosperity envisioned by countless generations of ancestors and parents, the world of enduring harmony and balance—and we would like to pass it on to our children and all those who follow.

PEACE PROMOTER

Sachi Kato, Los Angeles and Tokyo

Wa 和*—or Peace—will manifest when we eat brown rice.*
                                                    —MICHIO KUSHI

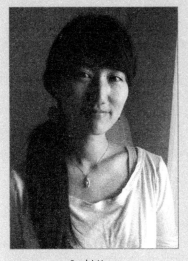

Sachi Kato

"Michio Kushi"—the first time Sachi Kato heard the name was at Inaka, a restaurant in Los Angeles. In the early 2000s, Inaka was the only macrobiotic restaurant in L.A., and Sachi was waiting tables to supplement her work as a freelance photographer. "It is a small family-owned restaurant that is like an oasis in the life of a big, busy city," Sachi recalled. "Many customers came to dine in this relaxing hideaway, and often we discussed macrobiotic philosophy and the correspondences between food and 'yin and yang.'" At first, she thought it was strange to consider food as energy, but soon she became intrigued by the concept. That is how she was first introduced to macrobiotics. Sachi couldn't understand very well at the time, but she had a gut feeling there was something important to it. This intuition strengthened her interest in macrobiotics and in meeting this *sensei*—Michio Kushi—one day.

Years later, Sachi pursued macrobiotic education. She took the Levels courses at the Kushi Institute of Europe, and soon learned that Michio Kushi was still teaching actively in her native Japan. She enrolled in Level 3 at the Kushi Institute of Japan in 2010 and looked forward to meeting and studying with him.

Sachi was surprised to find that the lectures in Level 3—the advanced course at the KIJ—were almost all about spirituality. They dealt with such subjects as, "Where did we all come from?" and "Where are we going after this life?" Michio presented these questions in many lectures, and the students discussed spirituality. He encouraged his listeners to meditate, empty their minds, and purify themselves. His message was unique, and Sachi strove to grasp everything he taught and not miss a single word. "He was often comical, making jokes and telling amusing stories," she observed. "I was impressed with how strong and capable a teacher he was despite his advanced age."

At the end of the final lecture of Level 3, Michio gently asked the students if they had any questions. The classroom grew silent. Michio said, "Okay, since there are no more questions, I will bid you so long. This may be the last occasion I will spend time together with you."

Then a sudden urge arose within Sachi to venture a question. She raised her hand and asked, "*Sensei,* what is the dream of brown rice?"

Michio had been lecturing about the dream of different foods. He taught that food was spirit, and that each food had its own unique dream. When we eat certain vegetables, their dreams live within us. Before this talk, it never occurred to Sachi that vegetables have a mind and a dream, or goal, in life. One part of her thought this idea was ridiculous, but another part was intrigued by the subject. "It was an eye-opening experience, and I began to see things in a totally different perspective," she later observed.

"What is the dream of brown rice?" At the very moment she asked Michio the question, strangely, the answer came to Sachi: "It was a revelation. A little voice echoed in my heart and whispered 'Peace.'"

Sachi was at a loss for words and tried to grasp what happened at the moment. The sensation was very strong and overwhelming. Then, a vision of a brown rice field appeared. "The tall brown rice straws were full of grains, bent over with full heads ready for harvest, and blowing in the wind. The golden fields were shining. It was a serene and peaceful scene, totally tranquil, and I could almost hear the sound of the straws touching and making waves." Then the message came to her that the rice grains don't speak a word, but are waiting for humans to eat them for the purpose of manifesting their dream of "Peace." The vision was very moving. "What an amazing and sacred dream the grains have! They just want us to make the world a peaceful place!"

The sensation was so overwhelming that in that split second Sachi burst into tears. Everyone in the classroom must have wondered what happened to her. But Michio remained sitting quietly without speaking.

Then finally Sachi said to Michio, "*Sensei,* I got it. The dream of rice is 'Peace,' isn't it?"

Michio didn't reply directly. Instead he quietly asked his wife, Midori, to come to the front of the lecture room and instructed her to write the Japanese word for "Peace" or *Wa* 和.

Michio gently said, "If you look closely at this word *Wa,* it contains two symbols. On the left is 'rice straw' and on the right, 'mouth.' This word *Wa* has a profound meaning: By eating rice we can manifest peace."

Until then, Sachi never knew that Japanese ideographs had such a deep meaning. Her appreciation deepened toward her ancestors who must have understood the concepts to compose those words. "This was one of my special moments with Michio *sensei* who taught me the essence of life," she said.

Michio's lecture was clear and very easy to understand. "I know now he just wanted us to understand the essence of life and how to live simply and meaningfully. He taught us how to live gracefully and eat well. If we understand more about the dreams of vegetables, rice, and other foods, we can appreciate better nature's gifts," Sachi said.

Michio emphasized eating well as the principal practice of macrobiotics because it enables people to manifest their dreams. He often said: "'The purpose of life is to play.' This means by eating in a balanced way, we are able to realize our potential and achieve our dreams. That is the ultimate freedom, and our lives become 'playful.'"

Sachi went on to become a macrobiotic teacher, counselor, and head chef at the Kushi Institute. She is cooking editor for the *Amberwaves* newsletter and has been active in non-GMO activities. She prepared the recipes for www.EbolaAndDiet.com, the Amberwaves' website offering macrobiotic dietary guidance during the Ebola epidemic in West Africa in 2014. Sachi teaches around the world and is co-author of the *Kushi Institute Cookbook* with Alex Jack.

Source

Remembering Michio by Michio Kushi's students, family, and friends. Kushi Institute, 2015, 93–96.

Conclusion
Realizing Our Endless Dream

In 1965, a year before he died, George Ohsawa came to America and visited Aveline and me at our home in Cambridge. One day, about noon, he went for a walk. When he returned, he announced that he had found the definition of happiness: "Happiness is endlessly realizing our endless dream."

Then he turned to me and said, "What do you think, Michio?"

Aveline and Lima, George's wife, were also listening. "Very poetic," they commented.

"It's very good," I said.

"Please try to change it," Ohsawa said.

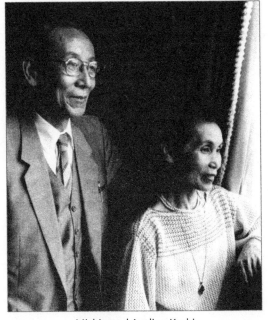

Michio and Aveline Kushi

Over the years, I have grown much older and have had many experiences, but I cannot make a better definition.

In realizing our endless dream, we must recover our endless memory. In addition to the future, we must change our past. The past guides us, too. It is always in front. We need to look at what has come before our time gratefully and see its bright side. Recovering our memory will take us into a peaceful future.

At one time, long before what is now called recorded history, there was a civilization in which all people were peacefully unified under one world government, practiced natural agriculture, and enjoyed lifelong health and happiness. This one world community was lost to various catastrophes and doesn't appear in our history books or our conscious knowledge. But deep inside, humanity has never forgotten that dream and has nurtured it through the thousands of years of war, conflict, and struggle that we call recorded history.

The memory of lost Paradise has inspired many prophetic visions, many utopian proposals and communities, many religious societies and secular movements, and many artistic and literary visions. In ancient Sumerian legend, Gilgamesh quested for Dilmun, the land without sickness, old age, and war. In the *Iliad*, the last world age on Achilles' shield depicted the Circle of the Dance, in which humanity was joined together in joyful song. In the Old Testament, the prophet Isaiah saw a vision of a future world in which swords were beaten into plowshares and there was no more war. In the New Testament, St. John the Divine saw a vision of the city of Jerusalem, in which all nations would be healed by the leaves of the Tree of Life and need no candle to light their way. Columbus saw his journeys to the New World as a fulfillment of the prophecies of Isaiah, and the Puritans founded their colony in New England as the New Jerusalem. Plato's *Republic*, Sir Thomas More's *Utopia*, Campanella's *City of the Sun*, and Samuel Butler's *Erewhon* were all textual attempts to recover this image. In his writings, Karl Marx envisioned human destiny leading inevitably to a classless society without war, poverty, and conflict. In the East, the legends of Shambhala, Horai-San (the Mountain Isles of the Blessed), Shangri-La, and the Pure Land sprang from this common source.

All of these images of a bright, happy, peaceful future flowed from a dim universal memory of the past and an intuitive understanding that history moves in a spiral. But because we have forgotten our common origin, modern humanity is divided into hundreds of competing countries, religions, and groups. The most dangerous chasm today is between the apocalyptic religionists and the proponents of globalization, who view the confrontation between tradition and modernity, religion, and science, as the last battle before the dawning of the new age. Actually, both sides want exactly the same thing—health, happiness, peace, and a better life for themselves and their children.

Through seasons of famine and hardship, fire and ice, war and pestilence, our common dream of One Peaceful World has endured. Today, it is facing its greatest challenge as we perfect the technological means to destroy ourselves internally and externally. Today, we live in an artificial, make-believe world, submitting ourselves to being illusory citizens of the United States, China, Russia, Japan, and other countries. We accept modern medicine, agriculture, education, and science, even though they are leading us to destruction. Our vision of Paradise has narrowed to a life of leisure insulated from the earth and sky, and our idea of utopia is an online shopping mall with an endless array of glittering consumer goods. Chasing fortune, fame, status, comfort, convenience, and other ephemeral goals, most of us are wasting our precious lives on this planet. Or if we are more socially and ideologically oriented, we are trying to impose our distorted images of reality—our limited view of Paradise or utopia—on others.

We have to change and wake up. We have to recover our universal dream and our memory, which are one.

The old world is passing away, and a new world is being born. We are in the last days of precessional winter before the arrival of precessional spring. Just before the warmth and light return with the rise of Polaris, the North Star, directly overhead, the cold and darkness are at their height. The dawning new world is being built by our dreams and aspirations, our memory and vision. If we can maintain harmony with nature and the environment, we can definitely survive winter's end and pass safely into spring. To enjoy this happy, peaceful world, we should:

1. Always eat human food—whole cereal grains and vegetables—as the main part of our daily sustenance;

2. Understand the Order of the Universe;

3. Be endlessly appreciative and grateful to others, including those who would be our enemies and those who would do us harm;

4. Give of ourselves endlessly in the spirit of "one grain, ten thousand grains," and

5. See not only the front (the visible world and its order), but also the back—the invisible, spiritual world and its order from whence we came and will return.

Understanding the world beyond space and time may be difficult in the beginning. I also found it difficult when I was young, but now when I do something, I know it was already imagined long ago, and my thought will be accomplished thousands of years from now. Thinking like this reaches infinite space instantaneously; pure thoughts, not trifling ones, are already realized in the world of vibration. For events to come to physical expression, to appear to our eyes, takes time. Everything depends upon our dream, our picture of reality, the image that guides us through life. When we have a dream, already in the world of spirit, it is realized; it only takes time to manifest in the relative world. When we are eating well and have a true dream, it does not even matter if we are still alive. One day, it will come.

The people of thousands of years ago dreamed true dreams. Our present world was conceived in their minds and consciousness, and so we were born; and our dream will be realized by our offspring for thousands of generations to come. We must understand this invisible succession. It is the actual source of all phenomena and other manifestations. The "biggest dream" of all, which everyone has in common, is the most genuine dream of health, happiness, and peace. We must keep and realize our universal, immortal dreams. We must not lose them, but continue to imagine and extend them into the future and past. By orienting our daily life toward our endless dream, it will never disappear. The dream of creating One Peaceful World was pursued by many people in ancient times who understood God or the infinite Order of the Universe. We are now realizing that eternal dream.

When we have practiced a more harmonious way of eating for a while and helped many people, true memories will start to come back. We will begin to discover our wonderful past as well as foresee our wonderful future. For that, we must keep a humble and modest spirit, endlessly distributing our understanding and knowledge to others. Then we can discover that our life is eternal and that we freely chose this time and place, this planet and this era, and all the adventures we are now experiencing. This we can understand, not as conceptual theory, but as actual experience.

This is the real purpose and practice of macrobiotics, opening ourselves to cosmological consciousness and together with our friends playing freely on all the planets in the universe. When we discover the true meaning of food as spirit and energy, then we can again join our many brothers and sisters and with them, spread the understanding of life, peace, happiness, and freedom throughout our world and through the whole spiral universe.

THE PEACEFUL REVOLUTION

Our eternal dream is always within us in the form of memory. The seed of One Peaceful World exists in every human heart and, when properly nourished and cultivated, grows and gradually extends to the family, the community, and the world as a whole. It doesn't matter where we are, whether we are healthy or sick, or what level of judgment we start from; the important thing is to begin.

Today, everyone—the religious and nonreligious, the sick and healthy, rich and poor, soldiers and civilians, children and elders—can participate in a peaceful biological revolution. Peace begins with each one of us. We must declare, "Yes, I will do it." By turning the spiral of our life, we turn the Spiral of History. We do not complain at the sorry state of the world. We take responsibility. We take action. We take charge of our kitchen. We change our cooking and bring health and peace to our own lives, to our families, and our community. Governments, religions, schools, and mass movements are not going to do it. But we can.

Present artificial borderlines between countries are maintained by force or they would collapse. Our "weapons" to eliminate these unnatural boundaries—and the national educational systems, industries, and armies that uphold them—are invisible ideas; food is universal and can easily penetrate national borderlines. Like the bloodstream nourishing the cells throughout the whole body, good-quality natural organic food will eventually reach each country. Changes may not be immediately apparent, but from the inside, changes will begin and eventually result in a safe transition to the Era of Humanity and the realization of One Peaceful World. No matter what happens in the flow of historical events, no matter what kind of revolutions or changes arise, our peaceful way will continue quietly, like water penetrating softly and steadily, changing individuals, families, and communities, until society as a whole changes.

In the early 1960s, my parents came from Japan to visit me in Boston. I had not seen them since I left Japan after the end of the war. For two weeks, they stayed at our home in Cambridge. During the days, I lectured, and Aveline gave cooking classes. At night, we packed brown rice and miso into small packages for our students and friends. I wondered what my parents must be thinking of their son, who was once a prize student in law and political science at Tokyo University. I knew they worried about me and couldn't understand my broken English. For many years in New York, I had been washing dishes, working as a bellboy, and engaging in small businesses to support my studies, while my former classmates had risen in banking, government, and industry.

One day, after watching and listening for about two weeks, my parents said they would like to talk with me that evening. I thought they might ask me to go back to Japan that night.

Father and Mother came to my room and closed the door. Kneeling down on the floor, they bowed to me and said that they had decided to become my disciples. Mother said, "I don't mind whether it succeeds or not, but please use me as a model, if you need to experiment. If I die, it doesn't matter." Father said, "If your students come to Japan, we will help them." How happy I was. Inside I was crying. I was the happiest person in the world. I knew from that day forward that I could attain my dream.

Several years later, Aveline and I returned to Japan. It was our first visit in over twenty years. In Ohtamura, my family's ancestral village, some two to three hundred villagers gathered and honored us at a banquet. About twenty elders were present, and we visited Dai Taiji, the Temple of Great Peace. The next morning, two elders came to my cousin's home, where we were staying, and took tea. They told us that after my talk the previous evening, the villagers had gathered in a council and had all decided to become macrobiotic. Once again, I was moved beyond words. In this beautiful natural setting, I knew that one day the world would again be one.

From our understanding of natural order, we know that during the next several thousand years, humanity will begin to synthesize the material and spiritual advances of preceding epochs. Violence and war will subside, and peace and harmony will gradually be established. The seeds that we plant in this generation—during the next ten, twenty, and thirty years—will one day bring forth a mighty tree of insight and understanding that will nourish and unify the planet.

The Buddha taught that the world of enlightenment and the everyday world are one. Jesus taught that the Kingdom of Heaven is spread over the earth, but we see it not. One Peaceful World already exists here and now, not in some remote future. By sharing the same quality of food, we start to share the same memories, same feelings, and same dream. Let us join together as brothers and sisters of one planetary family and enter the new Paradise together.

Appendix A

Menu and Recipes for One Peaceful World Day

by Sachi Kato

One Peaceful World Day is celebrated on May 17, Michio Kushi's birthday, and macrobiotic friends around the world rededicate themselves to realizing humanity's common dream of one healthy, peaceful world. Activities at this time take many forms, including public seminars, lectures, meditation, services, banquets, and festivals. At the Kushi Institute, the Kushi Peace Prize is awarded to an individual or organization for their outstanding contribution to health, peace, and sustainability.

At these gatherings, food is usually served, though some people may wish to observe the day in prayer and fasting. The following menu and recipes for One Peaceful World Day or similar occasions (such as the World Peace Days on August 6 and 9, the anniversary of the atomic bombings of Hiroshima and Nagasaki), include whole, natural foods based on the standard macrobiotic way of eating. Simple, yet elegant, they include a variety of everyday foods from East and West, North and South, and are easy to prepare, delicious, and satisfying. They may be used to prepare a sit-down meal or banquet, a buffet, a lunchbox, or a picnic basket. All recipes serve between four and six people. A few require pre-soaking or other advance preparation.

The foods give a very calm and peaceful energy. Enjoyed with a grateful mind and heart, they will help us experience peace within ourselves and within our family and community, contributing to greater happiness and harmony around the world.

ONE PEACEFUL WORLD DAY MENU

- Hummus
- Spring Miso Soup
- Shira-Ae: Tofu Salad with Land and Sea Vegetables
- Hiziki Stew
- Kimpira

- Sautéed Dandelions with Mushrooms and Corn
- Brown Rice with Quinoa
- Roasted Barley Tea
- Bancha Twig Tea
- Pear Compote

Hummus

Hummus, the tasty traditional dip or spread from the Middle East,
is one of the world's most popular snacks. It is made with chickpeas,
tahini (sesame seed paste), olive oil, lemon juice, and other seasonings.

YIELD: 4–6 SERVINGS

1 cup dried chickpeas, soaked overnight

1 stamp-sized piece kombu

$1/4$ cup lemon juice

2 teaspoons umeboshi paste

$1 1/2$ to 2 tablespoons tahini

1 clove garlic

Dash umeboshi vinegar

$1/8$ teaspoon sea salt (optional)

Bean cooking water, if necessary

TOPPING

$1/4$ cup saved cooked chickpeas

2 tablespoons extra virgin olive oil

powdered smoked paprika (optional)

1. Discard soaking water and place kombu and chickpeas in a pressure cooker.

2. Add water to $1/2$-inch above the beans.

3. Bring to a boil, uncovered, skimming off any white foam that may arise.

4. Cover the pressure cooker, bring to pressure, and simmer for 45 minutes.

5. Allow pressure to come down and open the pot. Let the beans cool to room temperature. They will have absorbed most of the water. Add a little more water if dry.

6. In a food processor, place all remaining ingredients and all but $1/4$ cup of cooked chickpeas.

7. Blend for about 2 to 3 minutes, or until smooth and creamy.

8. Add some bean cooking water if the mixture is too dry to blend.

9. Add topping and serve.

Variation: With the ingredients in the food processor, add $1/2$ cup basil leaves for herbal hummus.

Spring Miso Soup

Miso soup, made from fermented soybean paste, is a macrobiotic staple and enjoyed around the world. Miso is excellent to strengthen the flora in the small intestine, protect against digestive and circulatory disorders, and heal from disease.

YIELD: 4 SERVINGS

4-inch piece wakame, soaked until soft and finely diced

3 cups water

2 dried shiitake mushrooms, soaked in one cup water until soft, finely sliced (save the soaking water to add to the broth)

$1/2$ yellow onion, cut in thin half-moons

1 small carrot, cut in thin matchsticks

$1/2$ cup leafy vegetables (bok choy, collard greens, etc), finely sliced

4 teaspoons miso paste, or to taste

Scallions for garnish

1. In a medium saucepan, combine wakame, water, shiitake, and the shiitake soaking water and bring to a boil.

2. Add the remaining vegetables, and return to a boil. Reduce heat to medium-low and cook until the vegetables are soft, about 10 minutes.

3. Reduce heat to low. Remove a small amount of broth, use to dissolve the miso paste in a small bowl, and stir gently back into the broth.

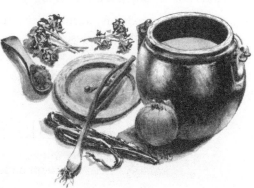

4. Simmer uncovered for 3 to 4 minutes to activate the enzymes. After adding miso, *do not* boil the broth in order to preserve the enzymes.

5. Serve with garnish.

Note: You can make miso soup all year round by using seasonal ingredients in addition to the leafy vegetables. For example, in springtime, use sprouts and celery; in summertime, corn kernels; in autumn, kabocha squash; and in wintertime, root vegetables such as burdock root.

Shira-Ae Tofu Salad with Land and Sea Vegetables

"Ae" means making harmony. Shira-Ae translates in Japanese to "harmony with tofu." In Japanese home cooking, there are many "Ae"-style dishes. This one is similar to tofu salad and features mashed tofu mixed with both land and sea vegetables.

YIELD: 5–6 SERVINGS

One 14-ounce package firm tofu,
boiled for 10 minutes and drained well

1/2 cup hiziki sea vegetable stew (*using the recipe below)

1 tablespoon walnuts, roasted and crushed

1 1/2 tablespoons white miso, or to taste

2 teaspoons tahini

Dash of umeboshi vinegar

1 cup mixed blanched vegetables: carrots,
cut into matchsticks; or mizuna or other summer greens

1 teaspoon lemon zest and scallions, for garnish

1. In a medium or large *suribachi* (Japanese mortar), place white miso, tahini seed butter, and a little water and grind well with a *surikogi* (pestle).
2. Add cooked tofu and grind all together until the texture becomes smooth.
3. Add other ingredients, including the hiziki stew below, and mix well with a spatula. Adjust flavor if desired.
4. Serve at room temperature or chilled in summertime.

Hiziki Stew

1 tablespoon sesame oil

1/2 cup onion, cut into matchsticks

2 tablespoons hiziki, soaked for 20 minutes in water and drained

1/2 cup carrot, cut into matchsticks

Shoyu, to taste

1. In a stew pot, heat sesame oil and sauté onions for 3 to 5 minutes or until the onions soften. Layer the hiziki and carrots on top of the onions. Add enough water to cover the onions.

2. Bring to a boil, cover, and simmer for 25 to 30 minutes.

3. Flavor with shoyu and cook uncovered until all liquid evaporates. You can then add the finished stew to the salad.

Kimpira

Kimpira is a Japanese word that means "golden pieces."
The assorted root vegetables are cut into matchsticks and, when cooked,
shimmer with a nice savory flavor and a golden yellow glow.

YIELD: 4 SERVINGS

1 tablespoon sesame oil

1 cup burdock, sliced into matchsticks

Several pinches sea salt

1 cup lotus root, sliced thin quarter moons

1 cup carrot, sliced into matchsticks

1 tablespoon shoyu, or to taste

1 tablespoon ginger juice (optional)

1 tablespoon of toasted sesame seeds, for topping

1. Heat sesame oil in a skillet over medium heat and sauté the burdock and sea salt for 3 minutes, or until the bitter, woody aroma transforms into a sweet aroma.

2. Add lotus root and carrot and sauté for 3 more minutes.

3. Lightly cover the bottom of the skillet with water. Bring to a boil, cover the skillet, and simmer about 15–20 minutes, or until the vegetables are 80 percent done and water is almost absorbed.

4. Add shoyu to taste and cover. Cook for a few minutes, uncover, and cook until liquid has evaporated. Add ginger juice, if desired.

5. Toss sesame seeds, mix gently, and serve.

Variation: For a gluten-free dish, use tamari instead of shoyu. However, since tamari is stronger than shoyu, use slightly less.

Sautéed Dandelions
with Mushrooms and Corn

*Dandelions are sometimes too bitter to digest, but this is a mild,
delicious way to prepare them. By sautéing them with onions,
the intense bitterness lessens and the umami flavor is enhanced
with mushrooms. The final flavor combines savory and sweet
with just a hint of natural bitterness.*

YIELD: 3–4 SERVINGS

1 tablespoon sesame oil

1 cup onion, sliced into thin half-moons

1 clove garlic, minced

$1/8$ teaspoon sea salt

1 cup mushrooms, sliced thin

1 bunch (about 3 cups) dandelion greens,
chopped into small 1/16-inch lengths

Water for steaming

1 teaspoon mirin (optional)

2 teaspoons shoyu

Corn kernels, blanched (for topping)

1. Heat sesame oil in a cast iron skillet. Sauté onion and garlic with sea salt for 3 to 5 minutes or until onion becomes translucent.

2. Add mushrooms and continue sautéing for another 3 to 5 minutes, or until mushrooms are cooked.

3. Layer dandelion leaves on top, cover the skillet, and steam with a little water sprinkled on the vegetables for 1 minute.

4. Take lid off the skillet and sauté until dandelions turn bright, about 3 to 5 minutes. Taste to make sure the dandelions are sautéed well and their bitterness is mild.

5. Season with mirin and shoyu. Adjust flavor if necessary.

6. Place corn kernels on top and serve immediately.

Brown Rice With Quinoa

Combined with brown rice, quinoa gives a light, fluffy texture to this dish and is especially appetizing for those who can't handle too much rice.

YIELD: 4–5 SERVINGS

1 cup short-grain brown rice, washed and soaked
in 2$^1/_2$ cups water for several hours

$^1/_4$ cup quinoa, washed and soaked in same water
as the brown rice for several hours

Pinch of sea salt

1. In a cast iron pot or a thick-bottom stainless pot, place the soaked grains together with the soaking water.
2. Bring to a boil on medium-high heat and sprinkle with sea salt.
3. Cover the pot and place a flame deflector underneath to prevent scorching.
4. Reduce the heat to low and cook for 50 to 60 minutes, or until all the cooking liquid is absorbed.
5. Remove from heat and let steam for 10 minutes. Open the lid and mix gently.

Variation: If you are using a pressure cooker, reduce the grain and soaking water ratio to 1:1$^1/_2$.

Roasted Barley Tea

Roasted barley tea is very cooling to the body and may be prepared cool or warm. It is often available in natural foods stores under its Japanese name, mugi cha. *It can also be made at home by dry-roasting unhulled barley or until a fragrant aroma is released.*

YIELD: 4 CUPS

1–2 tablespoons roasted barley

1 quart water

1. Place roasted barley and water in a pot and bring to a boil.
2. Reduce heat and simmer for 5 to 15 minutes, depending on the strength desired. Stir and shake the pot occasionally to prevent burning.

Bancha Tea

*Tea made from the stems and twigs of the tea bush is known as bancha
twig tea, or kukicha tea in Japan. It is picked at the end of the summer
or fall, when the caffeine has naturally receded from the tea plant.
It has a very soothing, peaceful energy and is the most common
daily beverage prepared in the macrobiotic community.*

YIELD: 4 CUPS

1 tablespoon roasted twigs

1 quart water

1. Place roasted twigs in water and bring to a boil. Keep unused twigs in an air-tight jar until needed.

2. When the water boils, reduce heat to low and simmer for several minutes. For a light tea, simmer 1 to 2 minutes. For a darker, stronger tea, simmer for 10 to 15 minutes.

3. To serve, place a small bamboo or metal tea strainer in each cup and pour out the tea.

Note: Twigs in the strainer may be returned to the teapot and reused several times. Bancha tea may be served hot year-round, as well as cool in the summer. It is usually drunk plain.

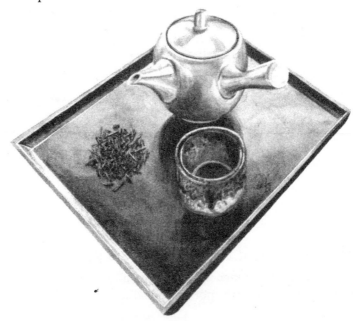

Pear Compote

This elegant dessert is simple to make and very delicious.

YIELD: 3–4 SERVINGS

2 pears, peeled, cored, and sliced diagonally
into quarters

1 cup apple juice

Few pinches sea salt

Few pinches cinnamon (optional)

1 heaping teaspoon kudzu,
diluted with 1 tablespoon water

1 tablespoon lemon zest

1 tablespoon lemon juice (optional)

1. In a medium saucepan, place pear, apple juice, sea salt, and cinnamon.
2. Bring to a boil, cover, and simmer for 20 minutes.
3. Remove the pear only and place in serving dishes.
4. Add the diluted kudzu to the pot. Keep stirring at a simmer until the sauce thickens and the texture becomes creamy.
5. Add the lemon zest and lemon juice.
6. Pour the sauce over the pear and serve.

Appendix B

Principles and Laws of the Infinite Universe

Seven Universal Principles

1. Everything is a differentiation of God or One Infinity.

2. Everything changes.

3. All antagonisms are complementary.

4. There is nothing identical to anything else.

5. What has a front (i.e., a visible side) has a back (i.e., an invisible side).

6. The bigger the front, the bigger the back.

7. What has a beginning has an end.

Seven Precepts for World Peace

1. We all share and are nourished by one planet—the earth.

2. Any threat of war can be changed into an opportunity for peace.

3. All factors in the modern world that appear antagonistic are actually complementary, contributing to overall future harmony.

4. The present world crisis offers a unique opportunity for establishing universal peace.

5. War, like peace, begins in the heart and in the home.

6. The greater the threat of war, the greater the opportunity for peace.

7. The use of war as a solution to world problems has reached its limit.

The Twelve Laws of Change

1. One Infinity manifests itself in complementary and antagonistic tendencies, yin and yang, in its endless change.

2. Yin and yang are manifested continuously from the eternal movement of one infinite universe.

3. Yin represents centrifugality. Yang represents centripetality. Yin and yang together produce energy and all phenomena.

4. Yin attracts yang. Yang attracts yin.

5. Yin repels yin. Yang repels yang.

6. Yin and yang combined in varying proportions produce different phenomena. The attraction and repulsion between phenomena is proportional to the difference of the yin and yang forces within them.

7. All phenomena are ephemeral, constantly changing their constitution of yin and yang forces; yin changes into yang, yang changes into yin.

8. Nothing is solely yin or solely yang. Everything is composed of both tendencies in varying degrees.

9. There is nothing neutral. Either yin or yang is predominant in every phenomenon.

10. Large yin attracts small yin. Large yang attracts small yang.

11. Extreme yin produces yang, and extreme yang produces yin.

12. All physical manifestations are yang at the center, and yin at the surface.

Appendix C
Standard Macrobiotic Guidelines

The Global Macrobiotic Guidelines that follow were especially prepared by Michio Kushi for *The Book of Macrobiotics* and have been replicated here. The following pyramid and pie chart are general, standard macrobiotic guidelines. The full guidelines (which can be found in *The Book of Macrobiotics* or online at www.kushiinstitute.org/what-is-macrobiotics) include dietary recommendations for ten regions of the world, including Temperate Regions, Central America, South America, the Mediterranean, Middle East, Africa, South Asia, Southeast Asia and the Pacific Islands, Cool Climates, and Cold Climates. The recommendations have especially been modified from past guidelines to take into account global warming, climate change, and the accelerated pace of modern life.

The guidelines include a food pyramid and a circular pie chart. The two graphics are substantially the same. However, the pyramid includes at the top a small amount of meat, eggs and poultry, and dairy food. This optional amount of strong animal food is primarily for those in transition to macrobiotics from the modern way of eating or who wish to consume a small amount of this food on an infrequent basis for social, cultural, or personal reasons.

The circular pie chart details relative proportions of food consumed on a daily basis. They do not represent the amount of food on a plate. This is a frequent source of misunderstanding and one of the reasons the pyramidal charts were developed. The percentages of food are listed in terms of weight, not volume. Hence, vegetables, which are more expansive and weigh less, will take up a larger volume of space on an actual plate than a comparable amount of grains or beans, which are more condensed and heavier. This too has been a source of confusion and another reason for the pyramidal charts. We hope the stereo view that these two different kinds of charts provide will complement each other and help unify vegans and those who consume animal food alike.

The key point in reflecting on charts is that the contemporary macrobiotic way of eating is not fixed and static, but flexible and ever changing. It is grounded in human biological and spiritual evolution (i.e., whole cereal grains are principal food for humans and their ancestors for millions of years except in special habitats) and then further modified for climate and environment, season and weather, social and cultural tradition and custom, ethical and environmental considerations, and finally for age, sex, gender, activity level, and personal condition and needs.

Macrobiotic Dietary Guidelines
for Temperate Regions

including North America, Europe, Russia, China, East Asia, and Moderate Regions
in Southern Africa, South America, Australia, and New Zealand

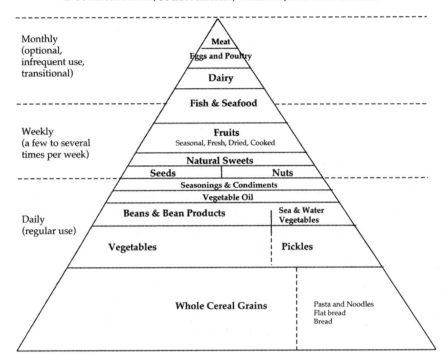

Monthly (optional, infrequent use, transitional)

- Meat
- Eggs and Poultry
- Dairy
- Fish & Seafood

Weekly (a few to several times per week)

- Fruits — Seasonal, Fresh, Dried, Cooked
- Natural Sweets
- Seeds / Nuts

Daily (regular use)

- Seasonings & Condiments
- Vegetable Oil
- Beans & Bean Products / Sea & Water Vegetables
- Vegetables / Pickles
- Whole Cereal Grains / Pasta and Noodles, Flat bread, Bread

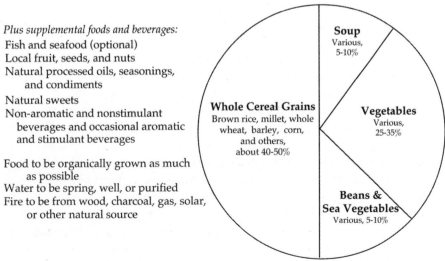

Plus supplemental foods and beverages:

Fish and seafood (optional)
Local fruit, seeds, and nuts
Natural processed oils, seasonings, and condiments

Natural sweets
Non-aromatic and nonstimulant beverages and occasional aromatic and stimulant beverages

Food to be organically grown as much as possible
Water to be spring, well, or purified
Fire to be from wood, charcoal, gas, solar, or other natural source

- **Soup** — Various, 5-10%
- **Whole Cereal Grains** — Brown rice, millet, whole wheat, barley, corn, and others, about 40-50%
- **Vegetables** — Various, 25-35%
- **Beans & Sea Vegetables** — Various, 5-10%

Copyright 2012 by Michio Kushi

Appendix D

One Peaceful Universe

by Edward Esko

Decades ago, George Ohsawa and Michio Kushi postulated a spirally formed fractal universe. They posited that creation was ongoing—without beginning or end—and that creation is an orderly, peaceful, and never-ending process. Many of the tenets of modern cosmology are diametrically opposed to this paradigm. Concepts like the Big Bang and the thermonuclear sun are not based on a peaceful universe. Rather, they are constructed around a universe of unimaginable violence. However, these modern tenets are increasingly being challenged as new information comes in from satellites, increasingly powerful telescopes, and deep space probes. Slowly but surely, hypothetical constructs such as the Big Bang and thermonuclear sun are facing serious challenges. The Ohsawa/Kushi cosmology may yet prevail, leading the way to a peaceful and harmonious view of the universe and a reflection of that reality on planet Earth. One Peaceful World is the realization of the reality of One Peaceful Universe among all people and beings on our beautiful planet.

BIG BANG

Following Einstein's equations and quantum theory in the early part of the twentieth century, modern physics began a departure from models based on actual experiment to purely theoretical models based on mathematics. Even Einstein himself conceived many of his ideas through his famous "thought experiments," rather than through actual experiments conducted in the real world.

One such model, based on Einstein's theory of relativity, is the so-called "Big Bang." The Big Bang claims that the entire universe began in a huge explosion about 13 billion years ago. Before the explosion, the entire universe, including all galaxies, clusters of galaxies, stars, planets, interstellar dust and gas, and all forms of life, were contained in a microscopic seed, known as a "singularity."

The Big Bang is a purely mathematical construct. It has yet to be proven or disproven through experiments or through observation of phenomena here on earth. Recent discoveries raise serious doubt. The discovery of gigantic filaments containing millions of galaxies (imagine giant Christmas trees with strings of lights, with each light being a galaxy, stretching over millions of light years) suggests that the universe is actually much older than 13 billion years, the date at which the Big Bang is supposed to have happened. Such enormous structures require far longer than 13 billion years to form:

• In 1986, astronomers discovered super clusters of galaxies 300 million light years long, 100 million light years thick, stretching 300 million light years across. Such structures require 80 billion years to form.

• In 1989, the Great Wall—a sheet of galaxies more than 500 million light years long, 200 million light years wide, and 15 million light years thick—was discovered. Such a structure would take 100 billion years to form.

• In 2003, astronomers discovered the Sloan Great Wall, a super cluster of galaxies 1.36 billion light years long. Such a structure would require 250 billion years to form.

Another challenge to the Big Bang comes from the study of quasars, or quasi-stellar objects. According to conventional astronomy, quasars are the most distant objects in the universe. Their high redshifts (long, low-frequency light waves that represent an object moving away from us) indicate they are receding with enormous velocity. (The higher an object's redshift, the higher its recessional velocity, according to standard astronomy.)

However, the discovery that high redshift quasars are linked to low redshift galaxies has undermined the "redshift equals velocity" argument. In his study of unusual galaxies, astronomer Halton Arp found that high redshift quasars were connected to nearby galaxies, and in fact, may have been emitted from active "parent" galaxies. Arp theorized that recessional velocity might not be the only factor determining redshift. Arp differentiated between the velocity component of the redshift and the inherent component. Through his study of unusual galaxies, Arp determined that the intrinsic component was a function of the age of the object. Thus, the high redshift quasars associated with low redshift galaxies are relatively young objects.

Far from being the most distant objects in the universe, quasars may in fact be part of the system of relatively nearby galaxies. These discoveries undermine the theory of an expanding universe that is the foundation of the Big Bang. (For more on this, read *The Big Bang Never Happened* by Eric Lerner, Vintage Books, 1991, and *Seeing Red: Redshifts Cosmology and Academic Science* by Halton Arp, Aperion, 1998.)

As shortcomings in the Big Bang became apparent, theoretical physicists patched together arbitrary mathematical explanations to make up for inconsistencies. They invented concepts like "dark matter" and "dark energy," as well as "black holes," "string theory," "wormholes," and others. As with the Big Bang itself, these imaginings may not be based in reality. They have yet to be proven or disproven through experiment, yet are accepted as fact by many in the scientific community as well as by the general public.

THERMONUCLEAR SUN

Another tenet of theoretical physics and cosmology (the science of the origin and development of the universe) is that the sun is a thermonuclear reactor. Modern cosmologists believe that the sun is a continually exploding hydrogen bomb in which, under great temperature and pressure, hydrogen is being transmuted into helium. (Hydrogen is the first element, helium the second.)

The thermonuclear star model is founded on Newton's idea of universal gravitation, in which the gravitational force of a star compresses its matter in on itself. As in a hydrogen bomb, tremendous centripetal or inward (yang) force produces great temperatures and pressures. These forces smash atoms into each other, causing them to fuse. This process releases tremendous energy, resulting in heat, light, charged particles, and radiation (yin).

In the gravitational model, the source of energy for the sun is the gravitational force of the sun itself. The sun is pulling mass toward its center. The sun will eventually exhaust its supply of nuclear fuel and then burn out.

However, the concept of a thermonuclear sun is facing a challenge from another model, called the Electric Sun hypothesis. This model is based on studies of plasma and electricity as well as satellite observations, such as those of Japan's Hinode spacecraft and NASA's fleet of Themis spacecraft. It is also based on observations of the sun's corona, solar wind, sunspots, penumbra, and dramatic occurrences such as solar flares, prominences, and coronal mass ejections.

The Electric Sun hypothesis postulates that the origin of the sun's energy is not the sun itself, but the electrically charged medium—the galaxy—that surrounds it. Thus, the sun is not a thermonuclear reactor powered by gravity, but a gigantic conductor of electricity. Critics of the gravity powered, thermonuclear sun point out that gravity is actually the weakest force in the universe—electrical energy is estimated to be 1039 times stronger than gravity.

Nearly seventy years ago, Dr. C.E.R. Bruce, an astronomer and electric researcher, presented a new hypothesis about the sun. He suggested that the sun was an electrical discharge phenomenon:

> It is not a coincidence that the photosphere has the appearance, the temperature and spectrum of an electric arc; it has arc characteristics because it is an electric arc, or a large number of arcs in parallel. These arcs quickly result in the neutralization of the accumulated space charge in their neighborhood and go out. They are not therefore stable discharges, but may rather be looked upon as transient sparks. Arcs thus continually appear and disappear. It is this coming and going which accounts for the observed granulation of the solar surface.

According to this hypothesis, most of the space in our galaxy contains plasma (electrically charged gas). Plasmas are made up of electrons, which have a negative charge and ionized atoms, which have positive charge. Every charged particle in the plasma has an electric potential energy or voltage. The sun is at the center of an immense plasma cell, called the heliosphere, that stretches far out—several times the radius of Pluto. The radius of the heliosphere is estimated to be 18 billion kilometers, or 122 times the distance of the earth to the sun.

The sun carries a more positive electric charge than the electrically charged space around it. Negative electrons enter the sun from the outside, while positive ions exit the sun, creating a plasma discharge exactly like those seen in electric plasma laboratories. The sun may be powered, not from within itself, but from the electric currents that flow from our arm of the galaxy in toward the sun. The sun's positive charge causes it to act as the anode in a plasma discharge. The negative charge, or cathode, originates far out in space at the edge of the heliosphere, in a region known as the heliopause (which, as we saw above, is about 18 billion kilometers from the sun). For more on this, read *The Electric Universe* by Wallace Thornhill and David Talbot, Mikamar Publishing, 2007.

Just as George Ohsawa and Michio Kushi taught, the energy powering the sun may actually be coming from the periphery of the solar system rather than from the sun itself.

THE OHSAWA/KUSHI UNIVERSE

Today's scientists have substituted mathematics for experiments,
and wander off through equation after equation as they
build a structure that has no relation to reality.

—NIKOLA TESLA

Alternative hypotheses such as that the Big Bang never happened and the Electric Sun-Electric Universe are much closer to Ohsawa/Kushi Cosmology than conventional concepts like the Big Bang and the thermonuclear Sun. In macrobiotic cosmology as defined by George Ohsawa and Michio Kushi, the universe is continually manifesting in the form of a logarithmic spiral originating in the infinite expansion. The oneness of infinity gives rise to space and time, beginning and end, front and back, and the countless sets of polarities that define our relative world. Polarization, which in macrobiotics we refer to as yin and yang, creates endless movement, energy, change, and evolution.

In essence, the universe is comprised of energy, waves, or vibrations that eventually condense into matter. Spirals form in an inward or centripetal direction. Pure, diffuse energy becomes increasingly yang or contracted, creating pre-atomic particles such as electrons, protons, and neutrons; the world of atoms or elements; the vegetable world; and finally, the world of animals and human beings.

In the macrobiotic view, the universe was not created at a fixed point in time, but is continually becoming manifest through what Ohsawa and Kushi named the "spiral of creation or materialization." The universe is at all times new. Galaxies, stars, and planets, appear, exist for a while, and then vanish in cosmic cycles governed by universal law. New galaxies, stars, and planets then appear and follow the same universal law. The universal law of change—yin changes into yang; and yang changes into yin—exists beyond time and space. The process of creation is going on throughout the universe at this very moment. The process has no beginning and no end.

Ohsawa understood that spirals form at the periphery, or outside, and wind inward toward the center. Here, they reverse course and begin an outward journey back toward the periphery. Galaxies exhibit this pattern, as does our solar system. Ohsawa, and later Michio Kushi, pointed out that the sun's energy did not originate within the sun itself, but from the periphery of the spiral at which the sun is the center. Proponents of the Electric Sun identify this spiral as the heliopause and agree that the energy that powers the sun originates at the periphery (yin) and not at the center (yang). They suggest that the energy powering the Sun is electrical and not gravitational or nuclear.

In macrobiotic cosmology, the solar system, galaxy, and universe itself are created from the outside in, and not from the inside out, as suggested by the Big Bang and gravitational sun models. As Alex Jack has observed, "The Big Bang and thermonuclear sun models are creation myths of the atomic age. They mirror the explosive violence of the early to mid-twentieth century that characterized the modern world and gave birth to these concepts. They reinforce the view that the universe is innately random, chaotic, and destructive."

Clearly, in order to progress from our current society (in which war and violence are universal) toward a future peaceful world, it is essential that we see the universe as it is—an endlessly manifesting, orderly, and peaceful reality.

Appendix E

Declaration of Planetary Commonwealth

The Declaration of Planetary Commonwealth was proclaimed in 2014 by Planetary Health, Inc., a nonprofit educational organization founded by Alex Jack and Edward Esko. Planetary Health is a grassroots movement of macrobiotic and holistic friends, families, businesses, and communities and sponsors of the Amberwaves campaign. Its goals are to keep America and the planet beautiful, and to preserve whole grains and other essential foods from genetic engineering, climate change, and other threats.

PREAMBLE

As the current Spiral of History ends in the early twenty-first century, a new spiral will form that will last for about the next twelve to thirteen thousand years. This new era has already begun to unfold as the old era draws to a close. The relationship of these two spirals is similar to an Olympic relay race, in which two runners run in parallel for a brief distance until the baton is safely passed. When a secure hold is established, the new runner accelerates and takes off on his or her lap while the old runner fades away. In the human race—the contest to preserve and develop our natural biological quality and spirit—this period of overlap extends from roughly 1980 to 2100, when the Pole Star arrives directly overhead. The two spirals will proceed in parallel for a while until the new orientation is strong enough to lead and the old orientation decays. Realistically, it may take the momentum of the past disharmonious factors two or three generations to fade away.

Thus, although worldwide modern civilization will continue to decline and fall over the next several decades, humanity need not necessarily disappear. At the same time that biotechnology is developing, a new orientation of civilization will arise among those people who have individually realigned their way of life according to the laws of nature and the Order of the Universe. Through their understanding and efforts, the construction of a new healthy and peaceful world will begin, by the unification of all antagonistic factors in human affairs.

As the new orientation spreads, existing political, economic, ideological, and cultural systems will be seen as complementary to one another and will be allowed to evolve naturally as civilization as a whole develops a more peaceful direction. The safe start of this new age will be signaled by the establishment of a world federal government or planetary commonwealth to oversee the final abolition of nuclear weapons, to preserve the earth's natural resources and wildlife, and to facilitate the biological, psychological, and spiritual health and happiness of humanity. The arrival of Polaris, the North Star, directly overhead in about 2100, will mark the safe entry into the new Era of Humanity and the beginning of a new cycle of peace and unity that can be expected to last for many thousands of years as the celestial influence of the Milky Way increases.

—Michio Kushi and Alex Jack, *One Peaceful World*

DECLARATION OF PLANETARY COMMONWEALTH

We, the undersigned, on behalf of all people, all species, and the planet itself, hereby establish a Planetary Commonwealth. The Planetary Commonwealth shall encompass all citizens of Earth, and represent and serve them, together with all species, and our natural environment on earth. As founding members of Planetary Commonwealth, we hold these truths to be self-evident:

There Is But One Universe

All men and women, all other species, and the planet itself originate within the infinite universe. All are manifestations of the infinite universe and all eventually return to the infinite universe. Thus, all men and women, all other species, and the planet itself share a common origin, a common existence, and a common destiny. As manifestations of the infinite universe, all men and women, all other species, and the planet itself possess independent sovereignty and self-regulating freedom. All human beings are infinitely free and absolutely sovereign.

Planetary Commonwealth exists within the infinite universe. Everything changes. The law of change is permanent and universal. The law of change is the law of peace, the law of harmony, and the law of love. The law of change is the one great law before which all other laws are relative and ephemeral. The law of change is the law of infinity. The law of change is the transcendent and universal law recognized by the Planetary Commonwealth.

There Is But One Planet

The earth is a singular undivided space, existing in time, under heaven, indivisible, and shared by all. The earth consists of rivers and mountains, forests and deserts, oceans and land, valleys and plains. The only "boundaries" that exist are those created by nature, such as mountains, rivers, oceans, and deserts, and these are fluid, not rigid. Human boundaries are artificial, produced not by nature, but by conceptual thought. We share our planetary environment with countless other species. Our destiny is their destiny. Their destiny is our destiny. Planetary Commonwealth shall represent all beings and all species. The earth is the one sovereign territory recognized by Planetary Commonwealth. On behalf of all species, we hereby declare the earth to be our sole sovereign territory. With the infinite universe as our witness, we vow to preserve, protect, cherish, and enjoy our planetary home.

There Is But One People

We share a common origin in the infinite universe. We share a common existence that encompasses birth, growth, change, death, and rebirth. We share a common destiny to return to the infinite universe. We are all the brothers and sisters, parents and children, husbands and wives, lovers and friends, neighbors and passersby of one infinite universe. We have descended from common ancestors and spread over the entire planet with an endless range of diversity. We have within ourselves the ability to realize endless health, peace, prosperity, and freedom on the earth, without outside intervention or assistance. Differences are minor in comparison to the things we all share.

In solemn yet joyful recognition of the above, we, the undersigned, hereby affirm the truth of One Universe, One Planet, and One People. We, the undersigned, hereby establish Planetary Commonwealth upon these self-evident truths. By our signature, we declare ourselves to be founders and citizens of Planetary Commonwealth.

AMENDMENTS TO THE DECLARATION

Planetary Commonwealth shall secure for all people and all species a clean natural environment, including clean air and water; safe, healthful, and nutritious food; adequate shelter; and basic education for life, health, happiness, and peace. Planetary Commonwealth shall establish a territory without hunger, pollution, poverty, ignorance, homelessness, and war.

Planetary Commonwealth shall strive for world unity, peace, and understanding, while respecting, protecting, and preserving the endless diversity of all human beings and all other species. All citizens of Planet Earth, together with all the natural species inhabiting the territory, are members of and shareholders in Planetary Commonwealth. Planetary Commonwealth shall not discriminate according to age, race, sex, religion, economic status, political affiliation, species, health condition, dietary history, species profile, or level of education.

Planetary Commonwealth shall recognize that, together with clean air, water, soil, and light, humanity's health and happiness is influenced by the quality of food. Planetary Commonwealth shall encourage adoption of a plant-centered diet based on whole grains, beans, and fresh vegetables, together with locally grown organic produce and other products of local agriculture. Adoption of this dietary pattern shall serve as the foundation for sustainable personal health and prosperity. Organic and natural farming, cultivation, food production, and processing shall be the cornerstone of Planetary Commonwealth.

We, the undersigned, do hereby ratify the Declaration of Planetary Commonwealth. We hereby declare the establishment of Planetary Commonwealth upon the earth and invite all citizens to join as founding members.

Appendix F

The Department of Peace

by Congressman Dennis J. Kucinich

In 2001, Dennis Kucinich—an Ohio representative who held a seat in Congress from 1997 to 2013—introduced legislation for a Department of Peace. Kucinich reintroduced this legislation every two years while he was in Congress. The Department of Peace's purpose would be to implement peace and eliminate war and violence worldwide. The following text is Congressman Kucinich's original description of the Department of Peace.

THE DEPARTMENT OF PEACE

There shall be established a Cabinet-level Department of Peace, which shall be of the Executive Branch of the Government. The Department of Peace shall hold peace as an organizing principle, coordinating service to every level of American society. It shall be oriented toward the development of human potential. It shall be enabled to strengthen non-military means of peacemaking. It shall endeavor to promote justice and democratic principles to expand human rights. It shall seek to create peace, to prevent violence, to divert from armed conflict, to use field-tested programs and to develop new structures in nonviolent dispute resolution. The Department of Peace shall be charged with taking a proactive, strategic approach in the development of policies which promote strategies for conflict prevention, nonviolent intervention, mediation, peaceful resolution of conflict and structured remediation of conflict. It shall address matters both domestic and international in scope. It shall endeavor to derive its strength from a structure which encourages the development of initiatives from local communities, religious groups, and non-governmental organizations. A Secretary of Peace shall be appointed by the President, with the advice and consent of the Senate.

Peacemaking

The Department of Peace shall be dedicated to peacemaking and the study of conditions which are conducive to peace. It shall be empowered in all matters pertaining to conflict resolution, including observation, analysis, control, cooperation, and prognosis of the dynamics of conflict at all levels, personal, interpersonal small groups, organizational, and mass conflict. It shall work proactively and interactively with all branches of government on all policy matters relating to conditions of peace. The act shall provide for the transfer of appropriate agency functions to the Peace Department.

Responsibilities

It shall be charged with the responsibility for monitoring and analyzing causative principles of conflict and to make policy recommendations for developing and maintaining peaceful conduct. It shall determine whether and which conditions call for peacemaking and shall be empowered to be proactive.

Administration and Policy Development

The Department of Peace shall call on the intellectual and spiritual wealth of the nation and seek participation in its administration and in its development of policy from civil rights leaders, religious leaders, labor leaders; non-government organizations; active duty enlisted military personnel and retired veterans of the military; educators, semanticists, and linguists; business executives; holistic practitioners, including those in medicine and nutrition; family physicians, school nurses, psychologists, and scientists; philosophers, anthropologists, and sociologists.

It shall further enlist the participation of writers, artists, including performing artists, coaches from high school, college and professional athletics, motivational speakers; and others at community levels, including neighborhood leaders and law enforcement personnel whose involvement in society has provided experience as to which conditions create peace or the absence of peace, and how peace may be maintained.

Domestic Application

The Department of Peace shall be empowered to develop policies which address domestic violence, including, but not limited to, spousal abuse, child abuse, and mistreatment of the elderly. It shall endeavor to create new policies which are responsive to the challenges of drug and alcohol abuse, and of crime. It shall analyze present policies, employ successful, field-tested programs; and develop new approaches for dealing with the implements of violence, including gun-related violence and the overwhelming presence of handguns in our society, school violence, gangs, racial or ethnic violence, violence against gays and lesbians, and police-community relations disputes. It shall be charged with making policy recommendations to the Department of Justice regarding civil rights and labor law. It shall assist in the establishment and funding of community-based violence prevention programs, including violence prevention counseling and peer mediation in schools. It shall counsel and advocate on behalf of women victimized by violence. It shall provide for public education programs and counseling strategies concerning hate crimes. It shall promote racial and ethnic tolerance.

Education

The Department of Peace shall develop a peace education curriculum, and, in cooperation with the Department of Education, it shall commission the development of such curricula and make it available to local school districts, to enable the utilization of peace education objectives at all elementary and secondary public schools in the United States. Such curricula include studies of the civil rights movement in the United States and throughout the world, with special emphasis on how individual endeavor and involvement have contributed to advancements in peace and justice. Peace education shall equip students to become skilled in achieving peace through reflection and meditation and instructed in the ways of peaceful conflict resolution. Peace education shall include the study of peace agreements and circumstances where peaceful intervention has worked to stop conflict. The Department of Peace, in cooperation with the Department of Education, shall offer incentives in the form of grants and training to encourage the development of state peace curricula and to assist schools in applying for such curricula.

The Department of Peace shall maintain a web page for the purposes of soliciting and receiving ideas for the development of peace from the wealth of political, social, and cultural diversity. It shall call forth America's youth, for the purposes of creative peacemaking, and shall proactively engage the critical thinking capabilities of grade school, high school, and college students via the Internet and other media. It shall issue periodic reports concerning such submissions. The Department of Peace shall provide for the funding of Peace Studies Departments in colleges and universities across the country and for the creation of a Peace Academy, which shall become coordinate in structure and in resources with existing military service academies.

International Application

The Department of Peace shall be coordinate and complementary to the Department of Defense and the Department of State on all matters relating to the national security, including the protection of human rights and the prevention of, amelioration of, and de-escalation of unarmed and armed international conflict. It shall provide for the training of all U.S. personnel who administer post-conflict reconstruction and demobilization in war-torn societies. It shall sponsor country and regional conflict-prevention and dispute resolution initiatives, create special task forces, and draw on local, regional and national expertise to develop plans and programs for addressing the root sources of conflict in troubled areas.

The Department shall provide for citizen exchanges and for exchanges of legislators. It shall encourage the development of international sister cities programs, pairing U.S. cities with cities around the globe for artistic, cultural, economic, and educational exchange. It shall be authorized to administer the training of civilian peacekeepers to support civilian police who participate in civilian peacekeeping. Together with the Department of the Treasury, it shall strengthen peace enforcement through hiring and training monitors and investigators to help with the enforcement of international arms embargoes and sanctions against terrorists and human rights abusers.

Consultation

There shall be established a formal process of consultation of the Department of Peace by the Department of State and the Department of Defense, prior to the initiation of any armed conflict between the U.S. and any other nation, or by the U.S. for any matter involving the use of State Department or Defense Department personnel within the U.S.

Peace Day

The first day of each year, January 1, shall be designated as Peace Day in the United States and all citizens should be encouraged to observe and celebrate the blessings of peace and endeavor to create peace in the coming year. The day shall include discussions of the lives of peacemakers.

The Department of Peace shall be financed based on a formula which is indexed at one percent of the total annual budget of the Department of Defense.

Appendix G

Nine Star Ki:
Danger of World War in 2022

by Edward Esko

In the 1980s, the world faced danger of nuclear war between the United States and the Soviet Union. In 1980, Michio and Aveline Kushi returned from a tour of Europe and reported that the mood there was tense and pessimistic. I'd never seen Michio so concerned. He stated that unless the situation changed, the chance of nuclear war was above 90 percent.

At that time I met leaders of peace groups in Boston, including the Union of Concerned Scientists and the Physicians for Social Responsibility (PSR). I went with a group of Michio's students to a PSR-sponsored gathering at the home of Dr. Helen Caldicott, the world-renowned advocate of nuclear disarmament and world peace, to meet with a peace delegation from the Soviet Union.

Through the efforts of these two organizations, together with the Nobel Peace Prize-winning International Physicians for the Prevention of Nuclear War (IPPNW), along with the efforts of like-minded people around the globe, a world-wide consensus opposing superpower confrontation and nuclear war began to emerge. Eventually, the call for nuclear disarmament and an end to conflict became a global mandate that influenced both the White House and Kremlin. Within several years, Ronald Reagan and Mikhail Gorbachev were negotiating deep cuts in the nuclear arsenals of both superpowers. By the end of the 1980s, the Berlin Wall fell and the Cold War faded into history. For the time being, it seemed the possibility of nuclear war had been averted. Everyone breathed easier and the focus shifted to concerns such as diet and health, energy, food quality (including GMOs), and the environment.

Fast forward to the present. According to PSR:

The nuclear weapons danger is real and growing. Nuclear terrorism, nuclear proliferation, and the thousands of weapons still on hair-trigger alert in the United States and Russia put the planet at risk.

What? Reality check? We thought we were home free regarding the possibility of nuclear war. A terrorist attack or a regional war for oil perhaps, but a global nuclear exchange, no. That threat ended with the fall of the Berlin Wall. Wrong. As we'll see, the threat is very much alive. The threat is real and perhaps imminent. Let's start by taking a look at the global inventory of nuclear weapons:*

12,000 (Russia)	240 (China)	80 (India)
9,400 (USA)	225 (UK)	80 (Israel)
300 (France)	90 (Pakistan)	10 (N. Korea)

*Nuclear weapons data is primarily from reports made by two experts, Hans Kristensen and Dr. Robert Norris, in *The Bulletin of the Atomic Scientists.*

The continuing threat of nuclear weapons is related to the Nine Star Ki cycle, as introduced earlier in this book. To recap, the earth goes through nine stages of energy during each nine-year period. This cycle (which finds resonance in the I Ching, the Aztec calendar, and other ancient cosmologies) divides people into nine star types: flexible 1 Waters; gentle 2 Soils; romantic 3 and 4 Trees; balanced 5 Soils; disciplined 6 and 7 Metals; visionary 8 Soils; and passionate 9 Fires.

Nine Star Ki allows us to develop insight into the movement of life energy, or Ki, at every level. All things exhibit a certain wave and vibration, and by understanding this rhythm, we can understand tendencies in individual character and personality, relationships within the family and among partners, weather and climactic conditions, and cycles of history and social change. Originating from the law of eternal change, the Nine Star Ki cycle shines a clarifying light on past events, present realities, and future probabilities, and is surprisingly accurate in predicting individual and social destiny.

As Michio Kushi has pointed out, in terms of international events, 5 Soil years are fraught with promise and peril. On one hand, the possibility for unity, consolidation, and peace are greatly enhanced. On the other, the chance of separation, violence, and destruction are also high. In the modern era, an extreme way of agriculture, food processing, and eating, as well as excesses in energy use, economies and financial networks, and other sectors prevail. Hence, the likelihood of chaos rather than order is enhanced during a 5 Soil year.

During these periods, the various sides in a conflict tend to harden in their view. Communication becomes difficult and the parties have trouble seeing the situation from the point of view of anyone else but themselves. If unleashed, destructive energies converge toward the center (5 Soil) with great force. These were precisely the conditions on the world stage in 1914, when cascading misunderstandings, miscalculations, and lack of communication led to a catastrophic war that none of the European powers sought or wanted.

The Ki flow for the year 2022 is illustrated in the Magic Square, as shown in Figure G.1. All energies are in their home positions, with 5 Soil in the center. In 2023, 4 Tree moves into the middle, and the other energies revolve accordingly (e.g., 5 Soil moves into the lower spot occupied by 6 Metal). The traditional direc-

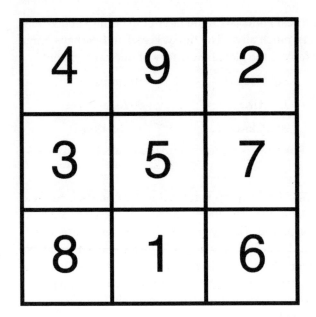

Figure G.1.
Nine Star Ki Magic Square.

Directional map of 2022. South is at the top; north at bottom. East at left; west at right.

tions associated with the energies in ancient China (on the basis of yin/yang classification and the five transformations) are South (top middle), North (bottom middle), East (left middle), and West (right middle). The inter-cardinal directions (e.g., northeast) fall in between.

The stakes are exponentially higher as we approach 2022, which is the next 5 Soil Year in the Nine Ki calendar. The peace and future well-being of the entire planet may be at stake. Is it possible that the current generation of politicians could actually be foolish enough to blunder into an all-out nuclear war? Remember that in 1914, what was essentially a regional conflict escalated into a protracted international struggle. Similarly, if full-scale war breaks out in the Middle East as we approach 2022, the possibility of conflict spiraling out of control is very real. The unthinkable could become thinkable.

As we know, 2022 will be a 5 Soil Year. The primary conflicts of the twentieth century—World Wars I (1914) and II (1941) and the Korean War (1950)—all went global in a 5 Soil Year. In the nineteenth century, the election of Abraham Lincoln in 1860, a 5 Soil Year, led to the outbreak of civil war the following April.

The 5 Soil Year follows the 8 Soil, 7 Metal, and 6 Metal years respectively. The trend lines all point in a downward, condensing, or hardening direction. The progressively yang or condensing energy of the 8, 7, and 6 years leads to increasing hardening and rigidity, and to an increasing sense that "I am right and you are wrong." Powerful gathering energy leads to the formation of blocs and alliances. When the 5 Soil Year arrives, each of the nine energies migrates to its home position. Opposing sides harden and act strictly according to self-interest.

Now, what geopolitical blocs are forming as we approach 2022? And, how is the situation similar to the lead-up to World War I? In 1914, the historic animosity between France and Germany led to the formation of two competing power blocs: Germany and the Austria-Hungary Empire versus France, Russia, England, and eventually the United States.

Similar patterns are appearing as we approach 2022. We now have two competing global power blocs. On one hand, we have the bloc composed of the United States, NATO (the North Atlantic Treaty Organization), and Israel. Opposing that bloc is the bloc composed of Russia, China, and Iran. Although the members of both blocs have overlapping interests in our increasingly global era—for example, the U.S. and China share trade, and the U.S. and Russia share space exploration—and other forms of economic, scientific, and cultural exchange, they are opposed to one another when it comes to policy in the Middle East. Russia, the United States, the NATO countries, China, and Israel possess the bulk of the world's 20,000-plus nuclear weapons. Clearly, war between these two blocs could lead to the destruction of civilization and an end to life on earth.

THE NATURAL CONTROL CYCLE

In the spring, rice seedlings are transplanted into the rice paddy. They have grown tall enough to project their stems above the water line. The water in the paddy serves to eliminate competition from weeds and keep the rice warm at night. The rice paddy is a perfect system of natural checks and balances.

The rice matures during the summer, and come fall, is harvested. At harvest, villagers move through the paddy wielding handheld metal scythes. They grab several stalks and cut. Cut rice is then stacked, bundled, and hung upside-down to dry.

In nature, the energy of metal (the scythe) is antagonistic to that of tree (the rice stalk). Metal saws fell giant oaks. On the cutting board, carrots and onions yield to the thrust of the vegetable knife. These are examples of what is known as the "control cycle" in Oriental philosophy (see Figure G.2). Condensed energy, or "metal," controls or overrides upward energy, or "tree" (shown in the chart as "wood"), water overrides fire, tree overrides soil ("earth"), fire overrides metal, and soil overrides water.

At the same time, going around the chart in a clockwise direction, we see that metal supports or nourishes water, water nourishes tree, tree supports fire, fire nourishes soil, and soil supports metal. Some relationships are complementary, others antagonistic.

The ancients who understood this cycle applied it to the progression of weather and atmospheric conditions through the seasons, daily and lunar cycles, and so on. Known as "Nine Star Ki," this system is codified in the Nine Ki calendar, believed by some to be older than the Mayan Calendar. The Nine Ki system recognizes the fact that in some years, the atmosphere is quieter, more stable, and

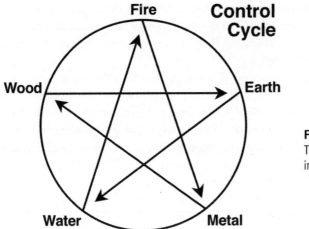

Figure G.2.
The Control Cycle
in Nine Star Ki.

settled. These years are labeled "soil" or "metal." In others, the atmosphere is more agitated, energetic, evaporative, and expressive. These years are labeled "tree" and "fire." Year after year, atmospheric conditions fluctuate between high and low, quiet and active, yin and yang. These changes occur in a repeating cycle of nine years and have an invisible but profound influence on human events.

ENRICHED URANIUM

The most recent 5 Soil crisis occurred in 2013. It centered on Iran's enrichment of uranium, as well as the release of chemical weapons in Syria. Iran, supported by Russia and China, insisted that the enrichment program is strictly for peaceful purposes, i.e., the pursuit of nuclear power and the production of radioisotopes for medical treatment.

Meanwhile, the United States, NATO, and Israel suspected that Iran was hiding a secret weapons program, even though Iran had signed the nuclear non-proliferation treaty and U.S. intelligence had not detected any such program.

A crisis triggered by uranium was totally predictable during a four-year 8 Soil to 7 Metal to 6 Metal to 5 Soil-sequence (2010 to 2013), during which energy moved downward and became more concentrated. Uranium (atomic number 92) is the heaviest element to appear in nature. It occupies the center of the spiral of elements and in that sense, it represents the terminus or completion of elemental formation. It is so saturated, dense, and heavy that it naturally decomposes, giving off radioactivity in the process. It is the quintessential heavy metal element. Left in the ground, uranium plays a role in the balance of nature and poses no threat. After millions of years, it will simply decay into a stable non-radioactive isotope.

On the other hand, isolated and concentrated uranium—especially "enriched" uranium (extreme metal)—overrides, works against, and threatens humanity's highest and most common ideals, including freedom, hope, understanding, peace, and survival itself, all represented by upward, branching out, expansive tree energy. (Refer once again to the "Control Cycle," in which the energy of metal is shown to cancel that of tree or "wood." The arrows moving across the circle show overriding or neutralizing influence, hence the name "Control Cycle.")

In the natural flow of energy, or "Ki," metal nourishes and supports water (the clockwise movement of energy around the cycle is one of nourishment and support.) In a healthy situation, clarity and focus, represented by metal, inspire confidence and courage, represented by water.

However, in the current unhealthy situation, Iran's underground enrichment of uranium (double extreme metal) fueled the negative aspect of water, which is fear. The danger is that this fear, no matter how irrational, could trigger anger, hysteria, and violence in a 5 Soil Year. Fortunately, through the intervention of Russian president Vladimir Putin, Syria dismantled its chemical weapons program. And through the persistence of U.S. President Barack Obama's administration, a deal was signed between Iran and the international community designed to prevent Iran from developing nuclear weapons.

As we move toward 2022, several key flashpoints have the potential to escalate into full-scale war.

1. *Syria.* With the entry of Russian planes and troops into the civil war in Syria in 2015, the danger of a direct air or land conflict between Russia and the United States, the two former Cold War adversaries, is extremely high. In addition, the region is becoming ground zero for holy war between Sunni and Shia Muslims, as well as tensions between Israel and its Arab and Persian adversaries. Millions of Syrian refugees seeking asylum in Europe have heightened tensions between Christians and Muslims and fostered the spread of anti-immigrant political parties.

2. *Iran.* Despite the nuclear deal, the election of a U.S. administration hostile to the accord could scuttle the deal and lead to a U.S. and/or Israeli attack on Iran's nuclear facilities, resulting in the death of Russian civilian personnel and the escalation of the Middle East conflict into global strife.

3. *Ukraine.* In the wake of Russia's annexation of Crimea and the outbreak of hostilities in East Ukraine, the potential for the U.S. and NATO to arm the Ukrainians or go head-to-head with Russia is high. Ukraine, the Breadbasket of Europe, has opened the country to Monsanto, Dow, and other biotech companies that have set up operations in Ukraine that threaten the food supply in Europe. Meanwhile, Russia has prohibited GMO cultivation and decided to move in a more organic agricultural direction, widening the divide between the two blocs.

4. *South China Sea.* Friction is increasing over the territorial rights to islands in the South China Sea claimed by China, Vietnam, Japan, Philippines, and other countries, heightening the potential for naval conflict between China and the U.S and its allies.

5. *Terrorist attacks.* Recruitment by the group Islamic State (ISIS) in Syria, Al-Quaeda, and terrorist networks in Africa have attracted international support, spreading terrorism worldwide, including the downing of airplanes, bombings in major European and American cities, and other acts of mass destruction.

As we enter this period of heightened danger, we urge all world leaders to pause and reflect on the path to peace. We urge an immediate reduction in the intake of meat, chicken, and eggs; dairy food; and fatty fish that—in concert with sugar, alcohol, and drugs—produce anger, short temper, and explosive reactions, especially among world leaders and those responsible for the welfare of their peoples. It is recommended that these dietary changes be implemented so as to facilitate a safe passage through this dangerous time and into a future of peace, health, and prosperity for all people.

Recommended Reading

Books

Akizuki, Tatsuichiro. *Nagasaki 1945*. London: Quartet Books, 1981.

Bhagavad Gita. Gorakhpur, India: Gita Press, 1964.

Bible, King James Version and other translations.

Butler, Samuel. *Erewhon*. New York: New American Library, 1960.

Campbell, T. Colin. *The China Study*. Dallas: BenBella, 2004.

Confucius. *The Analects of Confucius*. Trans. Arthur Waley. London: Allen and Unwin, 1938.

Davis, Garry. *World Government, Ready or Not!* Washington, DC: World Government House, 2003.

Dower, John W. *War Without Mercy: Race and Power in the Pacific War*. New York: Pantheon, 1987.

Dufty, William. *Sugar Blues*. New York: Warner Books, 1975.

Esko, Edward and Alex Jack. *Cool Fusion: A Quantum Solution to Peak Minerals, Nuclear Waste, and Future Metals Shock*. Becket, Massachusetts: Amberwaves Press, 2011.

Esko, Edward and Alex Jack. *Corking the Nuclear Genie*. Becket, Massachusetts: Amberwaves Press, 2014.

Esko, Wendy. *The Big Beautiful Brown Rice Cookbook*. Garden City Park, New York: Square One Publishers, 2013.

Fukuoka, Masanobu. *The One-Straw Revolution*. New York: Rodale, 1978.

Grossinger, Richard, and Lindy Hough, eds. *Nuclear Strategy and the Code of the Warrior*. Berkeley, California: North Atlantic Books, 1984.

Homer, *The Iliad*. Trans. Peter Green. Berkeley, California: University of California Press, 2015.

Homer, *The Odyssey*. Trans. Robert Fitzgerald. New York: Doubleday, 1961.

Hufeland, Christolph W. *Macrobiotics, or the Art of Prolonging Life.* (1796) London: Forgotten Books, 2012.

I Ching, or Book of Changes. Trans. Richard Wilhelm and Cary F. Baynes. Princeton, New Jersey: Bollingen Foundation, 1950.

Kervran, Louis. *Biological Transmutations.* Brooklyn, New York: Swan House, 1972.

Kojiki. Trans. Donald L. Philippi. Tokyo: University of Tokyo Press, 1968.

Kotzsch, Ronald E. *Macrobiotics: Yesterday and Today.* New York: Japan Publications, 1985.

Kushi, Aveline, with Alex Jack. *Aveline Kushi's Guide to Macrobiotic Cooking for Health, Harmony, and Peace.* New York: Warner Books, 1985.

Kushi, Michio, and Alex Jack. *Diet for a Strong Heart.* New York: St. Martin's Press, 1985.

Kushi, Michio, and Alex Jack. *The Gospel of Peace: Jesus's Teachings of Eternal Truth.* New York: Japan Publications, 1992.

Kushi, Michio, and Alex Jack. *The Macrobiotic Path to Total Health.* New York: Ballantine, 2002.

Kushi, Michio, and Aveline Kushi. *Macrobiotic Diet.* Edited by Alex Jack. Tokyo: Japan Publications, 1985.

Kushi, Michio, with Alex Jack. *The Cancer Prevention Diet.* New York: St. Martin's Press, 2010.

Kushi, Michio. *Macrobiotic Home Remedies.* Edited by Marc Van Cauwenberghe, M.D. Garden City Park, New York: Square One Publishers, 2014.

Kushi, Michio. *The Book of Macrobiotics,* revised edition. Edited by Alex Jack. Garden City Park, New York: Square One Publishers, 2013.

Kushi, Michio. *Your Body Never Lies.* Garden City Park, *New* York: Square One Publishers, 2006.

Lao Tzu. *Tao Te Ching.* Trans. Richard Wilhelm and H.G. Ostwald. London: Arkana, 1985.

Mencius. *Mencius.* Trans. W. A. C. H. Dobson. Toronto: University of Toronto Press, 1963.

Mizuno, Namboku. *Food Governs Your Destiny.* Trans. Aveline Kushi with Alex Jack. New York: Japan Publications, 1992.

More, Sir Thomas. *Utopia.* New York: Everyman's Library, 1978.

Needham, Joseph. *Science and Civilization in China* (5 vols). Cambridge, United Kingdom: Cambridge University Press, 1959.

Niwano, Nikkyo. *Buddhism for Today: A Modern Interpretation of the Threefold Lotus Sutra.* Tokyo: Kosei Publishing Co., 1976.

Northrup, F. S. C. *The Meeting of East and West.* New York: Collier, 1966.

Ohsawa, George. *Gandhi: The Eternal Child.* Trans. Kenneth G. Burns. Oroville, California: George Ohsawa Macrobiotic Foundation, 1986.

Ohsawa, George. *The Unique Principle.* Oroville, California: George Ohsawa Macrobiotic Foundation, 1973.

Qur'an. Channeled by Muhammad. Trans. M. A. S. Abdel Haleem. New York: Oxford University Press, 2008.

Sattilaro, Anthony, with Tom Monte. *Recalled by Life: The Story of My Recovery from Cancer.* Boston: Houghton Mifflin, 1982.

Schauss, Alexander. *Diet, Crime, and Delinquency.* Berkeley, California: Parker House, 1981.

Shakespeare. Collected works.

The Yellow Emperor's Classic of Internal Medicine. Trans. Henry Lu. Vancouver, British Columbia: Academy of Oriental Heritage, 1978.

Thoreau, Henry David. *Walden.* Mineola, New York: Dover Publications, 1995.

Tolstoy, Leo. *War and Peace.* Trans. Rosemary Edmonds. New York: Penguin Books, 1978.

U.S. Congress Senate Select Committee on Nutrition and Human Needs. *Dietary Goals for the United States.* Washington, D.C.: U.S. Government Printing Office, 1977.

Periodicals

Amberwaves (2001–present), Becket, Massachusetts.

Christina Cooks (1995–present), Philadelphia, Pennsylvania.

De Grosse Leben, Germany.

East West Journal (1971–1989), Brookline, Massachusetts.

Kushi Institute Study Guides (1980–1982), Brookline, Massachusetts.

Le Compass (1977–2008), Paris, France.

Macrobiotics Today (1984–present), Oroville, California.

MacroMuse (1982–1990), Rockville, Maryland.

Michio Kushi Seminar Reports (1973–1977), Boston, Massachusetts.

One Peaceful World Newsletter (1990–2002), Becket, Massachusetts.

The Macrobiotic (1966–1983), Oroville, California.

The Order of the Universe (1967–1982), Boston and Brookline, Massachusetts

Yin Yang, France.

One World Resources

Classes in macrobiotic education are offered by the following Kushi Institutes:

Kushi Institute of America
198 Leland Road
Becket, MA 01223
Phone: 413-623-5741
Website: www.kushiinstitute.org
The Kushi Institute of America is an educational center that offers the Way to Health program; Leadership Training program for future teachers, counselors, and cooks; International Macrobiotic Summer Conference; special seminars and workshops; macrobiotic consultations; shiatsu massage; Nine Star Ki sessions; personal menu planning; and more.

Kushi Institute of Europe
Weteringschans 65
1017RX
Amsterdam, The Netherlands
Phone: +31 20 625 7513
Website: www.macrobiotics.nl
The Kushi Institute of Europe offers cooking classes, seminars, workshops in shiatsu massage, and one-day programs at the Amsterdam location, as well as providing lectures across Europe based on demand.

Kushi Institute Extension in the U.K.
c/o Macrobiotic Shop
112 South Road
Haywards Heath
West Sussex
RH16 4LL
United Kingdom
Phone: 01444 628667
Website: www.macrobioticshop.co.uk

Working with the Kushi Institute of Europe, this extension in the U.K. offers intensive courses in subjects such as the Art of Cooking, Principles of Oriental Diagnosis, Macrobiotic Home Remedies, and more. Highlights of the courses include meditation exercises, Feng Shui, and Nine Star Ki astrology.

Kushi Macrobiotic School of Japan
3-14-16 Nishihara
Shibuya-ku, Tokyo 151-0066
Phone/fax: +81 3 6326 6746
Website: www.kushischool.jp

The Kushi Macrobiotic School in Japan provides a unique environment for macrobiotic students. The School holds lectures, workshops, and events that incorporate traditional wisdom with modern knowledge to promote a healthy lifestyle.

Other Organizations

Fortunate Blessings Foundation
409 Bantam Road Suite A-3
Litchfield, CT 06759
Phone: 860-567-8801
Website: www.fortunateblessings.org

Emergency relief organization founded by Bill Spear that sends teams to help children following natural disasters, war, and other traumatic events.

Planetary Health, Inc.
Box 2051
Lenox, MA 01240
Phone: 413-623-0012
Website: plantbasedmacrobiotics.org

A nonprofit educational organization founded by Alex Jack and Edward Esko that sponsors Amberwaves, a network to preserve brown rice, wheat, and other grains from genetic engineering, climate change, and other threats; and the Macrobiotic Research Institute, which sponsors scientific and medical research.

References

Chapter 4: Erewhon Revisited

1. Quoted in a report by Rik Vermuyten. *MacroMuse* 1984 (Fall/Metal): 39.

2. Levy, EM, et al. "Patients with Kaposi sarcoma who opt for no treatment." *Lancet* 1985, 2(8448): 223.

Chapter 6: The Order of the Universe

1. Bhagavad Gita. Vol. 3. Gorakhpur, India: Gita Press, 1964.

2. Toynbee, Arnold. *A Study of History.* New York: Oxford University Press, 1972. 89. Print.

3. *I Ching, or Book of Changes.* Trans. Richard Wilhelm and Cary F. Baynes. Princeton: Princeton University Press, 1967. 441. Print.

4. "Peace in the Old Testament." *The Interpreter's Dictionary of the Bible.* Ed. George Buttrick. Nashville: Abingdon Press, 1962. 704–705. Print.

Chapter 7: Lost Paradise

1. Cohen, Mark Nathan. *The Food Crisis in Prehistory.* New Haven, Connecticut: Yale University Press, 1977. 91–92. Print.

2. Bower, Bruce. "Hunting Ancient Scavengers." *Science News* 1985, 127: 155–157.

3. Trowell, H. C., and D. P. Burkitt. *Western Diseases.* Cambridge, Massachusetts: Harvard University Press, 1980. 15. Print.

4. Brody, Jane E. "Research Yields Surprises About Early Human Diets." *New York Times* 15 May 1979: Science Times section. Print.

5. Albala, Ken. "Food: A Cultural Culinary History." The Great Courses. 8 July 2013. Audio lecture.

6. Scott, Jim. "Diet likely changed game for some hominids 3.5 million years ago, says CU-Boulder study." *University of Colorado–Boulder News Center.* University of Colorado–Boulder, 3 June 2013. Web.

7. Ovid. *Metamorphoses.* Trans. Frank Justus Miller. Cambridge, Massachusetts: Harvard University Press, 1960. I.9.11. Print.

8. Falchi, F., et al. "The new world atlas of artificial night sky brightness." *Science Advances* 2, no. 6 (2016): e1600377.

9. Mortillaro, N. "Saving the night: Light pollution is a serious concern for human health and wildlife." *Global News,* http://globalnews.ca/news/748109/light-pollution-cause-for-concern. 2 Aug 2013.

10. Bennie, J., et al. "Cascading effects of artificial light at night: resource-mediated control of herbivores in a grassland ecosystem." *Philosophical Transactions of the Royal Society* B 370, no. 1667 (2015).

11. Spivey, A. "Light pollution: Light at night and breast cancer risk worldwide." *Environmental Health Perspectives* 118, no. 12 (2010): A525.

Chapter 8: The Origin and Causes of War

1. Harlan, J.R. "A Wild Wheat Harvest in Turkey." *Archaeology* 1967, 20: 197–201.

2. Wright, Quincy. *A Study of War.* 2nd ed. Chicago: University of Chicago Press, 1965. 648. Print.

3. Schiller, Ronald. "Where Was the 'Cradle of Civilization'?" *Reader's Digest* Aug. 1980: 67–71. Print.

4. Fried, Morton, Marvin Harris, and Robert Murphy, eds. *War: The Anthropology of Armed Conflict and Aggression.* Garden City: American Museum of Natural History, 1968. 94. Print.

5. Eaton, S. Boyd, and Melvin Konner. "Paleolithic Nutrition: A Consideration of its Nature and Current Implications." *New England Journal of Medicine* 1985, 312: 283–289.

6. Blainey, Geoffrey. *The Causes of War.* New York: The Free Press, 1973. 103. Print.

7. Ibid., 248.

8. Fried, Morton, Marvin Harris, and Robert Murphy, eds. *War: The Anthropology of Armed Conflict and Aggression.* Garden City: American Museum of Natural History, 1968. 213–236. Print.

9. Nicholas, FC. "The Aborigines of the Province of Santa Maria." *American Anthropologist* 1901, 3(4): 612.

10. Wright, Quincy. *A Study of War.* 2nd ed. Chicago: University of Chicago Press, 1965. 76–77. Print.

11. Ibid., 46.

12. Ibid., 63-64, 552–553.

13. Ibid., 224.

14. Tolstoy, Leo. *War and Peace.* Trans. Rosemary Edmonds. New York: Penguin Books, 1978. 1201–1202. Print.

15. Thomas, Hugh. *A History of the World.* New York: Harper & Row, 1979. 386. Print.

16. Tolstoy, Leo. *War and Peace.* Trans. Rosemary Edmonds. New York: Penguin Books, 1978. 1198. Print.

17. Cartwright, Frederic F., and Michael D. Biddiss. *Disease and History.* New York: Thomas Y. Crowell, 1972. 111. Print.

Chapter 9: Seeds and Civilization

1. Cohen, Mark Nathan. *The Food Crisis in Prehistory.* New Haven: Yale University Press, 1977.

Note: All dates in this chapter regarding early agriculture are taken from this source.

2. "India." *Encyclopedia Britannica.* 14th ed. 1929. Print.

3. Cartwright, Frederic F., with Michael D. Biddiss. *Disease and History.* New York: Thomas Y. Crowell, 1972. 11. Print.

4. Needham, Joseph. *Science and Civilization in China.* 5 vols. Cambridge: Cambridge University Press, 1959. Print.

5. Chang, K. C. *Food in Chinese Culture: Anthropological and Historical Perspectives.* New Haven, Connecticut: Yale University Press, 1977. 154. Print.

6. Mintz, Sidney. *Sweetness and Power: The Political, Social and Economic Effects of Sugar in the Modern World.* New York: Viking Press, 1985. 23. Print.

7. Spence, Jonathan D. *The Memory Palace of Matteo Ricci.* New York: Viking Press, 1984. 45–46. Print.

8. McNeil, William. *Plagues and Peoples.* Garden City, New York: Anchor Press/Doubleday, 1976. 207. Print.

Chapter 10: The Modern Age

1. McMullen, Roy. *Mona Lisa: The Picture and the Myth*. Boston: Houghton Mifflin, 1975. 179–180. Print.

2. Richter, Irma A. (ed). *Selections from the Notebooks of Leonardo da Vinci*. London: Oxford University Press, 1952. 279. Print.

3. Mintz, Sidney. *Sweetness and Power: The Political, Social and Economic Effects of Sugar in the Modern World*. New York: Viking Press, 1985. 43. Print.

4. Joyce, EJ. "Thomas Jefferson, Gardener." *Rodale's Organic Gardening* March 1986: 42. Print.

5. Mintz, Sidney. *Sweetness and Power: The Political, Social and Economic Effects of Sugar in the Modern World*. New York: Viking Press, 1985. 256. Print.

6. Ritchie, Carson I.A. *Food in Civilization: How History Has Been Affected by Human Tastes*. New York: Beaufort Books, 1981. 127. Print.

7. Mintz, Sidney. *Sweetness and Power: The Political, Social and Economic Effects of Sugar in the Modern World*. New York: Viking Press, 1985. 48. Print.

8. Zola, Emile. Quoted in *The Macrobiotic*. Oroville, California: G.O.M.F., n.d.

9. Philpott, Tom. "A Brief History of Our Deadly Addiction to Nitrogen Fertilizer." *Mother Jones*. Mother Jones, 19 April 2013. Web.

10. Flesch, Rudolf (ed). *A New Book of Unusual Quotations*. New York: Harper & Row, 1966. 95. Print.

11. Hay, William Howard. "Cancer: A Disease of Western Civilization?" *Cancer* 1927, 4: 299.

12. Sayen, Jamie. *Einstein in America: The Scientist's Conscience in the Age of Hitler and Hiroshima*. New York: Crown: 1985. 151. Print.

13. Nelson, Craig. "The Age of Radiance: The Epic Rise and Dramatic Fall of the Atomic Era." New York: Scribner, 2014. 220–221. Print.

Chapter 11: Increased Violence in the Twenty-First Century

1. *Bulletin of the Atomic Scientists*, 2013

2. U.S. Department of Energy Environmental Management. "Department of Energy Five Year Plan FY 2007-FY 2011 Volume II." March 2006. Retrieved 8 April 2007.

3. Thorp, Nick. "Uranium Metal from Fernald, O.H." *ToxiPedia*. Washington Nuclear Museum and Educational Center, 11 May 2011. Web.

4. Levitt, Tom. "Should Future Generations be Forced to Deal with our Nuclear Legacy?" *The Ecologist*. 13 May 2011.

5. Jack, Alex, and Edward Esko. "Ebola & Diet." *Amberwaves*, Planetary Health Special Report, 2015.

6. "Revealing the Link: SSRIs and School Shootings." *SodaHead*. SodaHead, 10 December 2011. Web.

7. Davey, Monica, and Gardiner Harris. "Family Wonders if Prozac Prompted School Shootings." *New York Times*. New York Times, 26 March 2005. Web.

8. Jack, Alex. *Imagine a World Without Monarch Butterflies*. Becket, Massachusetts: One Peaceful World Press, 2000.

9. Courter, Catherine, and Peter MacGill. "The Effects of Electromagnetic Fields." *new illuminati*, 2014 April 10. nexusilluminati.blogspot.com

See also Rees, Camilla, and Magda Havas. *Public Health SOS: The Shadows Side of the Wireless Revolution*. CreateSpace Independent Publishing, 2009.

10. Georgiou, George. "The Hidden Hazards of Microwave Cooking." *Journal of American Association of Integrative Medicine Online* (April 2006): n. pag.

11. Jack, Alex. *Food as Medicine: A Planetary Health Research Guide*. Becket, Massachusetts: Amberwaves, 2007.

12. U.S. Environmental Protection Agency (EPA). "Evaluation of the Potential Carcinogenicity of Electromagnetic Fields." Washington, DC, October 1990.

13. "Global Warming." *Wikipedia*. Wikipedia, 2015. Web.

14. Food and Agriculture Organization of the United Nations (FAO). "Livestock's Long Shadow." 2006. Web.

15. Jack, Alex. *America's Vanishing Nutrients: Decline in Fruit and Vegetable Quality Poses Serious Health and Environmental Risks*. Becket, Massachusetts: Amberwaves, 2005.

16. Loladze, Irakli. "Hidden shift of the ionome of plants exposed to elevated CO2 depletes minerals at the base of human nutrition." *eLife* 3 (3024):e02245.

17. Zaitchik, Alexander. "Global Warming, Global Violence." *Foreign Policy in Focus*. Institute for Policy Studies, 11 September 2011. Web.

18. Parenti, Christian. *Tropic of Chaos: Climate Change and the New Geography of Violence*. New York: Nation Books, 2011.

19. "2015: It is Three Minutes to Midnight." *Bulletin of Atomic Scientists*. Bulletin of the Atomic Scientists, 2015. Web.

20. Esko, Edward, and Alex Jack. *Corking the Nuclear Genie*. Becket, Massachusetts: *Amberwaves*, 2014.

21. Bobbitt, Philip. *Achilles' Shield: War, Peace, and the Course of History*. New York: Knopf, 2002.

Chapter 12: Diet and Decreased Violence

1. Pinker, Steven. *The Better Angels of Our Nature: Why Violence Has Declined*. New York: Viking Press, 2011. Print. All quotes are from this edition of the book.

2. Harari, Yuval Hoah. *Sapiens: A Brief History of Humankind*. New York: HarperCollins, 2015. Print. All quotes from this edition of the book.

3. U.S. Select Committee on Nutrition and Human Needs. "Dietary Goals for the United States." 1977. Web.

4. U.S. Department of Agriculture. "Nutrition and Your Health: Dietary Guidelines for Americans." 2000. Web.

5. U.S. Department of Agriculture. "Scientific Report of the 2015 Dietary Guidelines Advisory Committee." 2015. Web.

6. van Veghel, Hanneke. "Meat: China's demand to 2030." *University of East Anglia* 2013.

7. Rosenberg, SA. "Combined-Modality Therapy of Cancer." *New England Journal of Medicine* 1985, 312:23: 1512–1514.

8. *Second Opinion: Laetrile at Sloan-Kettering* (documentary). Dir. Eric Merola. Merola Productions, 2014. DVD.

Chapter 13: Preventing Violence and Mechanical Thinking

1. Green, Jesse (ed). *Zuni: Selected Writings of Frank Hamilton Cushing*. Lincoln, Nebraska: University of Nebraska Press, 1979. 302–303. Print.

2. Ibid., 3; Monte, Tom. "Is America Going Crazy?" *East West Journal* (1980): 42; and "The Diet-Behavior Connection." *Science News* (1983): 125.

3. Schauss, Alexander. *Diet, Crime, and Delinquency*. Berkeley, California: Parker House, 1981. 24. Print.

4. Schauss, Alexander. *Diet, Crime, and Delinquency*. Berkeley, California: Parker House, 1981. 5. Print.

5. Ibid., 14.

6. Ibid.

7. Wyden, Peter. *Day One: Before Hiroshima and After.* New York: Simon and Schuster, 1984. 28. Print.

8. Ibid., 56.

9. Ibid., 101.

10. Toland, John. *The Rising Sun: The Decline and Fall of the Japanese Empire, 1936–1945.* New York: Random House, 1970. 73. Print.

11. See Dower, John W. *War Without Mercy: Race and Power in the Pacific War.* New York: Pantheon, 1986.

12. Bergamini, David. *Japan's Imperial Conspiracy.* New York: William Morrow, 1971. 723. Print.

13. Ibid., 348.

14. Ibid., 864.

15. Douglas, Charles Noel (ed). *Forty Thousand Quotations: Prose and Poetical.* Garden City, New York: Halcyon House, 1940. 931. Print.

16. U.S. House of Representatives. "Hearings Before a Sub-Committee of the Committee on Appropriations of the House of Representatives." 1979. 323.

17. "The Links Between Sugar and Mental Health." *Mercola.* Mercola, 22 December 2009. Web.

Chapter 14: Politics: "Medicine Writ Large"

1. Pringle, Peter, and James Spigelman. *The Nuclear Barons.* New York: Avon Books, 1981. 41. Print.

2. Virchow, Rudolf. *Cellular Pathology.* 1858.

3. McAuliffe, Sharon, and Kathleen McAuliffe. "The Genetic Assault on Cancer." *New York Times Magazine.* The New York Times, 24 October 1982: 38–43.

4. Silbemer, J. "Aiming at Cancer." *Science News* 4 May 1985. 276.

5. Raymo, Chet. "The Human Body's 'Cell Wars' Defense." *Boston Globe.* 6 January 1986.

6. Saltus, Richard. "'Star Wars' Laser May Aid Medicine, MGH Scientists Say." *Boston Globe.* 13 September 1985.

7. Caldicott, Helen. *Missile Envy.* New York: Bantam Books, 1984. 350. Print.

Chapter 16: World Peace Through World Health

1. "N.H. Residents Celebrate a Nuclear Dump Victory." *Boston Globe.* 2 June 1986.

2. Hershaft, Alex. "Introductory Statement." *A Symposium on the National Impacts of Recommended Dietary Changes.* Toronto: American Association for the Advancement of Science, 4 Jan. 1981.

3. Stepaniak, Joanne, and Kathy Hecker. *Ecological Cooking.* Summertown, Tennessee: Book Publishing Co., 1992. Print.

4. Robbins, John. *The Food Revolution.* Berkeley, California: Conari Press, 2010. Print.

5. West, Nancy. "1986 ban on NH nuke waste burial was repealed in 2011." *New Hampshire Business Review.* McLean Communications, 10 December 2015. Web.

6. Cherfas, Jeremy. "Your Quinoa Habit Really Did Help Peru's Poor. But There's Trouble Ahead." *NPR.* NPR, 31 March 2016. Web.

7. Pinker, Steven. *The Better Angels of Our Nature: Why Violence Has Declined.* New York: Viking Press, 2011. Print.

About the Authors

Michio Kushi was born in Japan in 1926. He studied international law at Tokyo University and came to America in 1949. Influenced by the devastation of World War II, he decided to dedicate his life to the achievement of world peace and the development of humanity. Sponsored by Norman Cousins, he came to New York and furthered his studies at Columbia University and in personal meetings with Albert Einstein, Thomas Mann, Upton Sinclair, Pitirim Sorokin, and other prominent scientists, authors, and statesmen.

With the help of his wife, Aveline, who came to the U.S. in 1951, Michio introduced modern macrobiotics to the U.S. and founded Erewhon, the pioneer natural foods company, in Boston in the early 1960s. The Kushis went on to found the East West Foundation, the *East West Journal,* the Kushi Foundation, and other organizations to spread macrobiotics worldwide. For more than fifty years, Michio Kushi guided thousands of individuals and families to greater health and happiness, lectured to physicians and scientists, advised governments, inspired medical research, and served as a consultant to natural foods businesses and industries.

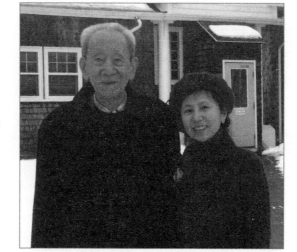

Michio and
Midori Kushi.

The author of many books, Michio Kushi received the Award of Excellence from the United Nations Writers Society. In recognition of his role in launching the modern health and diet revolution, the Smithsonian Institution opened a permanent Kushi Family Collection on Macrobiotics and Alternative Health Care in 1999. In Washington, D.C., he made a presentation on macrobiotics to the White House Commission on Complementary and Alternative Medicine and has spoken at educational, medical, and governmental institutions around the world.

Several years after Aveline passed away in 2001, Michio married Midori Hiyashi. They traveled frequently to Japan and, until his death on December 28, 2014, Michio taught and counseled actively at the Kushi Institute in America and Japan.

Alex Jack was born in Chicago and grew up in Evanston, Illinois and Scarsdale, New York. He edited the *East West Journal,* co-authored *The Cancer Prevention Diet* and many other books with Michio and Aveline Kushi, directed the One Peaceful World Society, and helped introduce macrobiotics to China, the Soviet Union, and other countries. He is the founder and president of Amberwaves, a network devoted to protecting rice, wheat, and other grains from genetic engineering; vice president of Quantum Rabbit; and chairman of the faculty of the Kushi Institute.

The author of more than twenty-five books, novels, and plays, Alex's writings include *The Cancer Prevention Diet, The Macrobiotic Path to Total Health,* and *The Gospel of Peace: Jesus's Teachings of Eternal Truth* (with Michio Kushi), *Aveline Kushi's Complete Guide to Macrobiotic Cooking* (with Aveline Kushi), *The Mozart Effect: Tapping the Power of Music to Heal the Body, Strengthen the Mind, and Unlock the Creative Spirit* (with Don Campbell), annotated editions of Shakespeare's *Hamlet* and *As You Like It,* and *Cool Fusion* and *Corking the Nuclear Genie* (with Edward Esko).

Alex has taught at the Leningrad Cardiology Institute, the Zen Temple in Beijing, Shakespeare's Globe Theatre, Rosas Dance Company in Brussels, the Ohsawa Center in Tokyo, and schools, hospitals, and religious centers around the world. He lives in the Berkshires.

Index

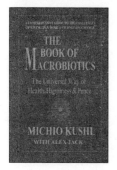

THE BOOK OF MACROBIOTICS
Michio Kushi with Alex Jack

The Book of Macrobiotics is a passport to a world of understanding. It has been studied by hundreds of thousands of people in search of a comprehensive approach to living in a world of constant change.

Now, after two decades, this classic has been revised and expanded to reflect refinements in Michio Kushi's teachings, as well as developments in the modern practice of macrobiotics. The standard macrobiotic diet has been simplified and broadened, and macrobiotic approaches to cancer, heart disease, and other disorders have evolved and expanded, as have basic home care and lifestyle recommendations.

$17.95 US • 432 pages • 6 x 9-inch paperback • ISBN 978-0-7570-0342-4

MACROBIOTIC HOME REMEDIES
Michio Kushi with Marc Van Cauwenberghe, MD

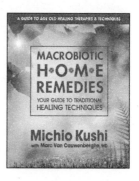

Macrobiotic Home Remedies is a comprehensive guide to effective natural home remedies that can be used alone or in conjunction with standard methods of healing. It explains macrobiotics and illustrates how food can be used to treat hundreds of common disorders, ranging from diarrhea to asthmatic coughing. It is also a guide to the use of external home remedies, including compresses, plasters, packs, baths, and lotions. Over 200 healing recipes are included.

$17.95 US • 208 pages • 7.5 x 9-inch paperback • ISBN 978-0-7570-0269-4

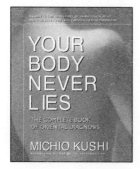

YOUR BODY NEVER LIES
Michio Kushi

Too often, conventional medicine fails to detect illness—especially when it first begins and is easiest to cure. But the ancient system of Oriental diagnosis can often discover physical problems before they even arise.

Your Body Never Lies begins by explaining the principles of Oriental medicine. It then shows you how to detect and understand health problems simply by looking at the mouth, lips, teeth, eyes, nose, cheeks, ears, forehead, hair, hands, feet, and skin. Clear diagrams and charts assist you in quickly recognizing the signs of illness so that you can work toward balanced well-being.

$16.95 US • 184 pages • 7.5 x 9-inch paperback • ISBN 978-0-7570-0267-0

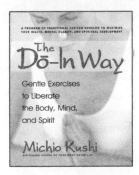

THE DŌ-IN WAY
Michio Kushi

Dō-In is an ancient traditional exercise for the cultivation of physical health and mental serenity. Over the last 5,000 years, it has served as the origin of such well-known disciplines as shiatsu, acupuncture, yogic exercises, and meditation. Offering many benefits, Dō-In promotes a release from troubling issues such as physical sickness, confusion, and intellectual and social disharmony.

The Dō-In Way is a comprehensive guide to an ancient system of motions designed to enhance every aspect of your health. It details the basic aspects of this exercise, including breathing, posture, and self-massage.

$15.95 US • 224 pages • 7.5 x 9-inch paperback • ISBN 978-0-7570-0268-7

EMBRACING MENOPAUSE NATURALLY
Gabriele Kushi

We are all too familiar with its symptoms: hot flashes, night sweats, and more. But while menopause triggers many physical changes, it also brings forth spiritual issues. To address the total impact of menopause, Gabriele Kushi has created a practical guide to dealing with this special time.

The author first provides a clear understanding of the overall process of menopause, from biological changes to emotional

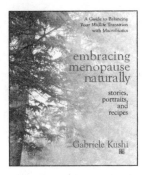

challenges. She then presents a way to deal with menopause through a diet of natural foods, and—in the heart and soul of the book—offers stories of twenty menopausal women.

$14.95 US • 160 pages • 7.5 x 9-inch paperback • ISBN 978-0-7570-0296-0

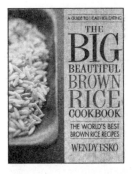

THE BIG BEAUTIFUL BROWN RICE COOKBOOK
Wendy Esko

When restaurants offer brown rice, the dish often appears bland and boring. But this grain can be as delectable as it is healthful. *The Big Beautiful Brown Rice Cookbook* features over 140 kitchen-tested vegetarian/vegan recipes spotlighting this nutritional powerhouse.

$16.95 US • 192 pages • 7.5 x 9-inch paperback • ISBN 978-0-7570-0364-6